Simply Keto

by
SUZANNE RYAN

Victory Belt Publishing Inc.

Las Vegas

First Published in 2017 by Victory Belt Publishing Inc.

ISBN-13: 978-1-628602-63-0

Cover Photographer: Jennifer Skog

Back Cover Photographers: Bill Staley and Hayley Mason

Cover Designer: Chelsea B. Foster

Illustrator: Colleen Pugh

Interior Designers: Yordan Terziev and Boryana Yordanova

Printed in Canada TC 0318

This book is dedicated to those who have ever felt stuck or

incapable of losing weight; to the people who feel unhappy

in their own skin or discouraged with their overall health;

and to those who have been struggling to find the inner strength

to stay motivated for the journey ahead.

Your power to realize your goals has not been lost.

It's never too late to begin again.

Change *is* possible.

So dig in your heels, turn the page,

and embrace this new chapter of your life.

In loving memory of James David Bunton.

TABLE OF CONTENTS

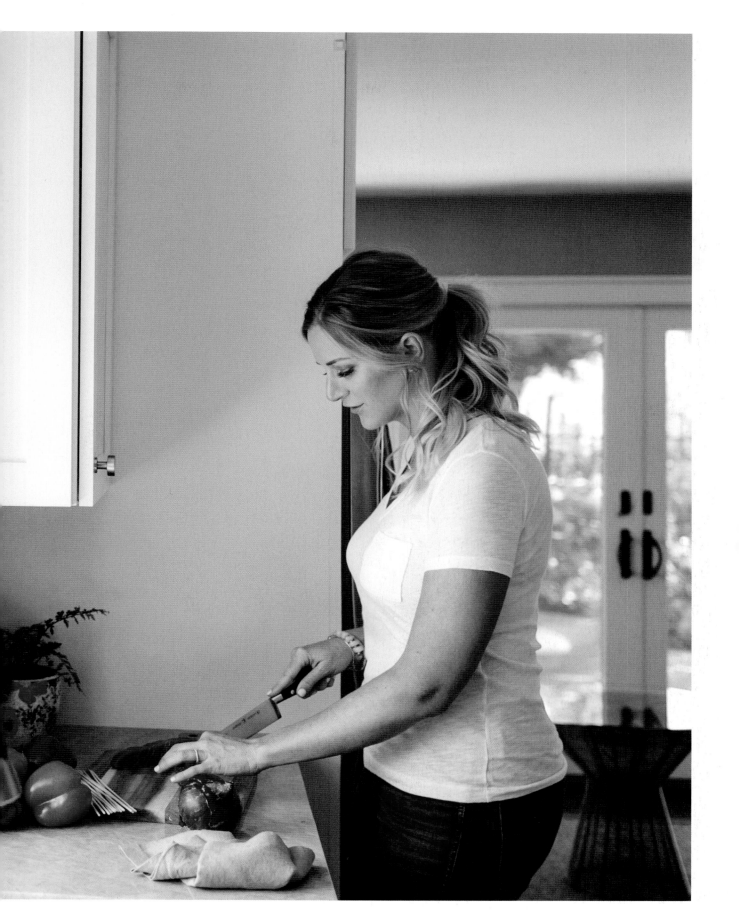

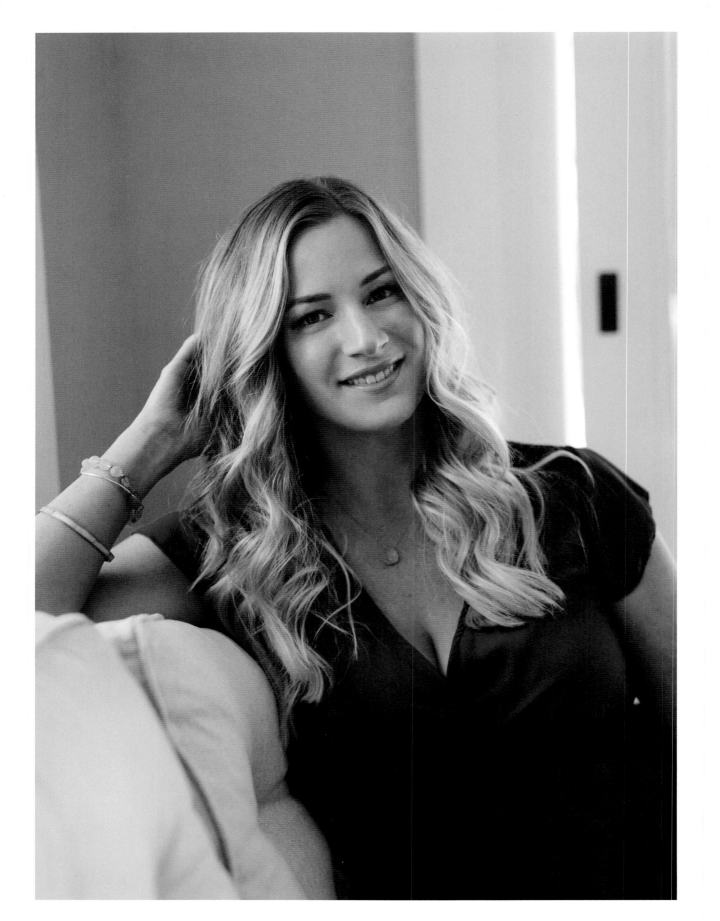

Introduction

Before I started the ketogenic diet in 2015, I did a lot of research, yet I was still confused about several topics. You'll soon find out that although there are some standard ideologies with the keto lifestyle, there are also *a lot* of gray areas. Let's face it, life just isn't black and white. Every person is different. Therefore, it's important to learn as much as you can and then decide which approach is the best and most livable one for you.

My goal in this book is to guide and encourage you through the ins and outs of keto in an easy-to-understand format. The last thing anyone needs when starting a new lifestyle is to feel overwhelmed or intimidated, hence *Simply Keto*.

But first, I want you to know that if you are struggling with your weight and feeling down, unsure about your ability to succeed, or just flat-out frustrated, I get you! I know how deeply that kind of emotional pain can hurt. One of the worst feelings is wanting so badly to change, but not knowing how or *if* you can really do it. Well, I'm here to tell you that change really is possible. I started and stopped more diets than I can count, and if you would have told me a few years ago that I would be where I am today, I would have told you that was absolutely impossible. The beauty in that reflection is recognizing that I was capable all along—I just had to get out of my own way. For far too long, I let fear take over and win. I let my past "failures" and ever-increasing weight define who I was. I gave up on myself—feeling like a failure—but through some pretty difficult periods in my life, I realized that the only way I would actually fail was if I stopped trying.

SO WHY KETO?

What's so special about it, and why am I so passionate about it? The short answer is, I fully believe that this lifestyle helped save my life, and I wholeheartedly believe that it can do the same for you and countless others. Prior to living a keto lifestyle, I was definitely on a path to major health problems, gaining more and more weight with each passing year. On top of being morbidly obese, I was depressed and lethargic, and completely out of ideas for how to make things better.

When I discovered keto on Reddit, something about it really resonated with me. Seeing *real* people getting *real* results, having absolutely nothing to gain from sharing their stories, made me do a double take. I guess you could say that after *years* of trying to buy my way out of obesity, I was maxed out and beyond sick of the multibillion-dollar weight-loss industry. I didn't want to purchase any special plans, join any programs, eat or drink any packaged meals or shakes, or take any pills. I just wanted to learn balance, buy real food, eat when I was truly hungry, and incorporate it all into a livable lifestyle change.

I knew that if I was really going to change, it needed to come from within. But there was one *big* problem: I was always hungry and completely addicted to food. As I started to dig a little deeper into this whole keto thing, I learned about sugar addiction and how eating high fat helps satisfy your appetite while significantly decreasing food cravings. I was in! I knew that this would be my last attempt to lose weight on my own; I remember telling myself that if it didn't work, then I would be off to see a weight-loss surgeon. (Thankfully, that day never came.)

A few weeks after starting keto, I felt a freedom from food like I had never experienced before. I was no longer thinking about eating all the time, and I felt excited and optimistic. With my new livable ketogenic lifestyle and the most amazing support system by my side, my life completely changed. After one year, I had lost 100 pounds. I fully believe that a combination of personal growth and this sustainable and freeing diet gave me the tools I needed to succeed.

Almost three years into the ketogenic lifestyle, I am maintaining my 120-pound weight loss and have no plans ever to go back to eating a high-carb, low-fat diet. My goal now is to pay it forward and help as many people as I can. I know firsthand how hard it can be to lose weight, and I hope that my journey, my struggles, and my pain can be turned into something positive. Change is possible!

MY STORY

My story begins unlike that of your typical cookbook author. Although I've always loved to eat, cooking wasn't something I enjoyed for most of my life. I was always put off by long lists of ingredients, the need for specialty kitchen tools, a lack of time, and let's not forget the dreaded pile of dirty dishes at the end of it all. Everything just seemed overly complicated. Little did I know that finding a simpler way of cooking would play a huge role in changing some pretty poor eating habits that I had developed throughout my life.

I grew up in a fairly dysfunctional family. After my parents divorced, my brother and I spent a lot of time going back and forth between the two. Although I always knew I was loved, we didn't have a lot of consistency in our lives, and nutrition wasn't a topic that we discussed. My dad knew how to make a few things, such as fried chicken fingers and mashed potatoes, but he never really learned how to cook. My mom would always joke that her dinner specialties were canned, microwave, and takeout. We frequented fast-food drive-throughs, lived for discount pizza night every Wednesday, and went for bagel breakfast sandwiches almost every morning. To say that sugar and carbohydrates made up the bulk of my diet is an understatement; they *were* my diet. My beverage of choice was soda (generally ginger ale or cola). The time of day had no bearing on this selection; I would drink soda with breakfast, lunch, and dinner. I remember going months at a time without drinking any water; instead, I drank only soda. In fact, it wasn't unusual for me to drink an entire two-liter bottle of soda in one day. That's about 840 calories and 234 grams of sugar! Drinking that much soda seems pretty crazy to me now that I happily thrive on less than 20 grams of net carbs a day.

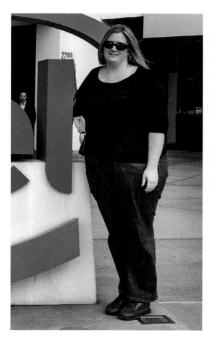

My weight started to become an issue when I was in middle school (as if middle school isn't already an awkward time for a young person). I couldn't fit into any of the clothes from the "cool" stores where the other girls shopped. My classmates teased me relentlessly about my weight. I was called every derogatory name you can think of, and after a while, I started to believe the things people were saying. My self-esteem grew worse by the day, but food was always there for me. In those sweet, delicious moments, I forgot about the problems at home, the teasing at school, and the anxiousness I felt throughout my body, and I just enjoyed the experience of eating.

I started my first diet in middle school. I stuck to it for three days before slipping up. This was the first of many—and I mean *many*—failed attempts to lose weight. I remember feeling strong and sure that I would succeed because I was doing so well the first two days. After a slip-up at breakfast on the third day, I figured I had ruined it, so I went back to eating poorly. I'm sure you have been there. You go "off-plan" for one meal, feel guilty, and then decide that because you've already "blown it," you might as well eat whatever you want for the rest of the day and start again tomorrow. I continued this cycle, gradually gaining more weight every year. I'm still reminded of those times when Facebook sends me memories of posts from prior years. Often those posts say things like "Day one in the gym" or "Starting <insert diet of the month here> today. So excited to finally lose weight."

By the time I got to high school, my weight issues had only gotten worse, and I felt secluded in a lot of ways. I decided to try out for the freshman basketball team. (Apparently, when you are a five-foot, eleven-inch tall woman, playing basketball is a requirement.) Although I wasn't very good, I somehow made the team. (And before you think I am being too hard on myself, our team won only one game that entire season.) I remember being so excited that I was *finally* going to be a part of something.

My excitement quickly turned to anxiety on uniform assignment day. When the subject of sizing came up, I could feel my heart pounding because I was mortified to say my size in front of everyone. At the time, I weighed between 200 and 230 pounds and wore a size 16/18. When it was my turn, I quietly mumbled my size while looking at the floor. The coach flipped through all the uniforms and handed me the largest one they had so that I could try it on. I could tell just by looking at it that it would never fit, yet I carried it into the bathroom anyway. I remember closing the stall door and struggling to put it on. Tears filled my eyes, and I stood in that bathroom stall for a while trying to compose myself; I didn't want to let anyone see me cry. I waited until most of my teammates had left and then handed the uniform back to my coach with a shake of my head. I couldn't even talk; I was mortified.

The coach found me a larger size in the new varsity team uniforms, and I was the only person on the freshman team that year with a uniform that didn't match everyone else's. Although that might not seem like a big deal, if you've struggled with your weight, you know how painful these sorts of moments can be. Each game, I wore a uniform that was different than the ones my teammates wore. People joked about the way I stood out, and yet again my weight made me feel like less of a person. I felt as though I could never be a normal part of something.

I remember thinking that *this* was going to be the thing that would make me lose weight. I was determined to drop enough pounds to fit into the same type of uniform that the rest of my teammates wore. I used to look online for ways to lose weight, and I would go into drugstores and read the labels on weight-loss miracle pills, hoping to find my solution inside one of those bottles. (Spoiler alert: I didn't.)

When I was a teenager, my brother, who was always thin and popular, would try talking to me about my weight. He said things like, "Well, stop eating so much," or, "Just lose the weight. It can't be that hard." Ugh, if only it could have been that simple, and yes, it *was* that hard. I knew he was trying to be helpful, and the things he said came from a place of love and concern, but I don't think *anyone* realized how incapable I felt. I'm not sure if he knew it then—or even now—but I always looked up to him. I was so proud to be his sister. He was everything I longed to be: smart, funny, popular, and fit. Although it wasn't his intention, I grew up in his shadow, never understanding why I couldn't be like him.

After graduating from high school, I moved away to attend college. I lost thirty pounds by eating a low-carb, low-fat diet, but I was hungry all the time. When I quit that diet, I gained every pound back, plus a few more. At that point, I felt as though I had tried everything. I had tried counting calories. I had tried to move more and eat less. I had tried a vegetarian diet and a juicing-only diet. I had even tried a medically supervised weight-loss program that involved appetite suppressant pills, vitamin B12 shots, and weekly weigh-ins. Each time I failed, I gave up on myself a little bit more. However, with every disappointment, food was there to comfort me, so I ate; I ate until I felt sick. I decided that losing weight wasn't in the cards for me, and I just felt bitter about everything. College didn't go so well. After a year, I ended up moving back home. I felt like a broken person. I didn't feel worthy, valuable, or capable of doing anything with my life.

Things only got worse after I returned home. I went through some extremely difficult times. I was in a deep depression, and on some days I questioned why I was alive. I hit rock bottom. I lost interest in everything. I kept to myself, didn't see my friends much, and spent most of my time in my room eating. Of course, this behavior only made me feel worse. At the time, however, I didn't see the connection.

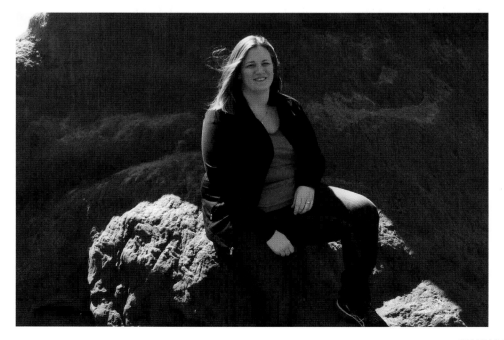

One day, I received a message on MySpace (yes, I feel old) from someone I didn't know. After a bit of hesitation, I opened the message, which was from a guy named Mick. He said that he had stumbled upon my page and just wanted to say hello. Little did I know that this person would eventually become my husband and would play a huge role in reigniting my passion for life.

Mick and I met face-to-face a few weeks after he sent that first message, and boy, was I nervous. I hadn't dated much, and I surely didn't think anyone would be interested in me. We ended up becoming friends and would talk for hours about life, love, politics, and just about everything else. Hours would go by in what felt like seconds. Mick had grown up with similar struggles regarding family, weight, and life. We connected in a way that I had never experienced before. He helped me through one of the most difficult times in my life, and with his support I started to pull my life back together.

New relationships have a honeymoon phase. As I was getting to know Mick, I gained even more weight. I think part of me was just so happy and in love that I didn't care about my size. I already "knew" that losing weight was impossible for me, and I thought, "Well, Mick loves me for exactly who I am, so I'll just enjoy the moment and not worry about how many pounds I've gained."

One morning when I was twenty-five, I woke up suddenly due to intense pain in my right side. Mick rushed me to the hospital, where an ultrasound showed that my gallbladder was infected and filled with stones and sludge. I was taken to surgery that same day, and my gallbladder was removed. A nurse told me that the typical gallbladder patient is female, fair-complexioned, fat, and forty. She let me know in a nice way that I fit all those categories except for not being forty. Ouch. Those things were always hard for me to face, but they were especially difficult to hear in a medical setting.

I was given a new diet to follow: a low-fat diet. I remember thinking, "Okay, this is it! This is my chance to lose weight and get healthy." I followed the doctors' recommendations more diligently than I'd followed any other diet I had tried, and guess what? I gained weight even faster than I had in the past. Once again, I felt like a failure. I was so dismayed that I just gave up. I truly had no idea how to lose weight, and it was a lot easier to put it off to deal with another day. Unfortunately, the days turned into months, and months turned into years. I was in the thick of low self-esteem and frustration, and I had lost all confidence in my ability to change.

A few years later, Mick proposed. At the time, I was a size 24/26 and weighed about 280 pounds. I remember thinking that *this* was finally going to be the key to losing weight. I was determined to lose weight for my wedding; it was the perfect goal!

Unfortunately, with all the engagement parties, bridal showers, cake tastings, and menu selections, I gained even more weight in the year leading up to my wedding. When it came time to select my wedding dress, the bridal

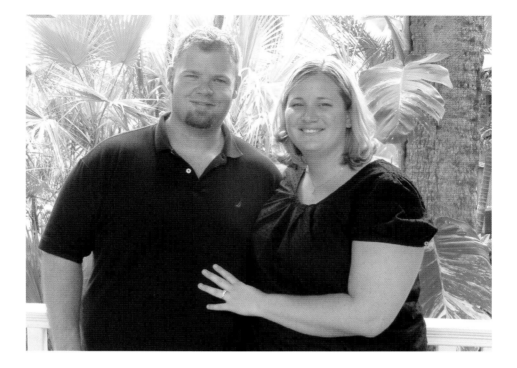

shops near my house only had sample dresses in size 10/12, so I drove an hour north from our small town in Florida to a bridal shop that had once been an ice skating rink. I was nervous, but the shop was filled with hundreds of dresses, so I just knew I would get to experience the "say yes to the dress" moment that you see on TV. Instead, I was shown the four dresses in my size that I could try on. Talk about a letdown! But I had no one to blame but myself. I tried on the dresses with my best friend by my side and found one that was okay. It was far from my dream dress, but at least it fit. I bought it and left feeling as though this was yet another moment in my life that was dampened because of my size.

I wish I could say that I was able to put my weight issues aside and enjoy my wedding day, but I was a bundle of nerves. I knew that there would be plenty of candid photos taken of me, and let's just say that a white strapless dress wasn't at all within my comfort zone. I didn't feel beautiful, and I surely wasn't comfortable wearing the world's tightest compression garments. I was so mad at myself for yet another failure to lose weight. I always thought that my wedding would be the motivation I needed to finally change, and when that didn't happen, I started to accept that change just wasn't in the cards for me.

After being married for a year, Mick and I decided that we would try to have a baby. A few months later, Mick was presented with an amazing career opportunity, and before we knew it, we were planning our move across the country to California. I remember thinking, "Okay, maybe I have another chance. I'm going to get a fresh start in a new place and *finally* lose this weight for good!"

A few days before our move, I was feeling really nauseated. To my surprise, I discovered I was pregnant. It was an exciting—and extremely scary—time because we were about to leave behind virtually everything we knew and loved. We finished packing and hit the road. I'm pretty sure I threw up in every single state between Florida and California. As luck would have it, I ended up developing hyperemesis gravidarum—a not-so-fun pregnancy condition with symptoms that include nausea, weight loss, vomiting, and imbalanced electrolytes. I had all the symptoms except—you guessed it!— weight loss. There were times when I wondered if something was wrong with me because I couldn't ever seem to lose weight, even when living on saltine crackers and oatmeal.

We settled in California, and my extreme nausea continued until the day our daughter, Olivia, was born. I looked into her eyes and knew instantly that I would do absolutely anything for her. It was a kind of love I had never felt before. When we left the hospital, I was filled with joy and anxiety. Hello, first-time-mom nerves and sleep deprivation.

My postpartum food choices weren't great; I pretty much grabbed anything that was readily available and focused entirely on Olivia. When she turned one and started walking, I remember thinking, "My goodness, how am I going to keep up with her?"

Even if I slept eight or nine hours a night, I would still wake up sore and exhausted. My joints would pop as I stood up, and I felt trapped in my body. As the scale tipped to more than 300 pounds, I started researching weight-loss surgery and reached out to a friend who had had a gastric bypass.

However, I had a strong feeling that gastric bypass surgery just wasn't for me. I knew I needed to work on *why* I was eating so much and what I needed to do to improve my sense of self-worth. I started looking at my weight as a symptom instead of a problem that I couldn't fix. I knew I needed to find a livable plan that I could stick to while uncovering past hurts and digging deep into why I hadn't followed through on previous diets.

One morning, I learned on Facebook that a friend's baby boy had received a terminal diagnosis, which is every parent's biggest fear. At that moment, I felt heartbreak for my friend and her family. I knew there was nothing I could do to ease her pain. I spent a lot of time reflecting on my own health and faced the fact that I was taking my health and life for granted. My friend's beautiful little boy would never get a chance to grow up, and here I was, living on the sidelines and feeling sorry for myself; I was simply existing. I felt ashamed. Something changed in me that day, and I decided to start fighting for my life and health. Enough was enough. If I wanted to be around to see Olivia grow up, I *had* to change. There was no more hoping, no more wanting. There was only action and consistency.

I decided that I needed to start small, so first I cut out soda. My stepsister, Joni, had been gently and lovingly nudging me to get healthier. She introduced me to a sparkling water that I loved, and I started buying that instead of soda. This one simple step helped me see that I could stick to something. I started losing a little weight and felt proud for doing it. To this day—years later—I still haven't had another regular soda. It's inspiring to look back now and see that small steps truly can lead to big, *big* change.

Then one evening, I was browsing around Reddit and stumbled upon someone's weight-loss progress photo. The photo caught my attention because this person wasn't selling anything. After years of trying to buy my way to weight loss, I was drawn in by someone talking about what worked for her and sharing her results with no strings attached. I started reading her story and discovered that she had lost all her weight naturally with the ketogenic diet. That day, I spent hours looking at photos and researching the ketogenic diet. Then I watched the documentary *Fed Up*, about the dangers of sugar and how it has contributed to the obesity epidemic in America, and shared it with everyone I knew. Finally, it all made sense: I was addicted to sugar.

New Year's was coming up, and I was excited to have a plan behind my annual resolution to lose weight. January 1, 2015, was the day, and I wish I could tell you that this was really it for me. I had a plan in place, I was pumped about it, and I desperately wanted to change. So what was the problem?

The big day came, and I wasn't prepared. I did okay with breakfast, but when lunchtime rolled around, I was hungry and craving carbs, and I had nothing in the house except my usual junk. As a creature of habit (and a sugar addict), I thought I shouldn't waste the junk food I had on hand. I could always start the diet again another day.

Almost two weeks went by, and I realized that this isn't about a single day. This is about my *life*. I was tired of waiting for tomorrow, for Monday, or for the first of the month or the first of the year to start taking care of myself. Those were nothing but tired excuses that had kept me stuck for years. I looked in the mirror and said out loud, "That's enough! I will not put this off another day." I grabbed my bag, went straight to the store, and came home with lots of keto-friendly foods.

I officially started the ketogenic diet on January 13, 2015, at 289 pounds. I'm five-eleven, so even after losing a little weight after I quit drinking soda, I was still considered morbidly obese. Some days, I felt like I had a mountain to move, and the task seemed daunting. I decided to tackle it one day—or even one meal—at a time, and I kept pushing through.

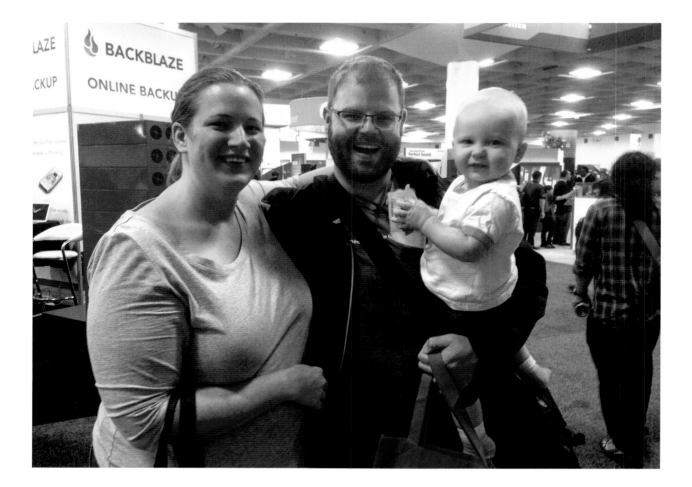

The first two weeks were definitely an adjustment, but I noticed pretty quickly that I wasn't overly hungry or obsessing over food like I had with other diets. My meals were delicious, filling, and easy to do at home, on the go, and out with friends. For the first time, I felt a freedom from my addiction to food. I also learned new ways to deal with stress, anxiety, and even happiness. Because food was at the center of every emotion in my life, I learned to ask myself whether I was I truly hungry or if emotional issues were driving my desire to eat. I believe the key to lasting weight loss is twofold:

- You must find a diet that is healthy and livable.

- You must take the time to work on the emotional components that trigger overeating and/or poor food choices.

When I was ten weeks into the ketogenic diet, I nervously sat down and filmed my first video for my YouTube channel, Keto Karma. I was so excited to share keto with whoever would listen. I knew it could change so many people's lives. I have always loved connecting with and helping people, and I wanted to turn my pain and struggles into something positive and useful.

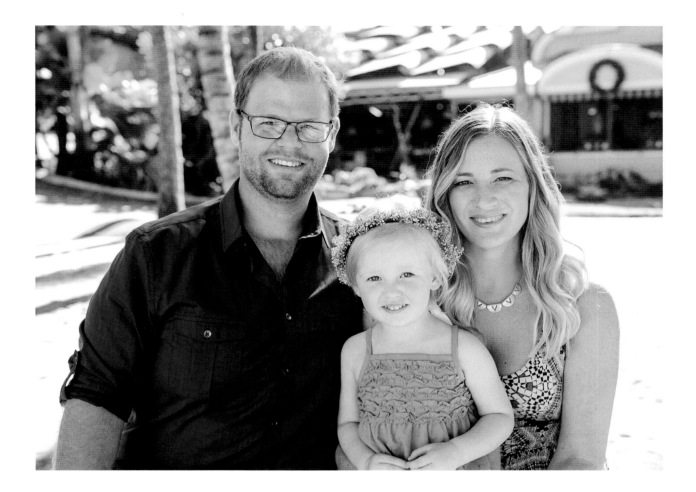

Little did I know what an amazing support system this would become. Every week for a year, I filmed a video with weigh-ins, tips, and advice, as well as chats about the emotional side of weight loss. Connecting with so many people on a personal level who had struggles similar to my own was healing in so many ways. I started my blog and social media channels so that I would have more ways to connect and share with others. Those support systems have been a tremendous help for my accountability and personal growth.

After one year of keto, I had lost a total of 100 pounds. I couldn't believe that the girl who couldn't stick to *anything* finally did. At the time of this writing, I have lost a total of 120 pounds, and I have been maintaining that new weight. My life has completely changed for the better. I wake up each day with a thankful heart and do my best to help as many people as possible. I have lots of energy to run around with my daughter and husband, and I can truly enjoy life. I am no longer a prisoner in my body. I try to keep challenging my comfort zones, and I know that this journey will be a lifelong one. I feel humbled and honored to be where I am today.

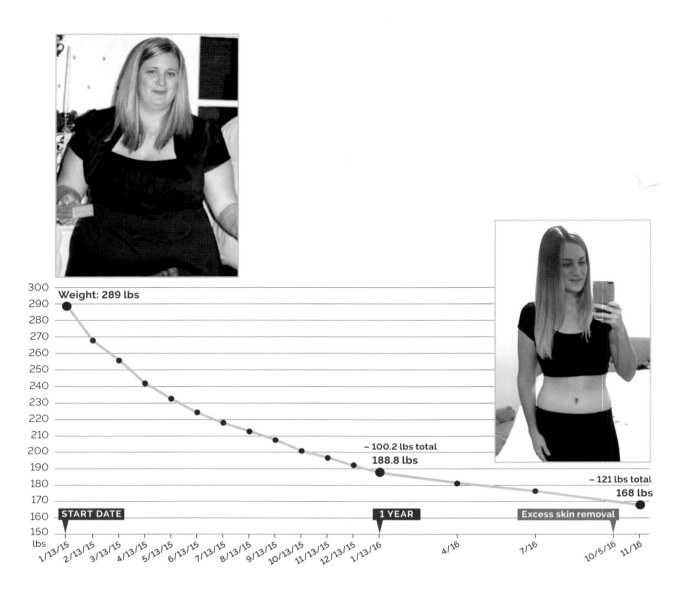

Weight: 289 lbs

– 100.2 lbs total
188.8 lbs

– 121 lbs total
168 lbs

START DATE

1 YEAR

Excess skin removal

300
290
280
270
260
250
240
230
220
210
200
190
180
170
160
150
lbs

1/13/15 · 2/13/15 · 3/13/15 · 4/13/15 · 5/13/15 · 6/13/15 · 7/13/15 · 8/13/15 · 9/13/15 · 10/13/15 · 11/13/15 · 12/13/15 · 1/13/16 · 4/16 · 7/16 · 10/5/16 · 11/16

I hope my story shows you that change truly is possible. No matter how many times you've tried and "failed," you can change. In fact, failure helps us learn and grow, even if that means learning what *doesn't* work. Your past doesn't define you, and you should never, ever give up on yourself. You are capable of amazing things, and the time to achieve them is now.

"Success consists of getting up just one more time than you fall."

—Oliver Goldsmith

ABOUT THIS BOOK

Simply Keto is so much more than a cookbook. It is a peek into my journey to find my inner strength and value. It's a practical and easy-to-understand guide to help you get started and be successful on your own path to self-improvement. It is inspiration and hope, especially for those who have struggled with their weight. And last but not least, it's a resource full of helpful information and tips that I've learned during and after my 120-pound weight loss on the ketogenic diet. In the following chapters, you will find

- The basics about the ketogenic diet, including an easy-to-understand breakdown of how it works (see page 28) and simple instructions for how to start and succeed on keto (see page 33)

- Information about key health topics (see page 39) and answers to the most frequently asked questions about the keto diet and my personal experience losing weight on keto that I receive (see page 44)

- Lists of some of the most popular ketogenic foods, with ideas for new ingredients to incorporate into your menus (see page 53)

- More than 100 easy recipes, with calorie counts and macros, including total and net carbs, for every recipe (beginning on page 64)

- Thirty days of preplanned meals to help you prepare for and visualize a full month of living a ketogenic lifestyle (see page 293)

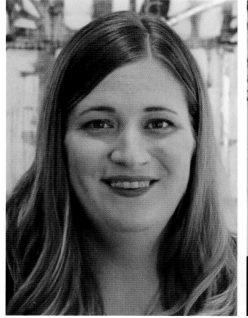

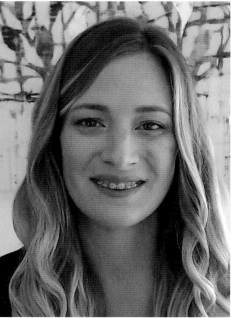

10 weeks after starting keto
–37 pounds

54 weeks after starting keto
–102.4 pounds

FROM THE KETO COMMUNITY

Over the past three years, I've had the honor of receiving thousands of messages from people all over the world who have been inspired by my story. Messages from incredible people like the ones below truly touch my heart. I feel so thankful and humbled that my journey has been a source of hope and inspiration to so many others. I want to thank all of you for your endless support, love, and kindness. My life is forever changed.

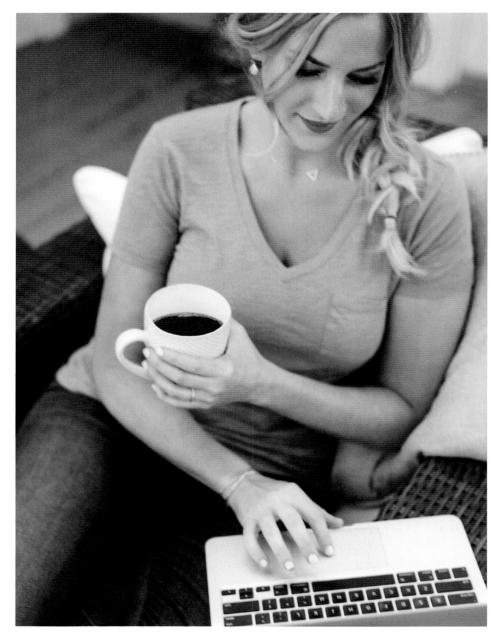

I remember exactly the day—September 27, 2016. A friend had mentioned the keto diet to me, and intrigued, I spent an entire evening scouring the hashtag on Instagram. I wanted to get a feel for the types of meals people were eating, and also to see some success stories. That's when I first found Suzanne. There was so much about her that instantly resonated with me. I think it was the combination of needing to lose about as much weight, being a stay-at-home mom, and the fact that we lived near each other [that] made her journey something that I could really relate to. I stayed up until 2 a.m. devouring Suzanne's Instagram feed, YouTube channel, and blog. Everything about her approach seemed so straightforward—she wasn't trying to sell anything and there were no gimmicks. Her photos were of real food that I would want to eat, and everything looked amazing. Her before and after pictures were jaw-dropping.

The very next morning I woke up determined to start the ketogenic diet immediately. From day one, I have heavily relied on her recipes, and I love how delicious and simple they are. Anytime I needed a dose of inspiration or self-love, or even just ideas of foods to buy at popular grocery chains, I would go to Suzanne's channels and find exactly what I needed. She's always showing her readers just how doable this lifestyle is; no pills, wraps, shakes, powders, or memberships were needed to succeed. I realized that I could simply believe in myself, keep keto, prioritize my care, and get results. I loved that her way of doing keto required nothing more than a local grocery store, and she never hesitated to share her insights with us. One year and 60 pounds later, I'm still completely smitten with this way of eating, and the cherry on top is that Suzanne has become one of my dearest and closest friends.

Suzanne is as beautiful on the inside as she appears on screen, and she has spent the last three years helping people navigate the ketogenic diet from a place of compassion and encouragement. She deeply believes that keto should be done as simply as possible for the best results. I am thrilled that she has written a book that includes all of her tips, tricks, and favorite recipes. Friends and family often ask me how to begin on the keto diet, and I am grateful that I can now hand them a copy of Simply Keto *and know that they will get all the information they need to have their own wildly successful journey, too.*

—Melissa L.

When I first decided to embark on my own keto journey, I came across Suzanne's blog and videos. She had started a few months before I did, but I could already see the progress she was making. I felt that if she could do it, I could do it too! Knowing that Suzanne made progress and healed her body through keto was enough for me to give it a shot. I've followed Suzanne's journey since then and it has been empowering for me, still on this journey to wellness. She's been an inspiration for me ever since, and it's wonderful to see her enjoy her life to the fullest!

—Lele J.

I first noticed Keto Karma (Suzanne Ryan) on an Instagram post with a side-by-side before-and-after picture. The dramatic weight loss transformation is what caught my sight at first. But then I started reading her posts. Suzanne was so honest about how she felt when she was overweight, both physically (feeling exhausted) and mentally (feeling defeated), [and her feelings] echoed my own. She knew what it was like to experience that negative inner dialogue of "I can't" and "I won't be able to," and she transformed it into one of strength and confidence. Slowly, after reading so many of her honest and encouraging posts, I began to believe I could do it, too. I remember one of her posts that really resonated with me. In it Suzanne discussed how before she started her journey she was "the girl who couldn't stick to anything, the girl who stopped believing in herself." But ultimately, she was the girl who did have the strength all along. She wrote, "Believe in yourself. YOU are capable . . . even if you've failed 100+ times before. I've been there . . . change is possible." Change IS possible. I started following Suzanne's Instagram page regularly for tips and inspiration. She made it so easy to follow a keto-friendly meal plan at home and out at restaurants with her simple pointers. She helped me find the strength to believe in myself. She inspired me to change my life, to adopt a new healthy lifestyle. I have so much gratitude for Suzanne for starting her journey and for sharing it with others so honestly.

—Sallie W.

When it comes to finding inspirational, healthy people on social media, the internet has thousands of fitness models and muscle-heads screaming into the camera with messages about feeling the fear and doing it anyway. The thing I love about Suzanne and her account is that she is a real person going through the very real struggle of how to maintain health and weight while being a mom and a wife and a real human being.

Suzanne is one of the kindest people I've ever encountered, and I'm proud to call her a friend. She is so transparent about her journey and has given hope to so many people who have never had a real champion before. She graciously answers questions and posts advice and feedback that is both actionable and sensitive to the real issues surrounding obesity, overeating, and healthy food consumption. For someone who has been told his entire life how impossible it is to lose weight and keep it off, Suzanne's example helps me believe that I can do this and do it forever.

—Tim B.

After having baby #3 I happened to find Suzanne's journey on Instagram. I immediately became inspired and knew keto was something I could do. I've lost over 45 pounds, and with many bumps in the road, she has always been there to encourage me. I think the main thing I have learned from Suzanne and her journey is to never give up. Thank you for having such a positive impact on my life and the lives of so many others.

—Melissa S.

When starting my own journey back in 2015, one of my goals was to build a support group of people going on similar journeys where we could encourage each other and share food ideas, and the biggest support came from Instagram. One of the first people I connected with was Suzanne. We began our journeys around the same time at the same weight. As we continued on our journeys we were losing weight at roughly the same pace. We began calling each other twins. From week to week we would always encourage, compliment, and support each other through all the victories and minor setbacks.

One thing that sticks out to me about Suzanne was her honesty, openness, and vulnerability throughout her journey. Each week on her YouTube channel she would weigh in, summarize her ups and downs for the week, and just be honest about the entire process. In addition to sharing her own story each week, she would spotlight someone else's journey, the weight they've lost, how they've done it and their favorite foods. Helping her viewers connect with others on similar journeys and sharing their success stories.

Lastly, Suzanne's blog, ketokarma.com, is a great reference guide for beginners and finding some yummy recipes. One of my favs, which my family and I thoroughly enjoy regularly, is her Twice-Baked Cauliflower Casserole recipe.

Suzanne, reflecting back on where you were back in 2015 to where you are now is nothing less than inspiring. Thanks for all the love, support, and encouragement throughout the entire process. I wish you nothing but the best in all you do.

—*Daniel T.*

I can't tell my keto story to others without mentioning Suzanne. I started in August 2014 and found her shortly after. She had such a level-headed approach and almost made keto look easier than it already is!

During some challenging moments or times of weakness I would often stop to look at her success. She never failed to recharge my motivation! I really respected that she continued to do the "right" thing and didn't let obstacles and difficult times disrupt her progress.

Suzanne is an absolute inspiration, and I'm so fortunate to have had her support. And I'm grateful for the wealth of knowledge she's shared along the way. I was able to lose over 40 pounds and felt better than I could ever remember!

—*Carisa G.*

"You must learn a new way to think before you can master a new way to be."

—Marianne Williamson

I have struggled with my weight all of my life, and always gave up diet after diet. In the spring of 2015, I came across Suzanne's YouTube channel, and I was instantly moved by her hard work and dedication. She introduced a new lifestyle to me—the ketogenic lifestyle—and it has changed my life. I maintain a low-carb, high-fat diet to keep my blood sugar under control (I am a type 2 diabetic), but the best part about this diet is that there are ways to beat the sugar cravings and still keep insulin levels low. Suzanne is not only very knowledgeable of the ketogenic diet but has showed her fans the results of such a great diet; her transformation is amazing!

Because of Suzanne's guidance and support, I was able to lose 25 pounds of fat effortlessly. Suzanne helps her fans realize that the ketogenic diet is a diet that is very easy to stick to, and consistency is key to losing body fat and staying healthy. Thank you, Suzanne, for helping me find myself after all these years. My newfound confidence is, without a doubt, due to your dedication to yourself and your fans. Cheers!

—Jon N.

I stumbled across Suzanne's YouTube channel around 11 months ago, and I'm so glad I did. I live in New Zealand and we tend to be a bit behind with trends, so it took me a while to hear about the ketogenic diet. I've been bigger my whole life and diligently followed the healthy eating guidelines, so the idea of eating fat and a lot of it sounded crazy to me! Then I remembered that old saying, "Insanity is doing the same thing and expecting different results." For years, I stuck to the same cycle of "healthy" eating and just kept getting bigger and sicker. It was time to try something new, and not really knowing where to start I did what everyone does and turned to Google. The day I found Keto Karma's videos was the kick in the butt I needed; I sat down and watched them from start to finish. It was amazing to see Suzanne's journey, not just in terms of losing weight but also watching her grow in confidence and maybe most importantly learning how to tune in to her body and gain control of her relationship with food. Suzanne always felt relatable, like a friend talking directly to me. She gave me faith to trust the process and helped me realize that time would be my friend if I just did little things consistently. It was only a matter of days after watching that I started keto myself. Since day one I've lost over 100 pounds, and even though I've still got a bit to go, for the first time ever I feel like this is a lifestyle change, not a diet. It's hard to put into words how life-changing Suzanne has been for me, but she really has made a huge impact. So here's a big THANK YOU from a grateful woman on the other side of the world.

—Colleen P.

"Change is the end result of all true learning."

—Leo Buscaglia

Suzanne is a true inspiration within the Keto community. Her devotion to a better life radiates from Suzanne, and her passion has influenced thousands of people to follow in her footsteps. I couldn't be more proud of Suzanne; her journey has been amazing and truly touching. The weekly videos motivated thousands of people (including myself) as it highlighted the fact that anyone can make a difference; you just need that dedication to better yourself. Even though we live in different continents with a time zone of 8+ hours, I am confident that Suzanne's loving and kind nature will always make time for me. She's not just another "keto girl on the internet," but a very close friend. Thank you for everything you do. I couldn't be more thankful of our friendship.

—Adam F.

After trying countless diets without success, I began following a ketogenic diet in January 2015. I finally felt like I had found a way of eating that I could adopt as a lifestyle and not just as a temporary fix to lose some weight.

Shortly after beginning this new phase of my journey, I began following Suzanne's weight loss Instagram page and YouTube videos. She was still pretty early on in her own journey as we had started at nearly the same time. Her transparency made her relatable and approachable. She was (and still is) always willing to offer her honest advice and words of encouragement. I have fallen short and felt as though I have let myself down many times, but because of those like Suzanne, I haven't given up on myself. I have continued to fight and believe in myself, and seeing what she has accomplished makes me want to try even harder today than I did yesterday.

Thank you, Suzanne, from the bottom of my heart, for continuing to cheer me and so many of us still fighting the good fight. Thank you for reminding us that we are worth it and that we can take control of our health. Thank you for sharing your journey with us and letting us have a glimpse into what it takes to bring us success. Thank you for inspiring me and countless others daily and for helping me to believe that I have the power within me to smash my goals!

—Andrea D.

"Owning our story can be hard but not nearly as difficult as spending our lives running from it. Embracing our vulnerabilities is risky but not nearly as dangerous as giving up on love and belonging and joy—the experiences that make us the most vulnerable. Only when we are brave enough to explore the darkness will we discover the infinite power of our light."

—Brené Brown

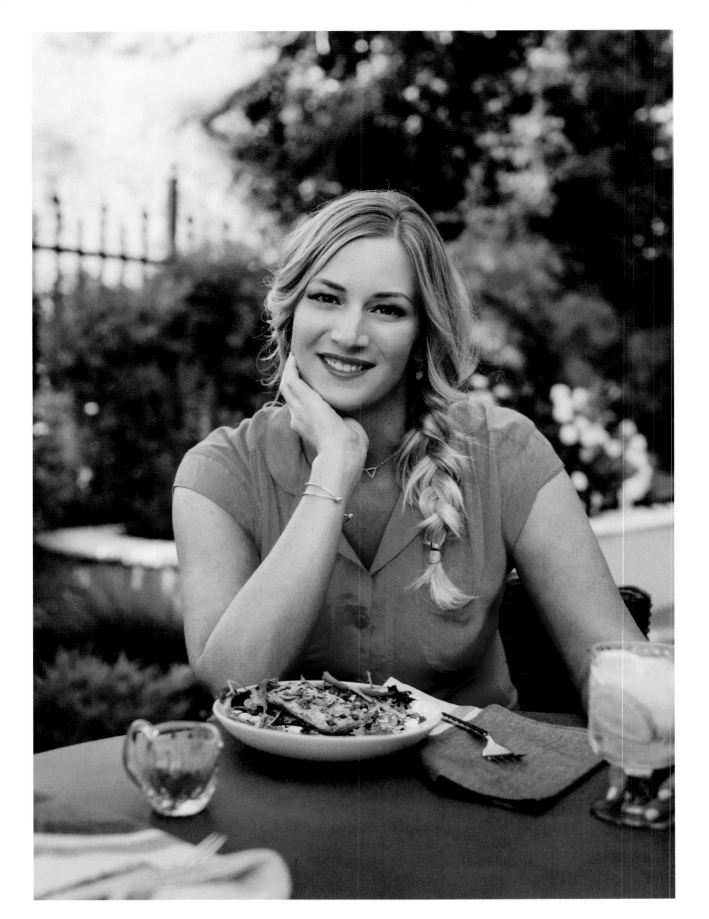

CHAPTER 1:
All About Keto

You probably have a lot of questions about the ketogenic diet and how to get started. In this chapter, I've provided answers to the most common questions that people tend to ask about keto.

KETO 101

The ketogenic diet (or "keto" for short) is a high-fat, low-carbohydrate, moderate-protein way of eating. Essentially, eating a ketogenic diet will naturally change your body's primary energy source from glucose (carbs/sugar) to ketones (fat).

What is nutritional ketosis, and how does it work?

Nutritional ketosis (also known simply as ketosis) is a natural metabolic state in which your body is utilizing fat and producing ketone bodies (ketones) within a range of 0.5 to 5 millimoles per liter of blood. This measurement can be found by testing for ketones, which I will get into later in this chapter.

On the Standard American Diet (a high-carb diet), carbohydrates (sugar and starches) are broken down during digestion into a simple sugar called glucose. Most of this glucose is released into the bloodstream; therefore, blood glucose levels rise, which stimulates the pancreas to secrete a hormone called insulin. Insulin helps regulate blood sugar and plays a key role in enabling glucose to enter cells to be absorbed and used for energy. Insulin also helps ensure a reserve of excess glucose in the liver and muscles, which is called glycogen or glycogen stores.

In contrast, on a ketogenic diet, you eat high fat, very little carbohydrate, and moderate protein, thereby avoiding foods that would likely cause a significant glucose and insulin response. Once your glucose levels drop and your body's glycogen stores are depleted, free fatty acids (from fat tissue) are released and are converted in your liver to ketones, which are used for energy.

HOW DOES KETOSIS WORK?

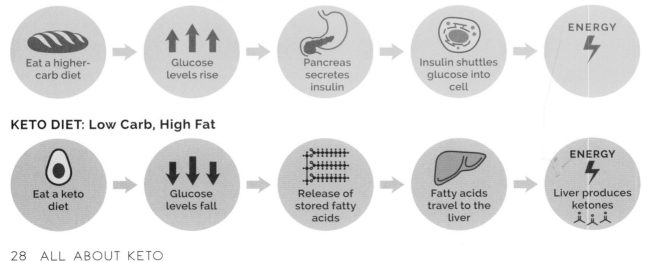

STANDARD AMERICAN DIET: Higher Carb

Eat a higher-carb diet → Glucose levels rise → Pancreas secretes insulin → Insulin shuttles glucose into cell → ENERGY

KETO DIET: Low Carb, High Fat

Eat a keto diet → Glucose levels fall → Release of stored fatty acids → Fatty acids travel to the liver → ENERGY Liver produces ketones

Why is keto a moderate-protein diet?

Simply put, when you eat more protein than your body requires, a natural process called *gluconeogenesis* converts a percentage of non-carbohydrate sources (in this case, protein) to glucose upon breakdown. Therefore, while it's not necessary to fear protein, and it's important to reach your protein goal to preserve your lean body mass, remember that consuming excessive amounts of protein can increase your risk of being kicked out of ketosis.

note: Gluconeogenesis also ensures that your body has the glucose it requires for normal function.

What are ketones, and where are they produced?

Ketones (ketone bodies) are a natural lipid-based energy source used by the body and brain. Ketones are produced in the liver as a result of the body breaking down fat for energy—a process known as *fat oxidation.*

There are three types of ketone bodies:

- **Acetone** is measured in the breath using a breath meter.
- **Acetoacetate (AcAc)** is measured in the urine using urine test strips.
- **Beta-hydroxybutyrate (BHB)** is measured in the blood using blood test strips—the most accurate method for testing ketones.

note: Acetone is technically a by-product produced during the breakdown of acetoacetate (AcAc), but it is often referred to as a ketone body.

How long does it take to get into ketosis after starting the ketogenic diet?

The timing varies from person to person, but it generally takes a few days to a week after dialing in your personal macros to get into ketosis.

What does it mean to be keto-adapted?

The term "keto-adapted" basically means that your body has been in ketosis for a consistent period to the point that it is fully adjusted and is now using ketones as its primary energy source. The amount of time it takes to become keto-adapted varies from person to person, but it generally takes a few weeks to a month.

What's the difference between diabetic ketoacidosis and nutritional ketosis?

People sometimes hear the word *ketogenic* and become alarmed because they are confusing nutritional ketosis with diabetic ketoacidosis. Let's go over the big differences between the two:

- **Diabetic ketoacidosis (DKA)** is a life-threatening condition sometimes seen in people with unmanaged diabetes (mostly type 1, but sometimes type 2). This condition is characterized by dangerously high levels of blood ketones (15 to 25 mM/L) and high blood sugar (above 200 mg/dl), as well as a very low blood pH. This condition causes the blood to become too acidic, which is a very serious medical emergency.

- **Nutritional ketosis** is a safe and natural metabolic state that produces "low-level" ketones (generally 0.5 to 5.0 mM/L) with blood sugars averaging from 60 to 120 mg/dl and normal pH levels.

What are the health benefits of the ketogenic diet?

While the ketogenic diet has been proven to be a very effective way to lose weight, weight loss is just one positive outcome in a long line of potential health benefits. Research is being done all over the world regarding the use of ketogenic diets to treat many conditions, including heart disease, cancer, Alzheimer's disease, epilepsy, Parkinson's disease, polycystic ovarian syndrome (PCOS), brain injuries, post-traumatic stress disorder, depression, acne, and so many more.

What are macros?

Macros is short for *macronutrients.* The three primary macronutrients found in foods and beverages are

- Fat

- Protein

- Carbohydrate

When people in the keto community talk about macros, they are referring to the breakdown of fat, protein, and carbohydrate in their meals or their overall diet. Macros are often expressed as percentages.

tip: If tracking everything you eat seems overwhelming, some people find it helpful to focus solely on keeping their net carbohydrates at or below 20 grams for the first one to two weeks. Once you get used to this step, you can begin tracking your other macros (protein and fat) as well as your caloric intake, if you choose. While there is no argument that not all calories are created equal, if you've struggled with overeating, like I have, tracking your caloric intake, even for a short time, can help you find a healthier balance.

What macros should I aim for on the ketogenic diet?

This (low-carb) pie chart is a great visual representation of how your meals and daily macros should look.

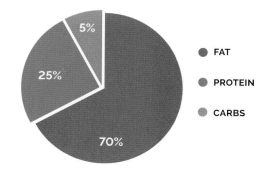

Carbs are kept to a minimum, at around 5 percent of total caloric intake (which typically translates to 20 to 25 grams of net carbs a day).

Protein is moderate, at around 25 percent of total caloric intake.

Fat (find out more about the different types of fat on page 42) is high, at around 70 percent of total caloric intake.

It is important to note that each person's ideal macronutrient percentages will be different; the above percentages are not set in stone. You can easily calculate your personalized macros by using the keto calculator on my blog, at ketokarma.com/macros. While macro calculators are a great place to start, you may need to make some adjustments to fine-tune your macros for optimal success.

What foods should I avoid on the ketogenic diet?

There are many delicious foods that you *can* enjoy on the ketogenic diet; see Chapter 2 for a comprehensive guide. The following foods, however, are to be avoided:

- **Foods that are high in sugar:** Soda, juice, cake, ice cream, candy, sugar, and so on

- **Grains and starches:** Wheat-based products, rice, pasta, cereal, and so on

- **Most fruit:** But see the lower-carb fruit options on page 55

- **Legumes:** Peas, kidney beans, lentils, chickpeas, and so on

- **Starchy veggies:** Corn, potatoes, beets, carrots, and so on

What are total carbs and net carbs?

Among people who follow low-carb diets, you'll often hear the terms "total carbs" and "net carbs." Here's a quick breakdown of what those two terms mean.

Total carbs is exactly what it sounds like: it's a calculation of all the carbohydrate in a food, including dietary fiber.

To arrive at the amount of *net carbs* in a food, you subtract dietary fiber (and sugar alcohols, if applicable) from the total amount of carbohydrate in that food, as shown in the example below. Dietary fiber and sugar alcohols (see page 57 for specific sugar alcohol recommendations) generally have a minimal impact on blood sugar; therefore, some people choose not to count them as part of their target carbohydrate intake. Instead, they focus on net carbs.

Total carbohydrates – Dietary fiber – Sugar alcohols = Net carbs

(In case you are wondering, I personally count net carbs.)

Here is an example of a food that contains both dietary fiber and sugar alcohols. As you can see from this nutrition label from Good Dee's Yellow Snack Cake low-carb baking mix, the total carbohydrate per serving is 13 grams. To calculate the net carbs, you subtract the 6 grams of dietary fiber and the 5 grams of sugar alcohols from the total carb count, which gives you only 2 grams of net carbs per serving.

NUTRITION FACTS	
Serving Size 1/12 pkg (22g mix)	
Servings Per Container 12	
Amount Per Serving	
Calories 70	Calories from Fat 50
	% Daily Value*
Total Fat 6g	9%
Saturated Fat 0g	0%
Trans Fat 0g	
Cholesterol 0mg	0%
Sodium 100mg	4%
Total Carbohydrate 13g	4%
Dietary Fiber 6g	24%
Sugars 0g	
Sugar Alcohol 5g	
Protein 2g	

Here's another example. 3 ounces of cauliflower has 4 grams of total carbs. When you subtract the 2 grams of dietary fiber, you get 2 grams of net carbs per serving.

Note that the nutrition information found on food labels may be calculated differently from country to country. In the United States, total carbs currently include fiber and sugar alcohols.

NUTRITION FACTS	
Servings Size 3oz (85g)	
Amount Per Serving	
Calories 20	Calories from Fat 0
	% Daily Value*
Total Fat 0g	0%
Saturated Fat 0g	0%
Trans Fat 0g	
Cholesterol 0mg	0%
Sodium 25mg	1%
Total Carbohydrate 4g	1%
Dietary Fiber 2g	8%
Sugars 2g	
Protein 2g	

STARTING THE KETOGENIC DIET

Now that we have covered what the ketogenic diet is and how it works, let's talk about how to get started and stay on track. These are the exact steps I used when I started keto. Remember, you don't have to be an expert in ketosis to be successful with this lifestyle. You can do this!

There are two main approaches that I recommend when starting the ketogenic diet, especially for weight loss. First I'll go over full tracking, followed by minimal tracking, aka Lazy Keto.

Full Tracking

Getting set up to track everything you eat on keto involves just three basic steps.

Step 1: Step on the scale and record your starting weight. But understand one thing: The number you see doesn't define you; it's simply your starting point. I remember stepping on the scale on the day I started keto and seeing 289 pounds. That number wasn't easy to face, but I felt empowered knowing that it would be the *last* time I would ever see a number that high.

I also highly recommend taking "before" photos and body measurements. I took photos and recorded measurements of my neck, waist, and hips in MyFitnessPal, a popular tracking app. (If you want to track other measurements in MyFitnessPal, you can add them by clicking My Home, then Check-In, and then Track Additional Measurements.) Measurements and photos can be very helpful in showing you changes in your body that the scale won't reveal. Remember, the number on the scale is helpful, but it doesn't tell the whole story; weight fluctuations can happen, and they don't necessarily mean you're doing anything "wrong." If at any point you feel that you've hit a stall with your weight loss, see pages 37 and 38 for advice.

Step 2: Set you your personalized macros in an online keto calculator. You can use the free calculator on my blog at ketokarma.com/macros or another online calculator of your choosing. Here is the process for setting up your personalized macros:

- Visit **ketokarma.com/macros** either on your phone or on your computer.
- **Enter your personal data:** This includes age, gender, height, and weight.
- **Set your activity level:** Select the activity level that fits your lifestyle best; this ranges from sedentary (the setting I chose) to athlete.
- **Choose your caloric deficit:** For weight loss, I recommend starting with a 20 percent deficit.

Now you have your very own personalized results! Save the information and update your stats in the keto calculator from time to time as you lose weight. I recalculated my macros after every fifteen- to twenty-pound loss, but a more common recommendation is to recalculate every two to three weeks. Remember, there is a lot of gray area when it comes to dialing in what works best for you, so do what feels right.

Step 3: Take your personalized macros from the keto calculator and set them up in your food tracker of choice. I use MyFitnessPal. In this app, you can track your macros with percentages for free or with exact target numbers in grams for a monthly or yearly fee. If you are the type who is okay with rounding things out, then the free version will probably be just fine, but if you would prefer to track your exact numbers, then you can upgrade to a premium account for more customized settings. I was able to get my macros very close to my goals by using the free percentage tracking. To change these settings in MyFitnessPal, go to My Home, then Goals, and then click the edit button next to Daily Nutrition Goals.

I decided to track both my macros and my caloric intake for the first year because I wanted to learn about the macros in different foods and about proper portion sizes. I also liked the accountability of seeing exactly what I was eating each day. I stopped tracking after a year, and now I am able to go off of what I learned during that time. I personally think that tracking is a valuable opportunity to learn, but it isn't something you have to do forever, unless you enjoy it. Do whatever works best for you. At this point, almost three years into living a ketogenic lifestyle, I basically just keep a rough estimate of the carbs I'm consuming each day, make sure my protein intake is moderate, and of course enjoy lots of healthy fats.

These three steps are the foundation of a great start on the ketogenic diet. Remember, the macros you have calculated are purely a starting point. See how you feel and be open to making adjustments as needed, such as if weight loss stalls (see pages 37 and 38). If you test your ketone levels (optional), then your results will be a good indicator of whether your macros are appropriately dialed in or need to be adjusted. If you don't plan on testing for ketones, ask yourself: how do I feel, what is my energy level (after the first 3 weeks), am I losing weight, how is my appetite, and so on, then adjust your macros as needed.

"Incredible change happens in your life when you decide to take control of what you do have power over instead of craving control over what you don't."

—Steve Maraboli

"Lazy Keto": Minimal Tracking

I get it; some people find tracking to be too time-consuming or stressful. With the Lazy Keto approach, you keep track of your carb intake (generally with the goal of consuming no more than 20 grams of net carbs daily) and eat a moderate amount of protein and high fat, but without logging your meals and snacks.

I recommend that even with this method, you calculate your personalized macros as outlined above and track what you eat for the first two to three weeks. Tracking in the beginning gives you an idea of what you're eating each day and helps you gauge proper portion sizes. You'll also learn a bit about the macronutrient breakdowns in various foods. (You'd be surprised by the amounts of carbs in some "healthy" foods!) Tracking for two to three weeks will give you a good feeling for what a typical day looks like when following a ketogenic diet. Remember, tracking isn't a punishment, but a tool to help you learn about food and your eating habits. If you do choose Lazy Keto, then I highly recommend testing your blood ketones from time to time (see the following section) to ensure that you are eating in a way that allows your body to be in ketosis.

All that's left to do is go shopping for food (see Chapter 2) and prepare for success!

TESTING FOR KETONES

Let me start by saying that unless you are doing keto for a specific health condition or have an immediate desire to test, testing isn't something you have to do right away. I recommend checking your blood ketones at some point (especially when you are dialing in your personalized macros or if your weight loss stalls), but the timing (if at all) is totally up to you! Here are the three options for checking your ketone levels:

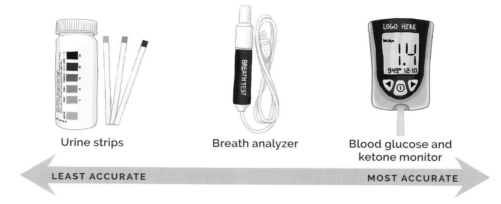

| Urine strips | Breath analyzer | Blood glucose and ketone monitor |

LEAST ACCURATE ←——————————————————→ **MOST ACCURATE**

- **Urine strips:** This method is the least accurate, especially after keto adaptation. Due to the number of false negatives and positives I've seen, I don't recommend using urine strips for ketone testing.

- **Breath analyzer (such as Ketonix):** This method is more reliable than urine strips, but still not the most accurate form of testing. A breath analyzer gives you a good range to determine whether you are in ketosis but does not tell you your exact ketone level.

- **Blood glucose and ketone monitor (I use the Precision Xtra):** Using a tiny blood sample is the most accurate way to measure ketones. It's easy to do at home and requires only a simple prick of your finger. Take it from me, I'm a complete wimp when it comes to anything involving pain or blood, and even I find it very easy. Here's a tip: when using the lancet, prick the side of your fingertip, as this area is a lot less sensitive than the pad of your finger!

THE IMPORTANCE OF HAVING A SUPPORT SYSTEM

Having a system of support is one of the most overlooked factors in successful weight loss. After years of failed dieting, my self-esteem and self-confidence were pretty low, and I didn't have many people in my life who truly understood how I was feeling. Although my loved ones meant well, there's no substitute for people in your life who totally get what you're going through. It's so helpful to surround yourself with like-minded people who are on a mission similar to your own.

Weight loss is mostly a mental battle. Having a support system in your corner will help you grow. It's a great way to get new meal ideas, learn new things, and keep yourself accountable. If you don't have a solid support system at home or if you desire more support, I encourage you to get involved with a few great (and free) communities online. See page 312 for suggestions.

note: Ketone levels are often lowest in the morning and peak later in the day. Try to test at the same time of day for a more accurate day-to-day comparison. When testing to determine whether a specific food affects your ketone levels, it's smart to test your blood ketones around two hours after consuming that food to check for changes.

Case in point: My friend Melissa called me one day, bummed out because her urine test strip had just shown that she wasn't in ketosis. She was frustrated because she felt she had been doing everything right. She knew I wasn't a big fan of urine strips, but she had purchased them due to the low price and ease of testing. I immediately drove to her house with my Precision Xtra monitor and let her check her blood ketones. A few seconds later, we had an accurate blood ketone reading of 1.3 mM/L! (Over 0.5 mM/L is in ketosis, if you missed that part, so Melissa had definitely achieved her goal.) This is a prime example of why, though I see the appeal of the ease and cost of urine strips, I don't recommend them. If you can't rely on them, why bother with them at all?

As a side note, Melissa has now lost more than 55 pounds and has her very own blood glucose and ketone monitor.

"They always say time changes things, but you actually have to change them yourself."

—Andy Warhol

DEALING WITH WEIGHT—LOSS STALLS

Quite often I receive messages from people that say something along the lines of, "HELP! I was doing great the first few weeks after starting keto, and now the scale isn't moving! What do I do?"

The first thing I want you to know is that weight-loss stalls happen to almost everyone at some point. Your weight can go up or down or stay the same for a number of reasons, including hormone fluctuations, stress, fluid retention, and food choices. I wouldn't classify myself as being in a stall until I had been at the same weight for two to three weeks. That being said, let's go over a few things that can cause stalls:

- **Too much or too little protein.** While it is important to eat enough protein to prevent muscle loss, the ketogenic diet is a moderate-protein diet, so you have to determine how much protein is best for your body and activity level. (Visit the keto calculator on my blog at ketokarma.com/macros to determine a good starting point for your protein consumption.) It's helpful to play around with your macros to see what works for you. Consuming excessive amounts of protein can actually kick you out of ketosis due to increasing your blood sugar via gluconeogenesis. (Find more on that on page 29.)

- **Too much dairy.** While some people do just fine with dairy, we are all different, and others find that too much dairy can slow or stall weight loss. Try cutting back or cutting out dairy to see if it is, in fact, causing issues.

- **Too much artificial sweetener.** This includes things like diet soda, low-carb and sugar-free desserts/candies, and sweetener in your coffee or tea. I very rarely drink diet soda, but if I do, I limit it to once or twice a month. I also try to consume only one or two artificially sweetened beverages per day, and it's my Morning Coffee (page 282).

- **Too many nuts/nut butters.** Yeah, peanut butter, I'm talking to you. Nuts and nut butters are easy to overconsume. Nut butters are especially sneaky, as most of us just grab a spoon and scoop out what we assume to be one serving, but may in fact be several servings' worth. Nuts and peanut butter can add up quickly in carbs and calories, so try to premeasure or limit consumption if you are in a stall.

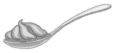

- **Too many calories.** Now, I know some people say that you don't need to worry about calories on keto, but I disagree. To me, it's very logical that while keto does help with food cravings, energy level, and overall health, calories in versus calories out will have an effect on weight loss. While I know that not all calories are created equal, as someone who has struggled with overeating, I find it helpful to have a guideline for sensible eating in a caloric sense.

- **Too many processed "low net carb" foods.** This adjustment is what I call getting back to basics. While I'm not against all processed foods, it is important to be honest with yourself and see if you can make some adjustments to eat more whole foods. As a mom who lives on a budget and has a hectic schedule, I understand that we don't always have the time or the money to have everything organic, pastured, fresh, or homemade. Part of this journey is being kind to yourself and learning what works and is livable for you. *Moderation* is a vague term, but try to set yourself up for success by doing some meal prepping and having healthy options on hand when you need to grab something and go.

  I also highly recommend testing your blood ketones when you try new foods to determine how they affect your ketones. This isn't necessary with every food, but I definitely recommend checking if you truly want to see whether a food you're eating is, in fact, knocking you out of ketosis. (Find out more about checking your ketone levels on page 35.)

- **Stress.** Check your emotional health. Are you stressed? Obsessing about the number on the scale? Stress is something we all deal with, but learning new ways to handle how you react to stress is life-changing. I love the quote "Life is 10 percent what happens to you and 90 percent how you react to it." When I'm feeling stressed, I try to refocus my energy on doing something productive. If I have the time, I listen to a guided meditation or go for a thirty-minute walk. Before starting keto, my go-to for stress relief was searching for food to eat, so replacing this habit was a crucial part of my success.

  Next, if you find yourself stressing or obsessing about the number on your scale, it may be smart to put the scale away and focus on your eating habits. There were times when I literally asked my husband to hide the scale so I wouldn't weigh myself more than once a week. It can be really easy to let the number on the scale define whether you think you're successful or not. It always helped me to remember that there are so many other factors in success, such as increased mental clarity, better-fitting clothes, fewer food cravings, and the ability to make smarter choices about food. I also periodically check various body measurements or look at progress photos so that I have other ways to visualize the positive changes.

- **Sleep.** Are you getting enough sleep? Think of sleep as nutrition for your brain. Try to get between seven and nine hours of sleep each night. I find that being well rested helps me feel more energetic and focused throughout the day, which in turn helps me make better choices.

- **Hydration.** Are you drinking enough water? Try this easy-to-remember rule: consume at least eight 8-ounce glasses of fluids a day. While it's best for the majority of your liquid intake to be water, this 64 ounces can include sparkling water, unsweetened tea, coffee, and other beverages as well (see page 59 for good drink choices).

KETO HEALTH TOPICS

Combating the Keto Flu

During the first few weeks of starting keto, it's common for people to have an electrolyte imbalance. If not properly managed, this imbalance can lead to a temporary condition known as the "keto flu." It is associated with unpleasant symptoms such as headaches, dizziness, brain fog, lethargy, constipation, and leg cramps. These symptoms occur primarily in the early phases of keto, and things often balance out once a person is keto-adapted. Even after keto-adaptation, some people (especially those who are very active) may require electrolyte supplements if they do not consume enough foods that are rich in electrolytes (see below). (Remember that it is important to talk with your doctor before taking supplements, especially if you have health issues.) On a ketogenic diet, the main electrolytes to focus on are sodium, potassium, magnesium, and calcium.

Here are a couple of key ways to prevent or minimize the symptoms of keto flu:

- **General keto flu symptoms:** Add sodium (salt) back into your diet. The general recommendation is to supplement with 2 to 7 grams of sodium each day: 2 to 5 grams for the average person or up to 7 grams for very active people. Adding sodium is easily done; simply drink 1 or 2 cups of bouillon or salted broth (see page 80 for my beef bone broth recipe) or add more salt to your food or beverages. Also, be sure to drink lots of water and other fluids! Dehydration can make you feel pretty awful, so be sure to stay hydrated.

- **Leg cramps:** Increase your intake of magnesium.

- **Constipation:** Drink more water and increase your fiber intake. Coffee sometimes does the trick, too!

Magnesium-rich foods:

- Avocados
- Broccoli
- Dark chocolate
- Fish
- Kale
- Mushrooms, especially white and portobello
- Nuts, especially almonds
- Seeds, especially pumpkin seeds
- Spinach

Potassium-rich foods:

- Artichokes
- Asparagus
- Avocados
- Broccoli
- Brussels sprouts
- Fish, especially salmon
- Kale/leafy greens
- Mushrooms
- Tomatoes

Calcium-rich foods:

- Almonds
- Bok choy
- Broccoli
- Celery
- Cheese
- Dark leafy greens (spinach, kale, collard greens, and so on)
- Sardines
- Seeds, like sesame and chia

Fun Fact: 100 grams of Hass avocado contains 485 milligrams of potassium, while 100 grams of banana (often touted as being the *source for potassium*) actually contains less, at 358 milligrams. Plus, in 100 grams of bananas, there are 21 grams of carbs! No wonder the keto community loves avocados!

Working Out on Keto

If you enjoy working out and/or have a livable exercise routine going, keep it up! Be sure to keep on top of your electrolytes and stay hydrated. If you're interested in building muscle, I highly recommend checking out the Ketogains subreddit on Reddit (www.reddit.com/r/ketogains/). The Ketogains community is a fantastic resource full of helpful and supportive people. Dr. Jacob Wilson's website (www.themusclephd.com) is another great resource.

If you're like me and struggle with working out, however, then this section is for you.

Here's the deal: We all know that exercise is good for us. The long list of physical and mental health benefits is pretty amazing, and it's smart to incorporate physical activity into your life. That being said, you don't have to live in the gym (unless you want to, of course). You can start simply by taking small steps to be more active—take the stairs instead of the elevator, go for a thirty-minute walk around your neighborhood, take a small hike around a park with friends, go for a swim, or ride your bike. When you make lifestyle changes, they have to be livable, so make plans that you can stick to consistently. There are many types of exercise—going to the gym, participating in outdoor activities or sports, doing CrossFit, attending group exercise classes, and exercising at home. Keep an open mind, and remember that as you lose weight, being active will become a lot more enjoyable. When I was pushing 300 pounds, I was tired all the time, everything hurt, and exercise seemed overwhelming and intimidating. Trust me, I know the journey seems daunting sometimes, but it really doesn't have to be. Day by day, little by little, small steps done consistently add up to *big* change.

Now, for the majority of my first year on keto, I didn't work out. There's a saying that you lose weight in the kitchen and tone/build muscle in the gym, and boy, have I found this adage to be true. In the past, when trying to lose weight, I would change *everything* right away . . . new eating plan, new gym, new workout clothes, new lifestyle. But guess what? I quit. Every. Single. Time. I collected gym memberships like stamps in the passport book of a world traveler. I eventually grew to despise the gym simply because no matter how long I stayed on the treadmill or how many weights I lifted, I never lost much weight. You see, you can't exercise your way out of a bad diet. This time around, I decided not to stress out and instead just focused on taking one reasonable step at a time. My first step was quitting soda, my second step was staying under 20 grams of net carbs, and my third step was tracking and sticking to my personalized macros (fat, protein, and carbs). The next thing I knew, a year had passed, and I had lost 100 pounds!

"Imperfections are not inadequacies; they are reminders that we're all in this together."

—Brené Brown

I can't even begin to tell you how much better I felt after losing that weight. I knew that the next step was to get more active, but I still dreaded the thought of going to the gym. What I've found works best for me is doing things that don't feel like "working out." For example, I love to chase my daughter around the park, go for a swim, take our dog for a walk, and go on hikes with family and friends. Currently, I've lost a total of 120 pounds, and the next step is to get a little more active, but still in a livable and maintainable way.

So my main message is to pace yourself— after all, Rome wasn't built in a day. If you're feeling overwhelmed, break things off into smaller, more manageable pieces. Take on one change, master it, and then keep adding onto it.

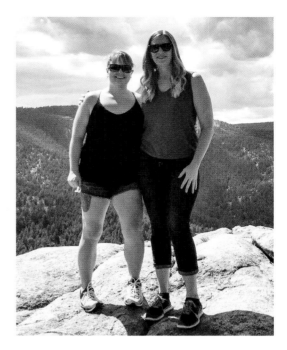

Considering Exogenous Ketones

Exogenous means "originating from an external source," and by now you know what a ketone is. There are currently two main forms of exogenous ketones (sometimes abbreviated as EKs and also known as ketone supplements): ketone salts (also referred to as beta-hydroxybutyrate salts or BHB salts) and ketone esters. Both are lab created.

While exogenous ketones show great potential as a treatment for various medical conditions, including epilepsy, cancer, Alzheimer's disease, and more, I do *not* believe that they should be marketed as weight-loss supplements. Sustainable weight loss will never come from a pill, wrap, or supplement; it comes from lifestyle change. If you are looking into these products for weight-loss purposes, I urge you to save your money. I've seen some pretty awful marketing and false information related to exogenous ketones, so please don't believe everything you read.

During my weight-loss journey, I never took ketone supplements, and I never obsessed over having high ketone levels. With the ketogenic diet increasing in popularity, there will be a lot of companies out to make money, so do your research before making any purchases. One of my favorite features of keto is that the only thing you need to buy to be successful is the right food. After trying to buy my way out of my weight problem for years, I know the feeling of wanting a quick fix, but real and lasting change can't be bought; it comes from within.

Healthy Versus Unhealthy Fats

While keto is a high-fat diet, it is important to educate yourself as to which specific types of fat are good to eat and which should be avoided:

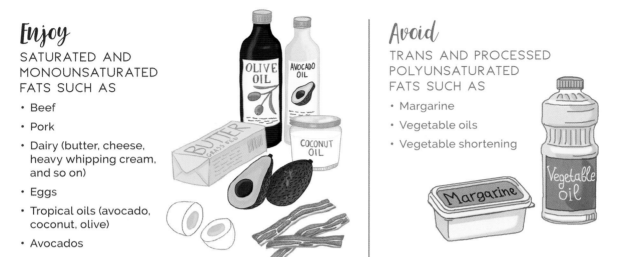

Enjoy

SATURATED AND MONOUNSATURATED FATS SUCH AS

- Beef
- Pork
- Dairy (butter, cheese, heavy whipping cream, and so on)
- Eggs
- Tropical oils (avocado, coconut, olive)
- Avocados

Avoid

TRANS AND PROCESSED POLYUNSATURATED FATS SUCH AS

- Margarine
- Vegetable oils
- Vegetable shortening

Like many of you, I was taught to stay away from saturated fat. I grew up with "I Can't Believe It's Not Butter," turkey bacon, vegetable oils, and a *lot* of sugar. It turns out that the majority of the medical community now considers trans fat to be one of the worst types of fat to eat. Trans fats have been linked with an increased risk of heart disease and have been shown to adversely affect cholesterol levels.

But saturated fat has been made the bad guy without proper cause for far too long. In fact, as Stephen Phinney and Jeff Volek point out in their excellent book *The Art and Science of Low Carbohydrate Living*, "Scientific evidence clearly shows that dietary intake of saturated fat compared to serum (blood) levels of saturated fat show little if any correlation."

They go on to say that some research has shown that an increase in dietary *carbohydrate* is linked with higher levels of saturated fat in the blood.

Starting in the late 1970s, the low-fat ideology was promoted by the healthcare industry, the food industry, the federal government, and the media. As you can see in the chart below, once these low-fat recommendations were implemented, the obesity epidemic skyrocketed. I guess you could say that the proof is in the low-fat, added-sugar pudding!

I'm sure you've heard the quote "Insanity is doing the same thing over and over and expecting a different result." Well, it's clear that this saying is a perfect fit for today's Standard American Diet (SAD).

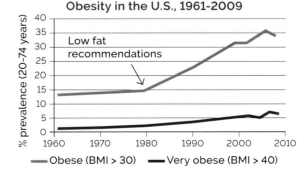

Obesity in the U.S., 1961-2009

Low fat recommendations

% prevalence (20-74 years)

— Obese (BMI > 30) — Very obese (BMI > 40)

The Role of Sugar

It's a well-known fact that sugar is extremely addictive. Sugar puts your body on a never-ending roller coaster ride of highs, lows, and endless cravings.

Before starting the ketogenic diet, I was hungry *all the time.* While eating breakfast, I would think about what I was going to have for lunch or dinner. I was literally obsessed with food and addicted to the food I was eating. Knowing what I know now, it makes perfect sense, because everything I ate and drank was full of sugar.

So let's talk about what happens in your body when you eat sugar:

First, you eat a cookie or two. It tastes good, and your brain's reward centers light up as the cycle begins. Next, your blood glucose starts to rise. Dopamine (a neurotransmitter that helps control the brain's reward and pleasure centers) is released, and you're feeling good. Meanwhile, your pancreas is busy releasing insulin (if you aren't diabetic) into your bloodstream to help regulate your blood sugar. Next, your blood glucose starts to decrease, and high insulin levels signal your body to store fat. You start to feel the sugar high dissipate . . . and then you glance over at that cookie tray again. You start to feel hungry, and your cravings kick into high gear. You find yourself daydreaming about those cookies, telling yourself that "just one more" can't hurt! So you grab another cookie, and the sugar roller coaster sets up for another ride.

1. YOU EAT SUGAR

- you like it, you crave it
- it has addictive properties

2. BLOOD SUGAR LEVELS SPIKE

- dopamine is released in the brain = addiction
- mass insulin secreted to drop blood sugar levels

SUGAR ADDICTION:
the perpetual cycle

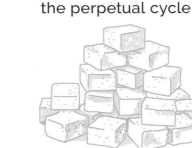

4. HUNGER & CRAVINGS

- low blood sugar levels cause increased appetite and cravings
- thus the cycle repeats

3. BLOOD SUGAR LEVELS FALL RAPIDLY

- high insulin levels cause immediate fat storage
- body craves the lost sugar "high"

FAQ

Due to the fact that there are many methods and ideologies within the ketogenic diet, I'm often asked to share my personal approach on various topics. With that in mind, I'll conclude this chapter with the most common questions and answers that people ask regarding my method or point of view. While I am happy to share my experience, I want to encourage you to find what works best for you, as we are all different!

Do you track your food and macros?

The first thing I did after hearing about keto was head to an online calculator to set up my personalized macros (see page 33 for the step-by-step process). From January 13, 2015, to January 13, 2016, I tracked every single thing I ate. This effort was so important for me because even though I had spent the majority of my life on one diet or another, keto was the first that really encouraged me to learn about what was in the foods I was eating so that I could make better choices. After a year, I had learned a great deal and was equipped with a solid understanding of keto nutrition, and I haven't fully tracked since. I still keep a rough tally of my carbohydrate and protein intake, but I no longer track what I eat at every meal.

It is important to note that not everyone will need to track their food for as long as I did. When I started keto, I needed not only a crash course in nutrition, but also some guidance as to what normal portion sizes looked like. I had spent most of my life overeating, and truthfully I needed to see what healthy eating looked like for me. While some may view tracking as restricting, I see it as a learning opportunity, and one that helped me change my life by equipping me with the knowledge to make good choices.

How do you view your macros goals?

Carbs should be tracked in terms of a daily maximum. I try to keep my carb intake as low as possible (20 to 30 grams of net carbs max—see the next question for more on net carbs versus total carbs).

Protein is a goal to reach. I make it a goal to consume my calculated amount of protein each day (see page 33 for more on how to make this calculation). It's okay if you go a little over your target on more active days, but in general you want to keep protein moderate to help your body remain in a ketogenic state—not too low (in order to spare muscle) and not too high (due to gluconeogenesis, a metabolic pathway in the body that converts some excess protein and other non-carbohydrate foods to glucose).

Fat is high and used to satisfy hunger. I've found that hitting my fat macro is pretty easy to do with so many delicious high-fat recipes out there. However, I never eat additional calories or consume foods like fat bombs at the end of the day just to get in more fat or to balance my macros. Plan your meals and add healthy fats like avocado, mayonnaise, butter, and ranch dressing for fat and flavor, but don't feel pressure to reach this macro at the end of the day if you aren't hungry. It's important to listen to your body! That being said, if you *are* hungry, fat is by far the best way to satisfy your appetite.

Do you count total carbs or net carbs?

I count net carbs. As explained earlier, counting net carbs involves subtracting fiber and sugar alcohols from the total carb count in a food. Typically, fiber and most sugar alcohols do not impact blood sugar; therefore, many people do not count them. (See the chart on page 57 for more on the Glycemic Index of various sweeteners to make informed choices about sugar alcohols.)

Counting net carbs works well for me, but I encourage you to do some experimenting and decide for yourself what works better for you.

Do you count calories as well as track macros?

In addition to tracking macros, I tracked calories during my first year on keto because I felt that I needed to learn about proper portion sizes for my body and lifestyle. I believe that when it comes to weight loss, calories in versus calories out will always matter. As mentioned previously, I know that not all calories are created equal, but because I had been overeating for most of my life, I found it to be very helpful to learn portion control through tracking.

Do you allow "cheat meals"?

Let me start off by saying that if you are doing the ketogenic diet for medical reasons, you should consult your physician regarding this topic. For the purpose of this book, however, I will share my personal experience.

When I started keto, I was very, very strict and stuck to my macros very closely. I felt that I needed to invest some serious time and energy into working not only on my food choices, but also on the emotional side of my eating habits.

About eleven months into keto, I had my first meal that wasn't ketogenic. (Notice I didn't say "cheat meal." I can't stand how so many terms in the weight-loss world are meant to make you feel bad about yourself or your choices.) My husband, Mick, and I were in Maui for our wedding anniversary, and we had reservations at a famous restaurant to celebrate. Before dinner, we had a long conversation about what exactly was livable for us. We talked about our plan for our food choices at dinner and how our views on food had changed since we'd started keto. I remember thinking that even the fact that we were thoughtfully discussing the subject was a big sign of growth. I have to admit that part of me was nervous before I ate that meal; after all, I was a pro at starting and stopping diets! But something felt truly different this time. I had lost almost 100 pounds, I was deeply invested in the ketogenic lifestyle (and I still am), and I had grown a lot as a person. The next day I had no trouble jumping right back into my normal ketogenic lifestyle.

Initially, though, I did not allow anything that wasn't keto, because I knew that I needed to dedicate some serious time and energy to working on my relationship with food. At a certain point in my journey, however, I realized that this lifestyle change wasn't dependent on an all-or-nothing approach. In fact, I started to feel like I had traded one addiction for another. I was so strict about what I could and could not eat that it started underscoring the idea that I didn't fully trust myself. Seeing how effortless it was to return to my normal way of ketogenic eating after that anniversary meal in Maui showed me that I really had come a long way. I know that I will always need to be mindful of my eating habits, but I feel like I have found a livable, sustainable, and healthy balance and relationship with food.

So, long story short, I happily stay on the ketogenic diet 90 to 95 percent of the time. The other 5 to 10 percent of the time, I allow myself to stray from keto, such as while traveling or for special events and occasions. That being said, I do have several rules in place for myself. For example, I decided some items that historically were very problematic for me, like regular soda, needed to stay in the past. Also, I should say that after being on a ketogenic diet for a while, your tastes do change. I find that I don't miss or even enjoy a lot of the foods that I used to eat (and thought I couldn't live without) prior to starting keto.

What do you use to test your ketones, and how often do you test?

I use the Precision Xtra Blood Glucose & Ketone Monitoring System, which allows you to test both blood glucose and blood ketones with the same meter. This device costs less than $30 and is a reliable way to track your ketones.

Due to the cost of ketone test strips (currently $1 to $3 each), I generally check my ketones only when trying new foods or adjusting my macro percentages, or just on occasion if I'm curious.

When did you start tracking your ketones?

I didn't check my ketones for the first few months because I wanted to give myself time to focus on my new lifestyle. While I find it helpful to know my ketone level from time to time, many people are very successful at losing weight on keto without ever checking their ketones, so do what works best for you. If you are following the ketogenic diet because of a particular health or medical issue, then it will be much more important to check your ketone levels to ensure that you are in fact in ketosis.

Did you take ketone supplements to lose weight?

No. I lost every pound simply by eating a ketogenic diet. For more information about ketone supplements, see page 41.

Did you work out as you were losing weight?

Although I became more active in general because I felt better and had a lot more energy, I didn't work out consistently while losing weight. There is a saying that you lose weight in the kitchen and tone/build muscle in the gym, and I couldn't agree more. If you enjoy working out, then by all means do so, but I felt the need to start by working on improving my eating habits and mind-set. Now that I'm at a normal body weight, I plan to incorporate more exercise into my health and wellness goals. (See the section "Working Out on Keto" on page 40 for more information.)

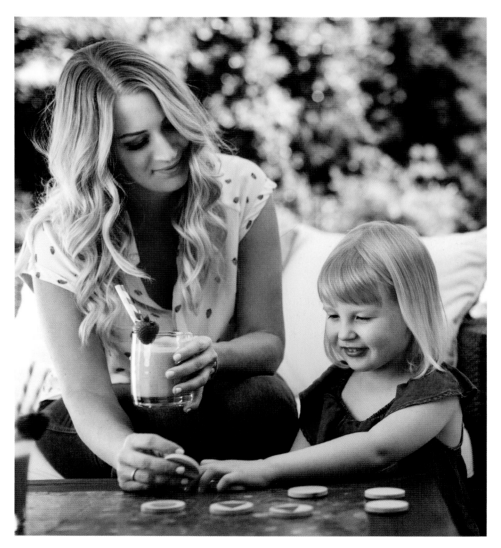

What adjustments did you make to your diet after you reached your goal weight?

I knew that I would remain keto after reaching my goal weight because I view this as a lifestyle change, not a temporary diet. All that was required was to change my deficit to 0 percent when using the keto calculator to generate my macros. I use these macros as a guideline, but I don't track anything in great detail. The nice thing about keto is that after a while, you really get a feel for how your daily meals should look, and it becomes a new normal with minimal effort.

After losing so much weight, do you have issues with loose skin?

After losing 110 pounds, I had a lot of loose skin (this can happen regardless of how fast you lose weight), and I opted to have some of that excess skin removed. In October 2016, I had a tummy tuck, lower body lift, and breast lift with fat grafting (a way to add volume to the breasts without the use of implants). My surgeon was Dr. Stephen Ronan of Blackhawk Plastic Surgery in Danville, California. During my surgery, Dr. Ronan removed 7.7 pounds of loose skin and tissue. You can see some of the before-and-after images on my blog, ketokarma.com, and on my Instagram page, @ketokarma.

After major weight loss, some people opt not to have their excess skin removed, which is perfectly fine and totally a personal choice. Please don't let the possibility of loose skin hold you back from losing weight. Your health is always the most important factor!

What is your opinion about cholesterol and eating a high-fat diet?

Cholesterol is a very complex subject, and there a lot of opinions and misinformation out there (even in the medical community). I have had my own cholesterol checked, and both my doctor and I are extremely happy with the outcome. In fact, my triglycerides dropped from 62 to 35 in just one year! I recommend that you do some research beyond the "standard" cholesterol guidelines and think outside the box—as that box might just be a stage for profit and fearmongering. The book *Cholesterol Clarity* by Jimmy Moore with Eric C. Westman is a great place to start, as are David Diamond's lectures (specifically *Dietary Sense and Nonsense in the War on Saturated Fat*, which you can watch for free on YouTube).

Can I eat high-fat/ketogenic without a gallbladder?

I had my gallbladder removed several years before I started keto. Right after my surgery, my surgeon told me to avoid eating fat. (Not so surprisingly, I gained even more weight when I followed that advice.) Since I started the ketogenic diet, I haven't had any issues eating high-fat without a gallbladder; in fact, I feel better than ever before! It should be noted that there may be a brief adjustment period immediately after having your gallbladder removed. It's always best to listen to your body and take things slowly if needed.

All that being said, I am not a medical doctor; I can only speak about my personal experience. Please talk with your healthcare provider about your individual situation.

Can I do the keto diet if I have kids or other family members in my home who don't eat low-carb?

The short answer is yes. In fact, when I started the ketogenic diet, I was the only one in my household eating this way. I found that overcoming temptations at home actually helped make me stronger. Weight loss is truly a two-step process: One part is a healthy and livable lifestyle change, and the other is a mind-set change. Real and lasting change requires both, because while a new eating plan is great, a mind-set change is needed to keep you accountable and grounded in your goals.

When faced with temptations, I've found it helpful to break things down into one meal or even one choice at a time. Before I eat anything, I ask myself two questions:

1) Am I truly hungry, or am I stressed, bored, emotionally eating, thirsty, etc.?

2) Is what I'm about to eat going to help me reach my goals?

I still use this process to ensure that I'm being mindful about my food choices and eating habits.

How often should I weigh in?

I recommend weighing in no more than once a week. If you find yourself obsessing over the number on the scale, then it might be a good idea to put the scale away for a few weeks and focus on your eating habits.

"We all make mistakes, have struggles, and even regret things in our past. But you are not your mistakes, you are not your struggles, and you are here NOW with the power to shape your day and your future."

—Steve Maraboli

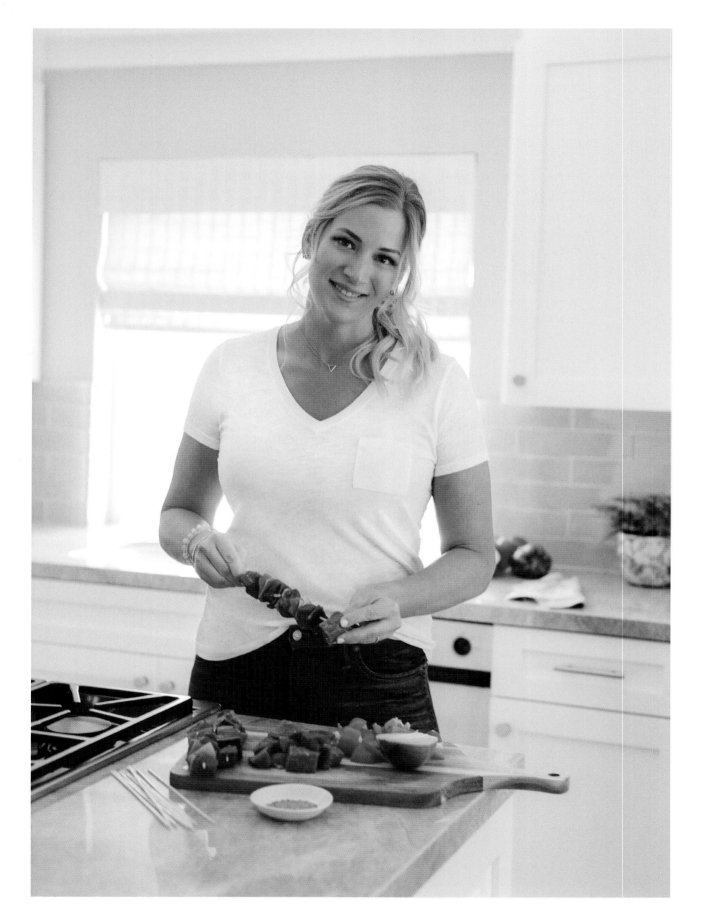

CHAPTER 2:

Ketogenic Food and Shopping Lists

This chapter lists the delicious foods that you'll enjoy when you switch to the ketogenic way of eating. My priority is to make the ketogenic lifestyle easy for you, so the last thing I want to do is tell you that you have to go out and hunt down hundreds of dollars' worth of expensive and hard-to-find ingredients. Thankfully, there's no need to do that! The majority of keto-friendly ingredients are whole, fresh foods found at all grocery stores. While shopping, you'll probably end up sticking mostly to the outer aisles, away from the highly processed foods that dominate the center.

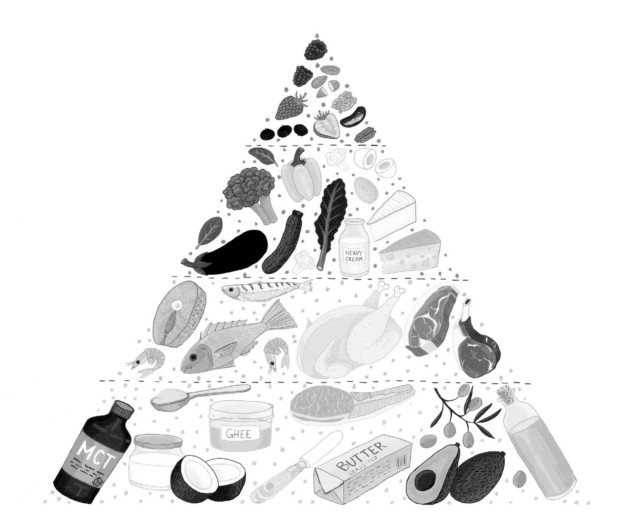

The Ketogenic Food Pyramid

FATS AND OILS

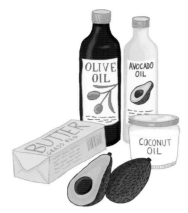

- Avocado oil
- Bacon fat
- Beef tallow
- Coconut oil
- Extra-virgin olive oil
- Ghee
- Lard
- Macadamia nut oil
- MCT oil
- Palm oil

What is MCT oil?

MCT is short for medium-chain triglycerides—a type of saturated fatty acid commonly found in and derived from coconut. MCT oil is a great way to add healthy fat to your diet while also acting as a natural energy source for your body and brain! If you find that MCT oil is hard to blend or gives you an upset stomach, MCT powder is a handy alternative.

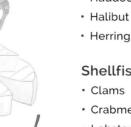

PROTEINS

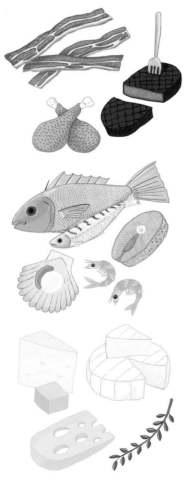

Red Meat
- Beef
- Buffalo
- Goat
- Lamb
- Pork

Poultry
- Chicken
- Duck
- Game hen
- Pheasant
- Quail
- Turkey

Wild Meats
- Bear
- Boar
- Elk
- Rabbit
- Venison (deer meat)

Eggs
- Chicken eggs
- Duck eggs
- Goose eggs
- Ostrich eggs
- Quail eggs

Fish
- Anchovies
- Bass
- Burbot
- Carp
- Catfish
- Cod
- Flounder
- Haddock
- Halibut
- Herring
- Mackerel
- Salmon
- Sardines
- Snapper
- Sole
- Swordfish
- Tilapia
- Trout
- Tuna
- Walleye

Shellfish and Other Seafood
- Clams
- Crabmeat*
- Lobster
- Mussels
- Octopus
- Oysters
- Prawns
- Scallops
- Shrimp
- Snails

Dairy
- Butter (salted and unsalted)
- Cheeses
  - Blue cheese
  - Brie
  - Camembert
  - Cheddar
  - Cottage cheese (watch the carb count)
  - Cream cheese (full fat)
  - Feta
  - Goat cheese
  - Gouda
  - Gruyère
  - Mascarpone
  - Mozzarella (whole milk)
  - Muenster
  - Parmesan
  - Provolone
  - Ricotta (whole milk; watch the carb count)
  - Swiss
  - Tilsit
  - Various other specialty cheeses (watch the carb count)
- Greek yogurt (full fat—use sparingly)
- Half-and-half
- Heavy whipping cream
- Sour cream (full fat)

*Avoid imitation crabmeat; it is not low-carb and has about 13 grams of carbs per 3 ounces.

See page 317 for a chart of safe cooking temperatures for meat and seafood, and make sure to invest in a quality meat thermometer!

VEGETABLES

One rule that never fails is to stick to leafy green cruciferous veggies. Think mostly nonstarchy veggies that grow above ground. Below are some common low-carb options:

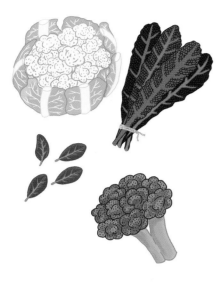

- Artichokes
- Arugula
- Asparagus
- Bok choy
- Broccoli
- Broccoli rabe
- Brussels sprouts
- Cabbage
- Cauliflower
- Celery
- Chard
- Chicory greens
- Endive
- Fennel bulb

- Garlic*
- Green beans
- Hot peppers (such as jalapeños)
- Kale
- Kohlrabi
- Lettuce (butter, romaine, radicchio, and so on)
- Mushrooms
- Onions*
- Radishes
- Seaweed
- Spinach
- Swiss chard
- Watercress

*Onions (especially red onions and shallots) and garlic should be eaten in moderation because of their carb content; see the chart below.

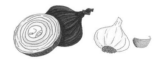

Onions and Garlic Macros per 100-Gram Serving

Type	Total Carbs	Fiber	Net Carbs
Green onions	7 g	3 g	4 g
White onions	9.4 g	2 g	7.4 g
Pearl onions	9 g	1.5 g	7.5 g
Yellow onions	9.5 g	2 g	7.5 g
Red onions	10.6 g	1.2 g	9.4 g
Shallots	17 g	3 g	14 g
Garlic	33 g	2 g	31 g

"The food you eat can be either the safest and most powerful form of medicine or the slowest form of poison."

—Ann Wigmore

FRUITS

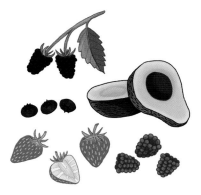

Often referred to as "nature's candy," fruit contains a natural sugar called fructose. Below are some fruits that are lower in carbs, but keep in mind that berries (see the chart below) and tomatoes should be eaten in moderation. Besides, we all know that avocado is the real MVP in this category!

- Avocados
- Bell peppers (all colors)
- Blackberries
- Blueberries
- Cucumbers

- Eggplant
- Lemons
- Limes
- Olives
- Pumpkin

- Raspberries
- Spaghetti squash
- Strawberries
- Tomatoes
- Zucchini

Berry Macros per 100-Gram Serving (Raw)

Type	Total Carbs	Net Carbs
Blackberries	10 g	5 g
Raspberries	12 g	5 g
Strawberries	8 g	6 g
Blueberries*	21 g	17 g

Because blueberries are on the high end, at 17 grams of net carbs (21 grams of total carbs) per 100 grams, it's best to limit them.

WHETHER OR NOT TO BUY ORGANIC PRODUCE

We know that organic food is generally best, but let's face it, a lot of us are on a budget, and buying all organic food can be very expensive. There are two lists that can help guide you as to which fruits and vegetables you should focus on purchasing organic. The Environmental Working Group's "Dirty Dozen" is a list of the produce that is best purchased organic due to pesticides and other chemicals, and the "Clean Fifteen" is a list of the produce that is generally safe to buy non-organic. Following are the keto-friendly options that made the lists. The EWG updates these lists annually; for the latest versions, visit www.ewg.org.

Low-carb produce from the Dirty Dozen list—recommended to buy organic:

- Strawberries
- Spinach
- Celery
- Tomatoes
- Sweet bell peppers

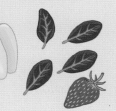

Low-carb produce from the Clean Fifteen list—okay to buy conventional:

- Avocados
- Cabbage
- Onions
- Asparagus
- Eggplant
- Cauliflower

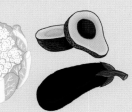

Although they aren't among the top twelve, cucumbers, cherry tomatoes, and lettuce are numbers thirteen through fifteen when it comes to pesticide residue. Exercise caution when buying these items as well!

NUTS, SEEDS, AND NUT BUTTERS

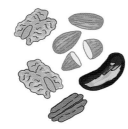

Feel free to enjoy nuts and seeds as a snack or in recipes. I recommend portioning out your desired amount instead of eating them straight from the bag or jar, as they are easy to overeat.

- Almonds
- Brazil nuts
- Cashews*
- Coconut (unsweetened shredded)
- Hazelnuts
- Macadamia nuts
- Peanuts
- Pecans
- Pili nuts
- Pine nuts
- Pistachios*
- Walnuts
- Chia seeds
- Flax seeds
- Hemp seeds
- Poppy seeds
- Pumpkin seeds
- Safflower seeds
- Sesame seeds
- Sunflower seeds
- Almond butter (unsweetened)
- Peanut butter (no sugar added; made from only peanuts and salt)

Pistachios and cashews are higher in carbs, so limit or avoid these.

HERBS AND SPICES

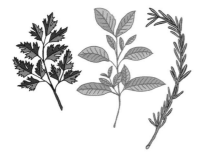

Fresh and dried herbs and spices can add a lot of flavor to your meals. These are the ones that I like to have on hand:

- Basil
- Bay leaves
- Chili powder
- Cilantro
- Cinnamon
- Cumin
- Curry powder
- Garlic powder
- Ginger powder
- Italian seasoning
- Mint
- Old Bay seasoning
- Onion powder
- Oregano
- Paprika
- Parsley
- Peppercorns
- Rosemary
- Salt (my favorites are pink Himalayan salt, various types of sea salt, and kosher salt)
- Steak seasoning (sugar-free)
- Taco seasoning (sugar-free; see page 82 for my recipe)

BAKING INGREDIENTS

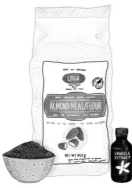

Here are some of my favorite baking ingredients:

- Almond flour (blanched and skin-free is my preference)
- Almond meal
- Baking powder (aluminum-free)
- Baking soda
- Cocoa powder (unsweetened)
- Coconut flour
- Flaxseed meal
- MCT powder
- Protein powder
- Psyllium husk
- Stevia-sweetened chocolate chips
- Unsweetened baking chocolate

SWEETENERS

These are the sweeteners that I personally use and recommend:

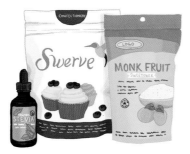

- Allulose
- Erythritol (I use the Swerve brand of erythritol blends, usually the confectioners' style but occasionally the granular style)
- Monk fruit
- Stevia (I like the liquid form best)
- Xylitol*

Animal lovers, take note: although xylitol is safe for human consumption, it is toxic for some animals, especially dogs. Be sure to keep items containing xylitol out of reach of your pets!

What Is the Glycemic Index?

The Glycemic Index (GI) is a scale that gives you an idea of how quickly a food will cause blood sugar to rise.

- Foods with a high GI should be avoided; they cause a rapid spike in blood glucose.

- Foods with a low GI are ideal; they have a slow and steady effect, or even no effect, on blood glucose. Selecting foods with a lower GI has been shown to aid in weight loss.

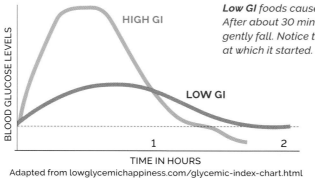

TIME IN HOURS

Adapted from lowglycemichappiness.com/glycemic-index-chart.html

Low GI foods cause blood sugar to rise gradually. After about 30 minutes, blood sugar begins to gently fall. Notice that it returns to the same level at which it started.

High GI foods cause blood sugar to rise rapidly. After about 30 minutes, blood sugar begins to plummet. Notice that it falls below its starting point. When blood glucose falls below normal levels, foggy thinking, tiredness, and depression can result.

The GI range is zero to 100, with 100 being pure glucose (sugar). On the other end of the scale is erythritol, which has a GI of zero.

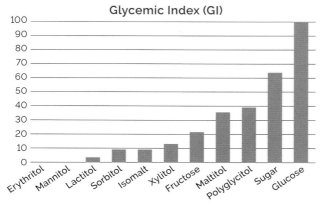

Glycemic Index (GI)

note: Maltitol is a sugar alcohol that is used in some low-carb bars, ice cream, candy, and chocolate. As you can see in the chart, maltitol has a pretty high GI of 36. I highly recommend that you stay away from maltitol and pick a lower-GI sweetener.

DRESSINGS AND SAUCES

A lot of dressings and sauces contain added sugar, so be sure to read the labels. When dining out, I usually play it safe and ask for sauces on the side or substitute something that I know is low-carb, like ranch dressing or mayonnaise. Here are some keto-friendly sauces that can be added to meals for more fat and flavor:

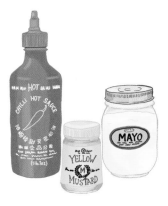

- Aioli (page 72)
- Alfredo sauce (page 68)
- Béarnaise
- Blue cheese dressing
- Buffalo sauce
- Caesar dressing (page 74)
- Gorgonzola sauce (page 164)
- Hollandaise (page 76)
- Hot sauce
- Italian dressing (check labels, but most are low-carb)
- Ketchup (sugar-free)
- Marinara sauce (no sugar added)
- Mayonnaise
- Mustard, yellow and Dijon
- Pesto (page 70)
- Pizza sauce (no sugar added)
- Ranch dressing
- Soy sauce (there are gluten-free options, if desired)
- Sriracha
- Sriracha mayo

FLAVORING INGREDIENTS AND OTHER PANTRY ITEMS

When purchasing these items, always check the labels and choose the products that are lowest in carbs, especially with tomato-based products.

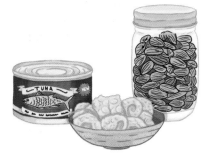

- Anchovy paste
- Apple cider vinegar
- Artichoke hearts
- Banana peppers
- Bouillon cubes (great for electrolytes!)
- Broth
- Canned tuna and other fish
- Capers
- Chocolate (sweetened with stevia or erythritol; stay away from maltitol)
- Coconut milk (full fat)
- Fish sauce
- Olives
- Pickled jalapeños
- Pickles
- Pork rinds
- Protein powder (sugar-free and low-carb; I like Quest brand)
- Red curry paste
- Red wine vinegar
- Sardines
- Sauerkraut
- Tomato paste
- Vanilla extract

DRINKS

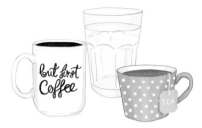

Drinking enough water has always been one of my biggest struggles. If you aren't a huge fan of plain water, try sparkling water or sugar-free flavored water.

- Almond milk (unsweetened, plain and vanilla-flavored)
- Bone broth (page 80)
- Cashew milk (unsweetened)
- Coconut milk (full fat)
- Coffee
- Sparkling water (LaCroix is my favorite, or you can purchase a SodaStream and make it at home)
- Stevia- or erythritol-sweetened sodas (Zevia is my favorite)
- Tea (unsweetened, iced or hot)

note: Although unsweetened coconut milk is keto-friendly, coconut water is not low in carbs and should be avoided. Coconut water averages 15 grams of sugar per 11.1-fluid-ounce serving.

Low-Carb Alcohol

Whether or not to drink alcohol is a personal choice. If you do choose to imbibe, keep in mind that alcohol should be consumed responsibly, and limiting quantities is smart. I enjoy a drink on occasion (not daily), but I limit myself to a max of one or two drinks. Keep in mind that keto is a lifestyle change, so find a livable balance that works for you. In my opinion, it's okay to enjoy an occasional drink that is low in carbs, but make sure you keep your health and goals in mind when deciding how much or how often. Moderation is key!

Wine

Wine is generally my go-to option when it comes to low-carb alcoholic beverages. With Napa Valley only two hours away from my home, I enjoy a variety of wines and find that wine rarely affects my ketone levels. Be sure to stay away from dessert wines, however, as they are loaded with sugar! The following are some of my favorite wine choices.

Serving size is 5 ounces.

RED WINE	Calories	Carbs
Pinot Noir	122	3.4 g
Merlot	123	3.7 g
Cabernet Sauvignon	123	3.8 g
Syrah	123	3.8 g
Petite Syrah	126	3.9 g
Zinfandel	131	4.2 g

WHITE WINE	Calories	Carbs
Pinot Blanc	121	2.8 g
Brut Champagne	119	2.9 g
Pinot Grigio	122	3 g
Sauvignon Blanc	121	3 g
Chardonnay	123	3.1 g
Albariño	143	3.5 g

Liquor

The majority of liquors contain zero net carbs as long as they are unflavored and unsweetened. Check each brand to be sure. The following chart shows the averages seen across most brands per 1½-ounce serving.

LIQUOR	Calories	Carbs
Brandy	103–126	0–3 g*
Gin	100	0
Rum	72–105	0
Tequila	96–104	0
Vodka	97–105	0
Whiskey/Scotch/ Bourbon	96–105	0

*Check labels for added carbs.

Stay away from the majority of liqueurs and mixers, as most are not low-carb. Here are some low-carb mixer options:

- Flavored unsweetened sparkling water (such as LaCroix)
- Stevia- or erythritol-sweetened soda (such as Zevia)
- Sugar-free energy drinks (check macros and look for brands sweetened with erythritol or stevia)
- Sugar-free water enhancers
- Lime juice (pair with tequila and the sweetener of your choice for a low-carb margarita)

Beer

In my opinion, beer should be your last choice as far as alcoholic beverages are concerned, especially if you are trying to lose weight. Most beer contains gluten, and beer is often referred to as "liquid bread." Again, keto is a lifestyle change; I don't expect that you will never drink a beer again if you enjoy beer. Keep in mind, though, that beer has the potential to affect ketosis more so than other alcoholic options. I personally enjoy a low-carb beer on occasion, but for the most part I stick to wine.

If you do choose to have a beer once in a while, here are some lower-carb options. Serving size is based on a single-serving can or bottle.

BEER	Calories	Carbs
Budweiser Select 55	55	1.9 g
Miller 64	64	2.4 g
Rolling Rock Green Light	83	2.4 g
Michelob Ultra	95	2.6 g
Budweiser Select	99	3.1 g
Miller Lite	96	3.2 g
Busch Light	95	3.2 g
Natural Light	95	3.2 g
Michelob Ultra Amber	95	3.2 g
Beck's Premier Light	64	3.9 g
Miller Chill	100	4.1 g
Coors Light	102	5 g
Amstel Light	95	5 g
Keystone Light	104	5 g
Budweiser Light	110	6.6 g
Heineken Light	99	6.8 g

"The most authentic thing about us is our capacity to create, to overcome, to endure, to transform, to love and to be greater than our suffering."

—Ben Okri

HIGH-CARB TO LOW-CARB SUBSTITUTIONS

Instead of

Eat this

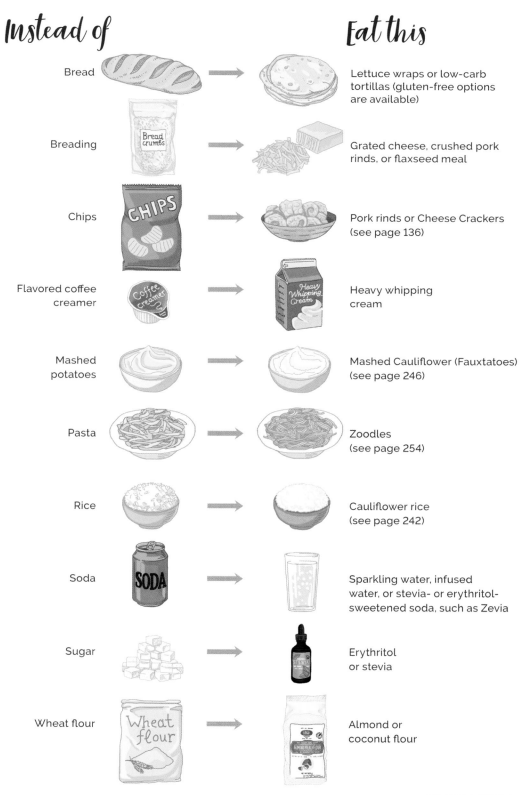

Instead of	Eat this
Bread	Lettuce wraps or low-carb tortillas (gluten-free options are available)
Breading	Grated cheese, crushed pork rinds, or flaxseed meal
Chips	Pork rinds or Cheese Crackers (see page 136)
Flavored coffee creamer	Heavy whipping cream
Mashed potatoes	Mashed Cauliflower (Fauxtatoes) (see page 246)
Pasta	Zoodles (see page 254)
Rice	Cauliflower rice (see page 242)
Soda	Sparkling water, infused water, or stevia- or erythritol-sweetened soda, such as Zevia
Sugar	Erythritol or stevia
Wheat flour	Almond or coconut flour

GROCERY SHOPPING

These are just a few of my favorite items from several common grocery stores in my area. For more grocery shopping ideas, check out my keto grocery haul videos on my YouTube channel: YouTube.com/ketokarma2015

Costco

- Almonds
- Avocados
- Bacon
- Bone broth
- Cheeses
- Chicken salad
- Coconut oil
- Coffee
- Cream cheese
- Eggs
- Guacamole cups
- Heavy whipping cream
- Kerrygold butter
- Macadamia nuts
- Meats
- Nonstarchy veggies
- Pork belly
- Rotisserie chicken
- Sausages
- Seafood

Safeway

- Aidell's Italian meatballs
- Aidell's sausages (check the carb count on each flavor)
- Almond flour (blanched)
- Avocados
- Bacon (nitrate-free)
- Cheeses
- Coconut oil
- Dairy products (butter, cream cheese, sour cream, and so on)
- Fresh veggies
- Low-carb condiments such as ranch dressing, mayonnaise, and hot sauce
- Lunchmeat (nitrate-free)
- Meats
- Quest bars
- Rotisserie chicken
- Seafood
- Sparkling water
- Spices
- Stevia
- Zevia

Trader Joe's

- Almond meal
- Avocados
- Bacon (the thick applewood smoked is my favorite)
- Blanched almond flour
- Cauliflower (whole heads, fresh riced, and frozen riced)
- Cheese bites
- Cheeses
- Chicken fajitas (refrigerated section)
- Chili lime chicken burgers (frozen section)
- Coconut flour
- Coconut oil
- Coconut oil spray
- Dairy products (butter, cream cheese, sour cream, and so on)
- Eggs
- Everything but the Bagel sesame seasoning blend
- Frozen large shrimp
- Grass-fed frozen burgers
- Greens for salads
- Hard-boiled eggs
- Heavy whipping cream
- Kerrygold butter
- Marinated goat cheese
- Meats
- Mini Brie bites
- Nonstarchy veggies
- Premade hollandaise
- Prosciutto
- Quest bars
- Seaweed snacks
- Zucchini spirals (frozen section)

Whole Foods

- Avocado oil
- Dairy products (butter, cream cheese, sour cream, and so on)
- Epic Bacon Bars
- Epic Pork Rinds
- Fresh seafood
- Freshly ground natural peanut butter
- Guacamole (produce section)
- Hot bar for quality on-the-go meals
- Lily's Stevia Sweetened Chocolate
- Meats
- Natural Calm
- Nonstarchy veggies
- Precooked bacon pieces (perfect for Twice-Baked Cauliflower Casserole, page 252)
- Quest bars
- Sparkling water
- Spices and specialty ingredients from bulk bins
- Swerve (sweetener)

HELPFUL TOOLS AND TIME-SAVERS

You don't have to have a professionally equipped kitchen to make delicious keto meals, but it does help to have some basic cooking tools and gadgets on hand. Here are some of my go-tos:

- Baking dishes (8-inch square, 9-inch square, 13 by 9 inches)
- Baking sheets, rimmed and unrimmed
- Blender
- Cast-iron skillet
- Chocolate molds for fat bombs (silicone ice trays often work, too)
- Cutting boards
- Digital food scale
- Food processor
- Garlic press
- Hand mixer
- Ice pop molds
- Large pot
- Measuring cups and spoons
- Meat thermometer (see page 317 for a chart of safe cooking temperatures for meat and seafood)
- Milk frother
- Mixing bowls in a variety of sizes
- Muffin pan
- Multi-cooker (such as an Instant Pot)
- Parchment paper or reusable baking mats
- Roasting pan or deep baking dish
- Salad spinner
- Saucepans
- Skewers (wood or metal, for kabobs)
- Slow cooker
- Spiralizer
- Strainer
- Tongs
- Waffle maker
- Whisk

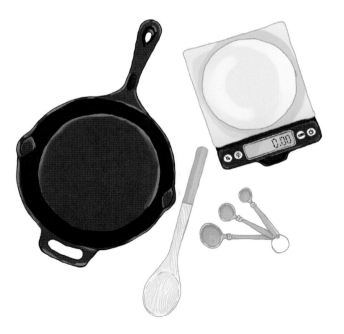

"The harder the struggle, the more glorious the triumph. Self-realization demands very great struggle."

—Swami Sivananda

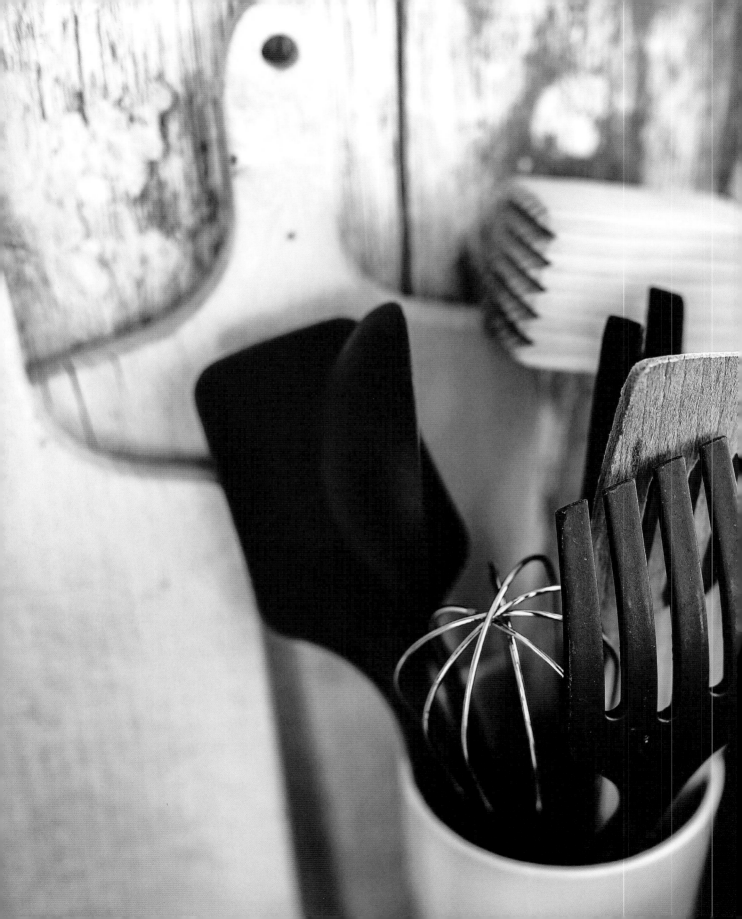

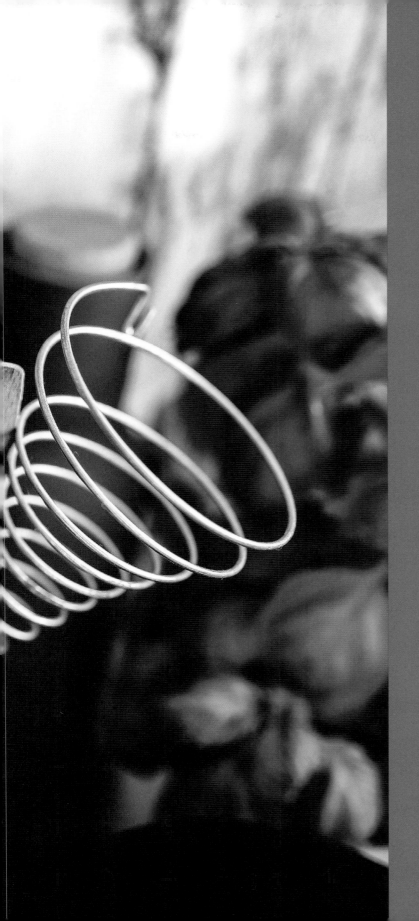

CHAPTER 3:
Recipes

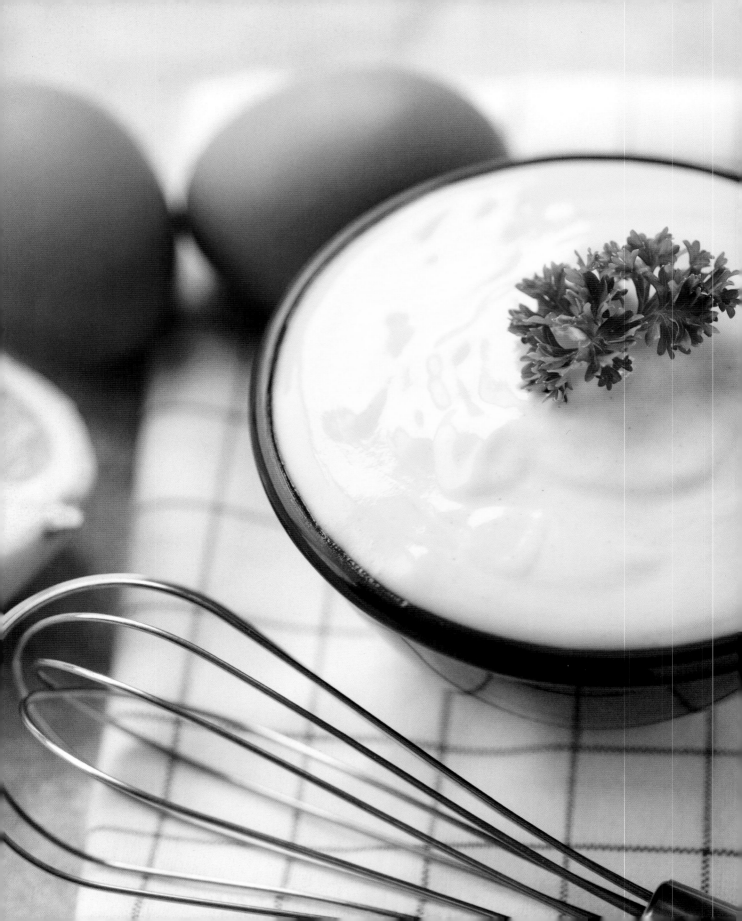

BASICS

ALFREDO SAUCE

PREP TIME: 5 MINUTES • COOK TIME: 15 MINUTES
YIELD: 2 CUPS (¼ CUP PER SERVING)

Alfredo sauce is great over zucchini noodles or broccoli with chicken, or even low-carb meatballs! If you're dining out, chicken Alfredo is a great dish to order; simply substitute broccoli or zucchini for the pasta!

⅓ cup unsalted butter

2 cloves garlic, pressed

4 ounces cream cheese, cut into cubes

1 cup half-and-half

½ cup grated Parmesan cheese (freshly grated is best)

½ teaspoon dried ground oregano

½ teaspoon salt

½ teaspoon ground black pepper

1   Melt the butter in a medium-sized saucepan over medium heat. Add the garlic and sauté for 20 to 30 seconds, until fragrant.

2   Add the cream cheese while whisking constantly. Once melted, slowly pour in the half-and-half and whisk until smooth. Gradually add the Parmesan cheese ¼ cup at a time, while whisking continuously.

3   Add the oregano, salt, and pepper and stir to combine. Simmer for about 1 minute to allow the flavors to blend; do not let the sauce boil. Check for seasoning and add more salt and pepper if needed.

4   Remove from the heat and serve. Store leftovers in an airtight container in the refrigerator for up to 4 days.

per serving:

CALORIES: 184 | FAT: 17.4 g | PROTEIN: 4.4 g | TOTAL CARBS: 2.3 g | NET CARBS: 2.3 g

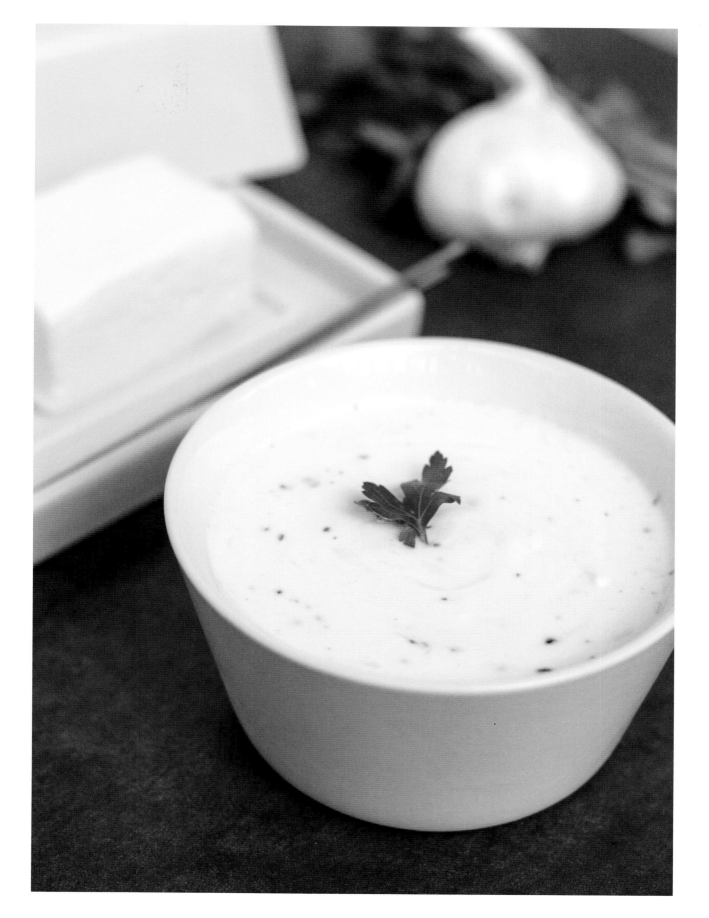

EASY PESTO

PREP TIME: 5 MINUTES • YIELD: 1 CUP (2 TABLESPOONS PER SERVING)

This quick and easy pesto sauce is a great way to add fresh flavor to a variety of dishes, such as chicken, shrimp, zucchini noodles, or a caprese salad (page 232).

¼ cup pine nuts

3 cups packed fresh basil leaves

½ cup grated Parmesan cheese

2 cloves garlic

Juice of ½ lemon

⅓ cup extra-virgin olive oil

Salt and pepper

1 In a food processor, finely chop the pine nuts.

2 Add the basil, Parmesan cheese, garlic, and lemon juice and pulse until well blended, then slowly drizzle in the olive oil while pulsing. Season with salt and pepper to taste.

3 Store in an airtight container in the refrigerator for up to a week.

tip: *You can freeze pesto in ice cube trays! Once the cubes are frozen, transfer them to a zip-top plastic bag and store in the freezer for up to 4 months.*

per serving:

CALORIES: 140 | FAT: 14 g | PROTEIN: 3.5 g | TOTAL CARBS: 1.6 g | NET CARBS: 1.3 g

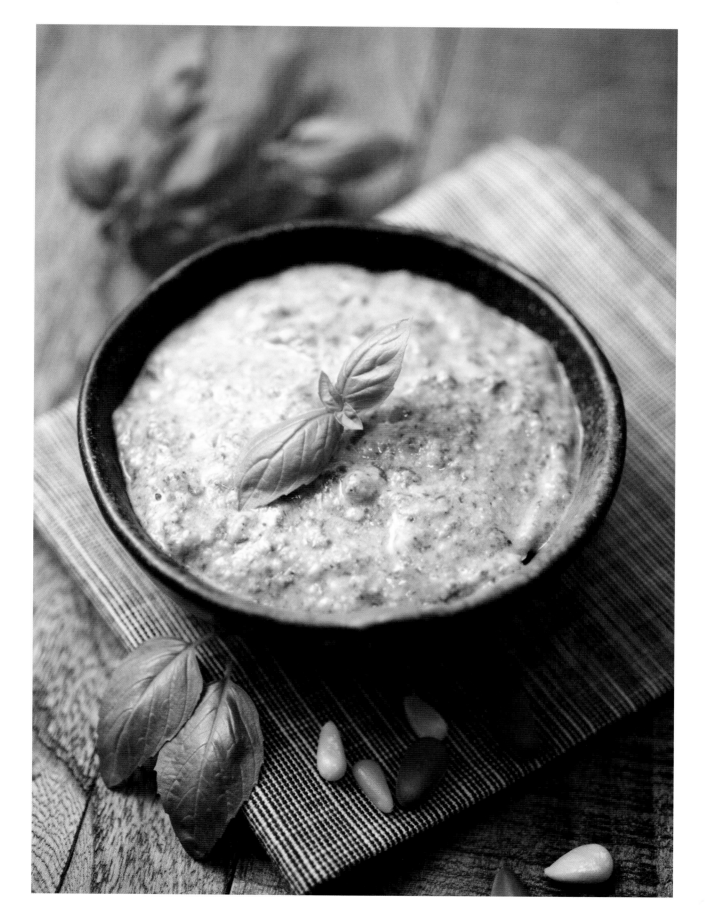

AIOLI

PREP TIME: 5 MINUTES, PLUS 1 HOUR TO CHILL

YIELD: ¾ CUP (2 TABLESPOONS PER SERVING)

If you're looking for a sauce with a little more flavor than regular mayonnaise, then this aioli might be just the thing! It pairs perfectly with Low-Carb Crab Cakes (page 222), bunless burgers, or veggies, or you can use it as a spread on a lettuce-wrapped sandwich.

3 cloves garlic, minced or pressed

¾ cup mayonnaise

1 tablespoon fresh lemon juice

Salt, to taste

1   Place all the ingredients in a small bowl and stir to combine, then cover and place in the refrigerator to chill for 1 hour before serving.

2   Store in an airtight container in the refrigerator for up to a week.

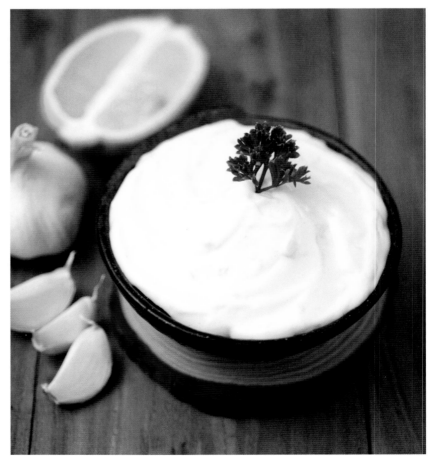

per serving:

CALORIES: 183 | FAT: 20 g | PROTEIN: 0.2 g | TOTAL CARBS: 0.7 g | NET CARBS: 0.7 g

KETO HONEY MUSTARD

⏱ 🚫 🥛 PREP TIME: 5 MINUTES • YIELD: ¾ CUP (2 TABLESPOONS PER SERVING)

Honey mustard was one of my favorite condiments before I started the ketogenic diet, so re-creating it to be keto-friendly was a must! This recipe has all the flavor of regular honey mustard, without the unnecessary carbs. It pairs well with Simple Chicken Tenders (page 202), or you can use it as a glaze for baked salmon.

½ cup mayonnaise

2 tablespoons prepared yellow mustard

2 tablespoons Swerve confectioners'-style sweetener

1 tablespoon Dijon mustard

1 Combine all the ingredients in a small bowl and stir until smooth and well blended.

2 Serve right away or store in an airtight container in the refrigerator for up to 2 weeks.

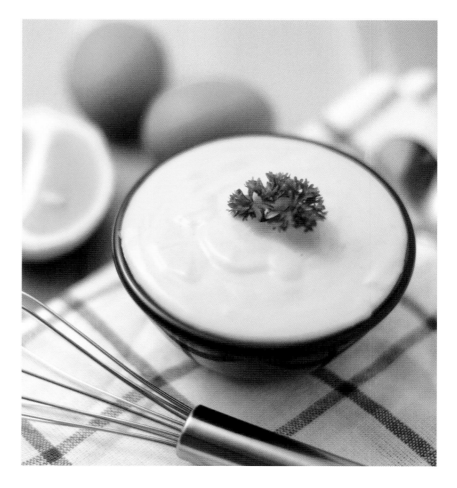

per serving: CALORIES: 126 | FAT: 13.5 g | PROTEIN: 0.2 g | TOTAL CARBS: 3.3 g | NET CARBS: 0.3 g

QUICK AND EASY CAESAR DRESSING

🕐 ⊘ PREP TIME: 5 MINUTES • YIELD: ¾ CUP (2 TABLESPOONS PER SERVING)

Caesar salad is one of my favorite meals. While most store-bought Caesar dressings are keto-friendly, nothing compares to homemade! This easy dressing comes together in only 5 minutes, and it will take your Caesar salads to the next level. Although the dressing tastes great without the optional MCT oil, the oil thins it a bit.

¾ cup mayonnaise

⅓ cup grated Parmesan cheese

1 large clove or 2 small cloves garlic, pressed

1 tablespoon MCT oil (optional, for a thinner dressing)

1 teaspoon anchovy paste

1 teaspoon fresh lemon juice

½ teaspoon Dijon mustard

½ teaspoon ground black pepper (or to taste)

Place all the ingredients in a medium-sized bowl and stir well until blended. Serve immediately or store in an airtight container for up to a week.

tip: When dining out, a Caesar salad is a great option, with a couple of simple modifications: skip the croutons and add chicken, shrimp, steak, and/or avocado! A lot of salad dressings contain a fair amount of sugar, so it's best to stick with Caesar, ranch, or blue cheese.

per serving:

CALORIES: 227 | FAT: 24 g | PROTEIN: 2.3 g | TOTAL CARBS: 0.3 g | NET CARBS: 0.3 g

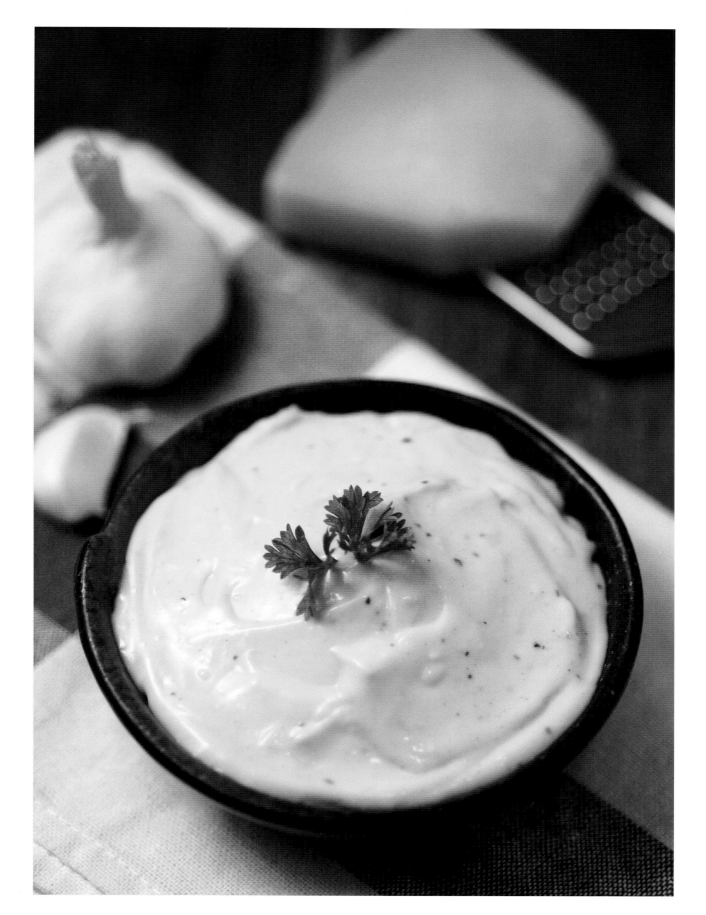

SIMPLE HOLLANDAISE

PREP TIME: 5 MINUTES • COOK TIME: 30 SECONDS • YIELD: ½ CUP (4 SERVINGS)

This quick and easy hollandaise sauce makes a yummy topping for an Easy Egg Scramble (page 102), Eggs Benedict (page 104), or even veggies such as asparagus!

2 large egg yolks

1½ teaspoons mayonnaise (optional, for a thicker sauce)

½ teaspoon fresh lemon juice

Pinch of cayenne pepper, or a dash of hot sauce

Small pinch of salt

¼ cup (½ stick) unsalted butter, melted

tip: Some grocery stores, such as Trader Joe's, sell premade hollandaise, which is a great alternative if you're in a hurry or want only one serving of hollandaise.

1 Whisk the egg yolks, mayonnaise (if using), lemon juice, cayenne or hot sauce, and salt in a microwave-safe bowl until smooth.

2 Slowly pour the melted butter into the egg yolk mixture while whisking until smooth.

3 Heat the butter and egg mixture in the microwave for 15 seconds, then whisk well. Microwave for an additional 10 seconds and whisk well. If you want the hollandaise a touch thicker, microwave for 5 more seconds and whisk once more before serving. (Note that the sauce will thicken as it cools, so don't allow it to become too thick in the microwave!) The cooking time will differ with each microwave; adjust as needed.

4 Store in an airtight container in the refrigerator for up to 2 days.

per serving, with mayonnaise:

CALORIES: 142 | FAT: 15 g | PROTEIN: 1.3 g | TOTAL CARBS: 0.3 g | NET CARBS: 0.3 g

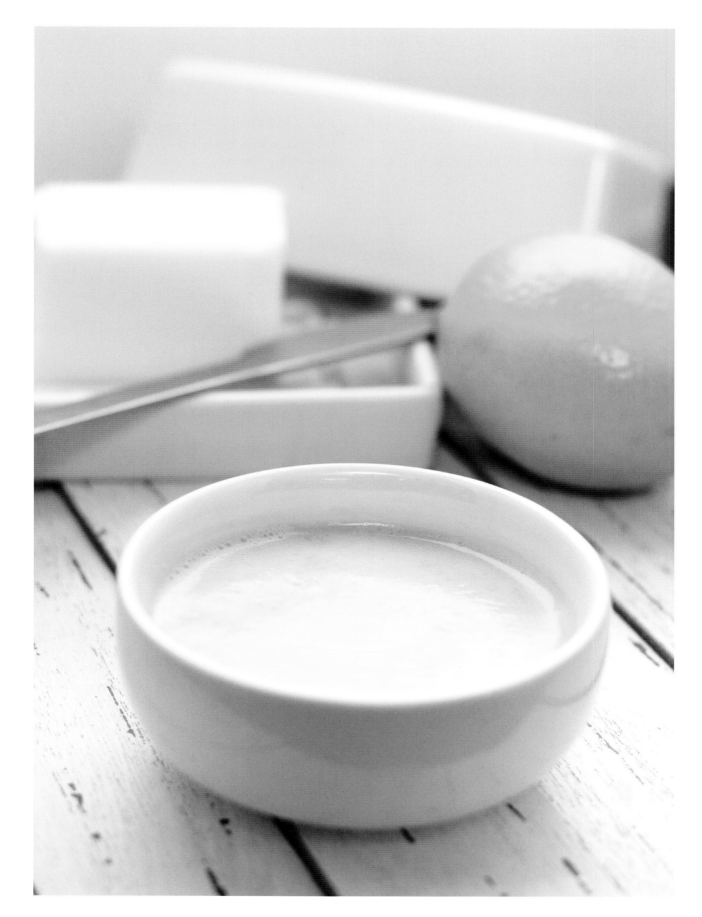

MICK'S SPICY AIOLI

PREP TIME: 3 MINUTES • YIELD: ¼ CUP (2 SERVINGS)

My husband, Mick, developed this sauce, and it's a big hit in our house! This spicy aioli reminds me of the "yummy yummy" sauce you typically find in Japanese restaurants. It pairs well with chicken, steak, seafood, Fried Cauliflower Rice (page 242), and veggies!

¼ cup mayonnaise

1 teaspoon Sriracha sauce

¼ to ½ teaspoon Swerve confectioners'-style sweetener, depending on desired sweetness

¼ teaspoon garlic powder

1 In a small bowl, mix together all the ingredients until well blended.

2 Serve right away or chill in the refrigerator before serving. Store in an airtight container in the refrigerator for up to 3 weeks.

note: *You can double or triple the recipe for a larger batch.*

per serving:

CALORIES: 206 | FAT: 22 g | PROTEIN: 0 g | TOTAL CARBS: 2.5 g | NET CARBS: 1.5 g

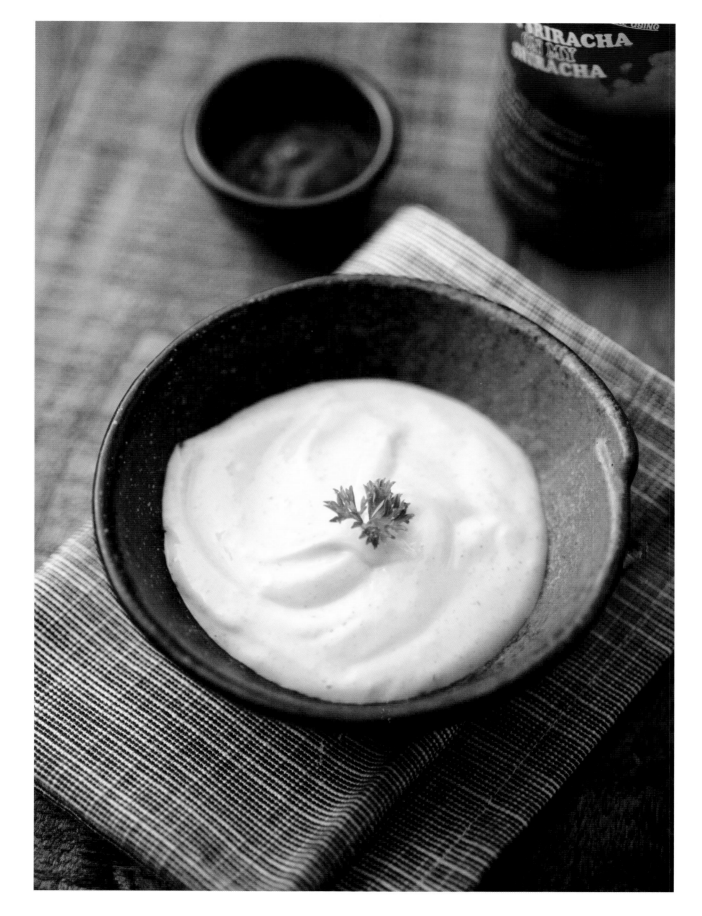

SLOW COOKER BEEF BONE BROTH

PREP TIME: 15 MINUTES • COOK TIME: 10 TO 15 HOURS
YIELD: 6 TO 8 CUPS (1 CUP PER SERVING)

Bone broth is a great base for a variety of recipes, or as a drink to help restore electrolytes.

3 to 4 pounds pastured beef bones

3 stalks celery, quartered

1 large yellow onion, quartered

4 cloves garlic, smashed with the side of a knife

2 tablespoons apple cider vinegar

3 bay leaves

1 tablespoon black peppercorns

Filtered water

Pink Himalayan salt and ground black pepper

1   Place the bones, celery, onion, garlic, vinegar, bay leaves, and peppercorns in a 6-quart or larger slow cooker. Fill the slow cooker about two-thirds full with filtered water, just enough to submerge the bones. Cover and make sure the slow cooker is in a safe spot on the counter, not too close to the edge and not touching any other items. Cook on low for 10 to 15 hours. (I often let my broth simmer overnight.) During cooking, add more water if needed to keep the bones submerged.

2   Use tongs to remove the bones and large vegetable pieces. Strain the broth through a fine-mesh strainer. Season with salt and pepper to taste.

3   Store the broth in an airtight container in the refrigerator for up to 5 days or in the freezer for up to several months.

per serving:

CALORIES: 65 | FAT: 4 g | PROTEIN: 6 g | TOTAL CARBS: 2 g | NET CARBS: 1 g

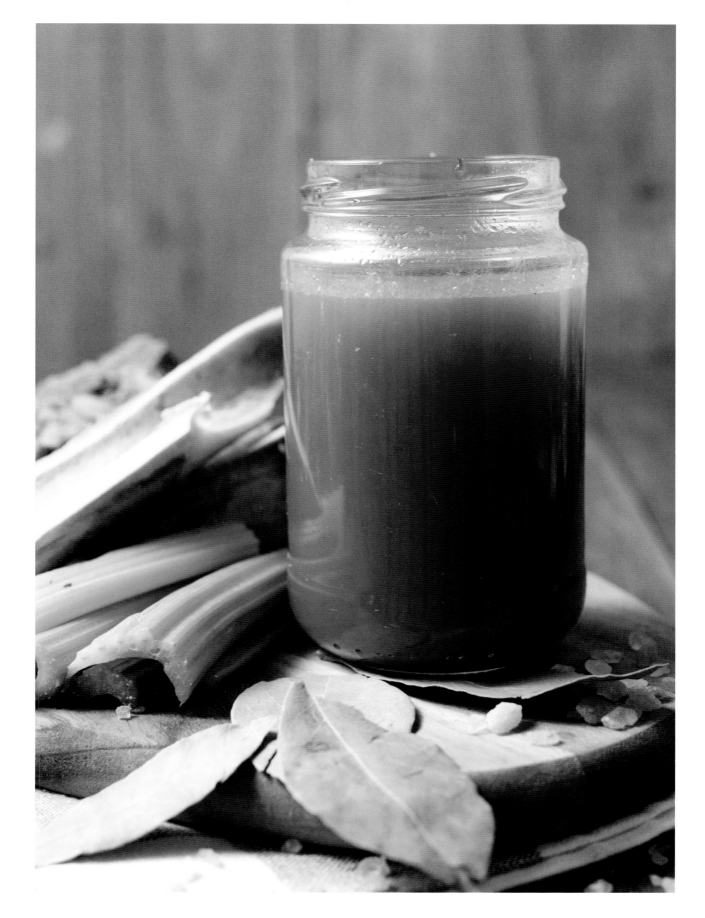

SUGAR-FREE TACO SEASONING

🕐 ∅ 🚫 🧂 PREP TIME: 5 MINUTES • YIELD: ABOUT ½ CUP (2 TABLESPOONS PER SERVING)

Taco seasoning is one of the seasonings that I choose to mix at home for two reasons: one, because most of the ingredients are common household spices, which means that I likely have them on hand with no special trips to the store; and two, because I want to avoid added sugar and unnecessary additives.

¼ cup chili powder

2 tablespoons ground cumin

2 teaspoons onion powder

2 teaspoons smoked paprika

2 teaspoons dried oregano leaves

1½ teaspoons garlic powder

1 teaspoon salt

½ teaspoon ground black pepper

In a small bowl, mix together all the ingredients. Store in an airtight container for up to a year.

notes: Feel free to double the recipe.

To make taco meat, use 2 tablespoons of taco seasoning and ¼ cup of water for every 1 pound of ground beef. After browning the meat, drain the fat, add the seasoning and water, and stir well. Allow to simmer and reduce for 3 to 5 minutes.

per serving:

CALORIES: 51 | FAT: 1.8 g | PROTEIN: 1.8 g | TOTAL CARBS: 7 g | NET CARBS: 3.7 g

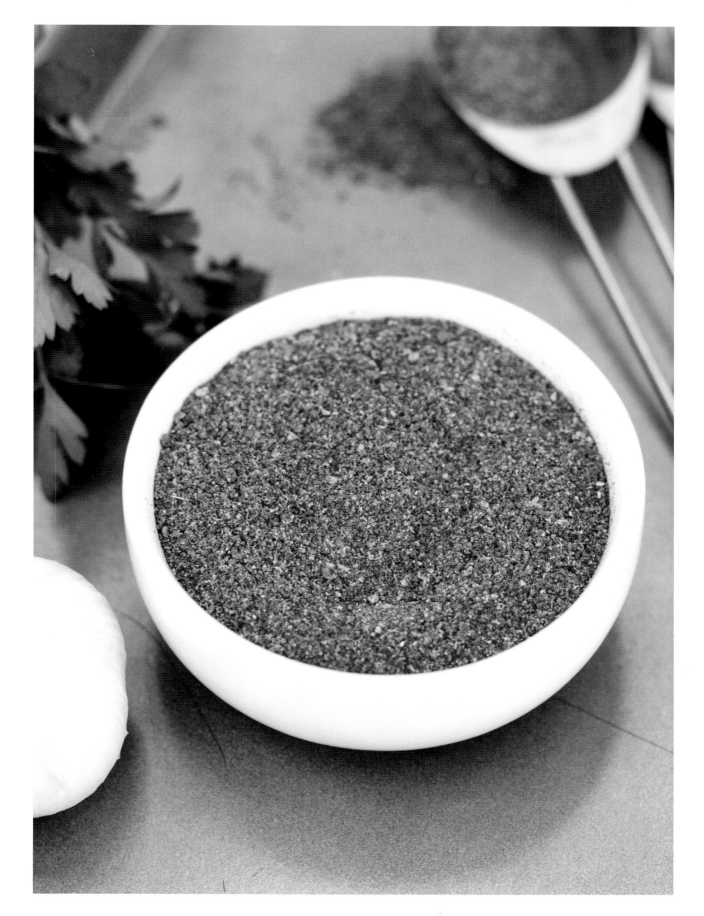

TZATZIKI SAUCE

PREP TIME: 10 MINUTES, PLUS 1 HOUR TO CHILL • YIELD: 1¼ CUPS (8 TO 10 SERVINGS)

I love the spices and flavors of Greek food, and tzatziki sauce has always been a favorite of mine. This creamy sauce pairs perfectly with Gyro Lettuce Wraps (page 172), chicken, or lamb.

⅓ cup peeled and grated cucumber (about ½ large cucumber)

½ cup sour cream

2 tablespoons crumbled feta cheese

1½ teaspoons chopped fresh dill

1 teaspoon fresh lemon juice

1 teaspoon extra-virgin olive oil

1 small clove garlic, pressed, or ¼ teaspoon garlic powder

Salt and pepper, to taste

1 Press the grated cucumber with a paper towel to remove the excess liquid.

2 Combine the cucumber with the remaining ingredients in a medium-sized bowl.

3 For the best flavor, cover and chill the tzatziki in the refrigerator for 1 to 2 hours before serving. Leftovers will keep for up to 3 days.

per serving:

CALORIES: 44 | FAT: 4 g | PROTEIN: 1 g | TOTAL CARBS: 1.6 g | NET CARBS: 1.3 g

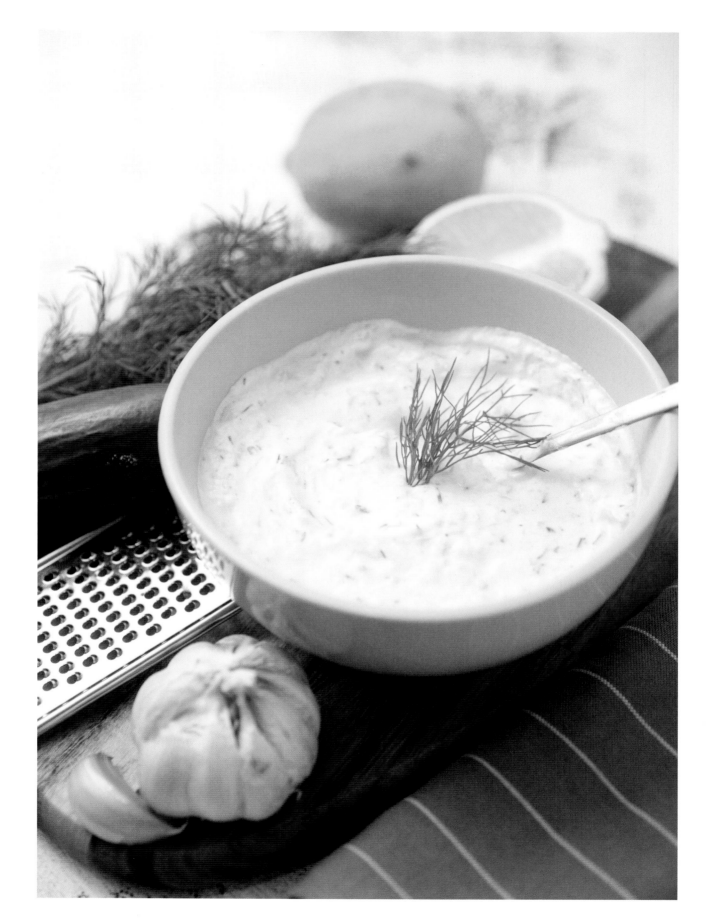

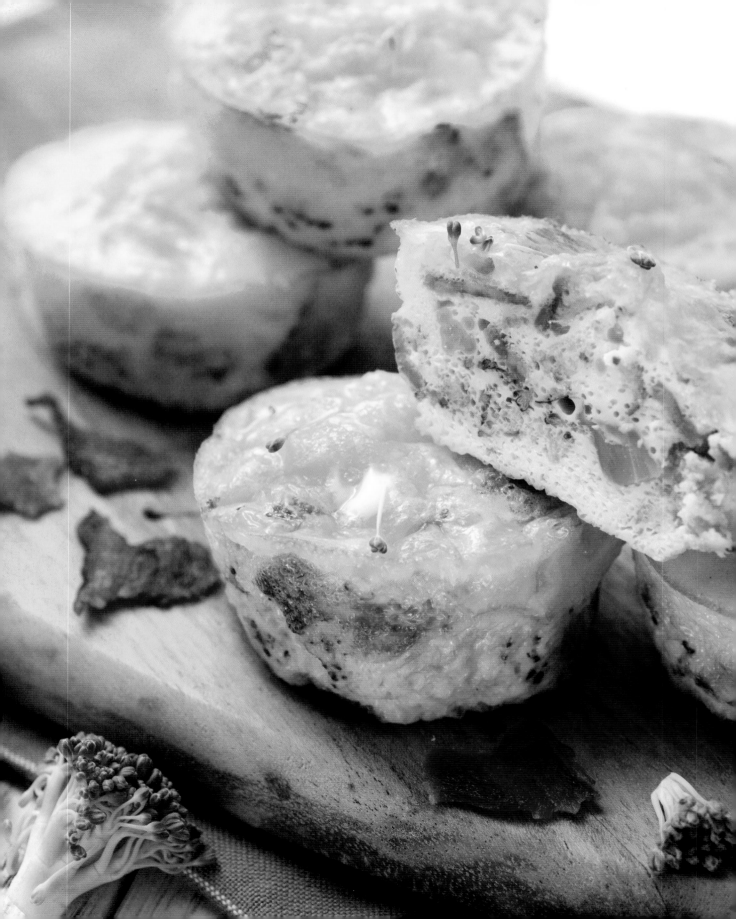

BREAKFAST

60-SECOND MUG BISCUITS

🕥 PREP TIME: 2 MINUTES • COOK TIME: 1 MINUTE • YIELD: 4 BISCUITS (2 PER SERVING)

These fluffy biscuits are ready to enjoy in less than 5 minutes. They are perfect for Biscuits and Gravy (page 96) or Eggs Benedict (page 104), or you can enjoy them plain with butter.

1 large egg

3 tablespoons blanched almond flour

1 tablespoon coconut flour

1 tablespoon unsalted butter, softened

1 teaspoon avocado oil

¼ teaspoon baking powder

Pinch of salt

1 Place all the ingredients in a microwave-safe mug and mix with a fork until smooth. Use the back of a spoon to smooth the top.

2 Microwave for 1 minute (you might need to adjust the cook time based on your microwave).

3 Carefully remove the mug from microwave—it will be hot—cover with a plate, and turn upside down to allow the biscuit to slide from the mug onto the plate. Set the muffin on its side and cut into 4 even slices.

per serving:

CALORIES: 182 | FAT: 16.5 g | PROTEIN: 6 g | TOTAL CARBS: 4.5 g | NET CARBS: 2 g

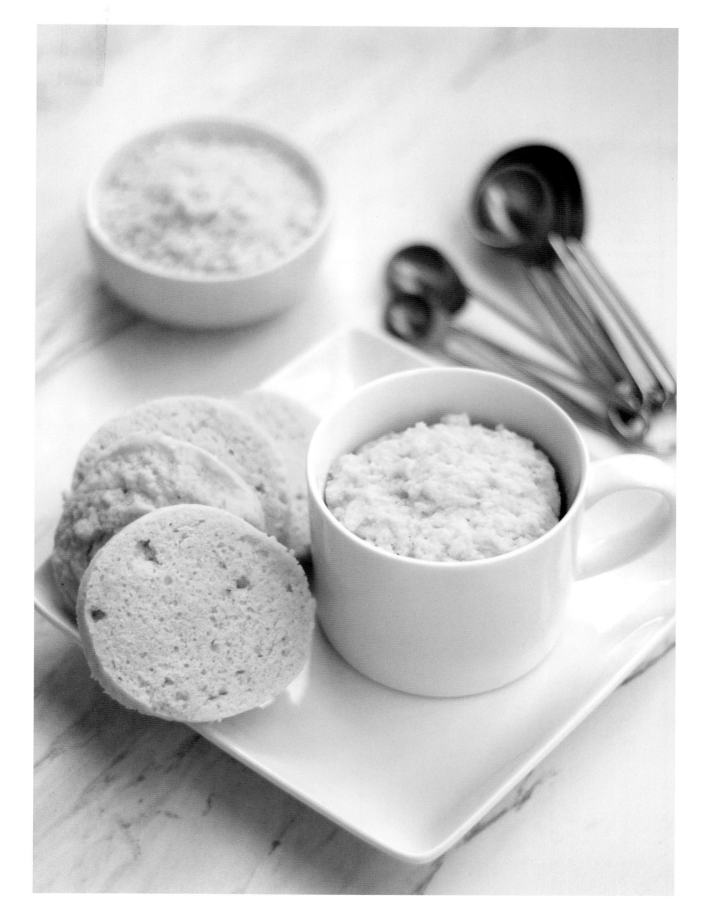

BLUEBERRY MUG MUFFIN

(30) PREP TIME: 5 MINUTES • COOK TIME: ABOUT 1 MINUTE • YIELD: 1 LARGE MUFFIN (1 SERVING)

I love a good mug muffin! Sometimes it's nice to have a simple and quick recipe that doesn't involve large amounts of specialty flours or dirty dishes! Enjoy this muffin warm and topped with butter, all in under 10 minutes!

3 tablespoons blanched almond flour

1 tablespoon coconut flour

1 tablespoon Swerve confectioners'-style sweetener

¼ teaspoon baking powder

Pinch of salt

1 large egg

1 tablespoon unsalted butter, softened

1 teaspoon avocado oil

¼ teaspoon vanilla extract

8 blueberries

Salted butter, for serving (optional)

1   Place the almond flour, coconut flour, sweetener, baking powder, and salt in a medium-large microwave-safe mug and blend with a fork.

2   Add the egg, butter, avocado oil, and vanilla; mix well.

3   Gently stir in the blueberries. Use the back of a spoon to press the batter down and smooth the top.

4   Place the batter-filled mug in the microwave and heat for 1 minute 15 seconds. (The cooking time may vary depending on your microwave. If the muffin is not fully formed after 1 minute 15 seconds, continue cooking in 15-second increments.) Carefully remove the mug from the microwave—it will be hot—flip it upside down over a plate, and allow the muffin to slide out of the mug onto the plate. Place the muffin on its side and slice in half.

5   Spread with butter, if desired, and enjoy!

per muffin, without spread of salted butter:

CALORIES: 372 | FAT: 33 g | PROTEIN: 12 g | TOTAL CARBS: 20 g | NET CARBS: 6 g

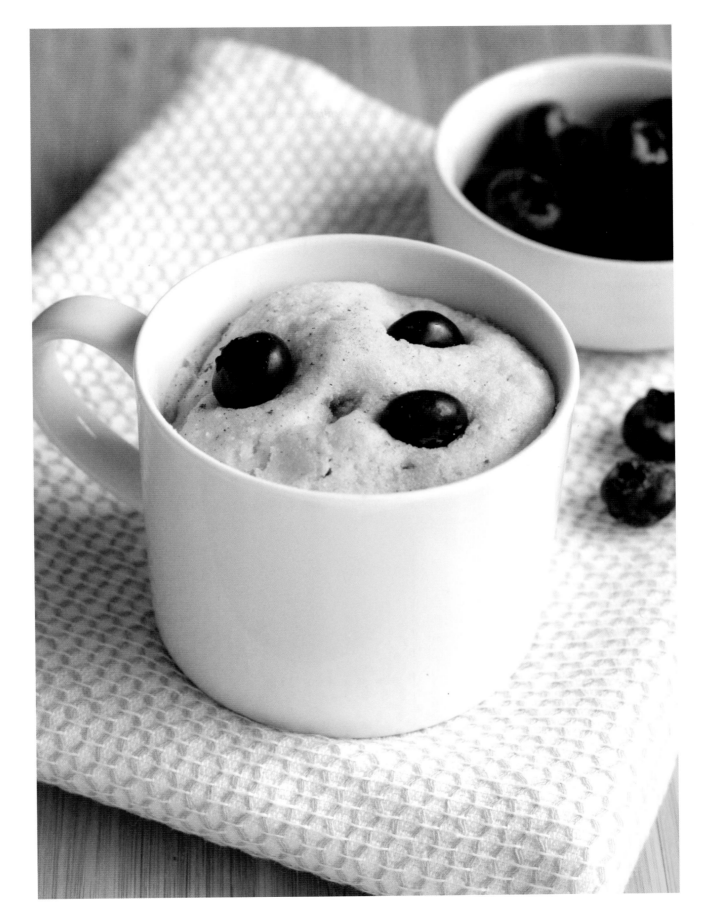

CHILI EGG SCRAMBLE

🕐 🥚 PREP TIME: 5 MINUTES • COOK TIME: 5 MINUTES • YIELD: 2 SERVINGS

One morning my husband decided to make breakfast. Instead of cooking plain eggs, he added some leftover Keto Chili. At the time I was skeptical, but after tasting it, I realized that he is actually a flavor genius! Just don't tell him I said that or it will go to his head.

4 large eggs

1½ teaspoons unsalted butter

½ cup Keto Chili (page 156), warm

Salt and pepper

½ avocado, sliced

¼ cup shredded cheddar cheese

¼ cup sour cream

½ green onion, finely chopped, for garnish (optional)

1 In a medium-sized bowl, whisk the eggs.

2 Melt the butter in a medium-sized skillet over medium heat. Add the eggs and scramble until almost fully cooked. Add the warm chili and use a spatula to incorporate it into the eggs as they finish cooking.

3 Season with salt and pepper to taste. Serve topped with the avocado, cheese, and sour cream, garnished with green onion, if desired.

per serving, without green onion garnish:

CALORIES: 443 | FAT: 37.5 g | PROTEIN: 35.4 g | TOTAL CARBS: 7.6 g | NET CARBS: 4.3 g

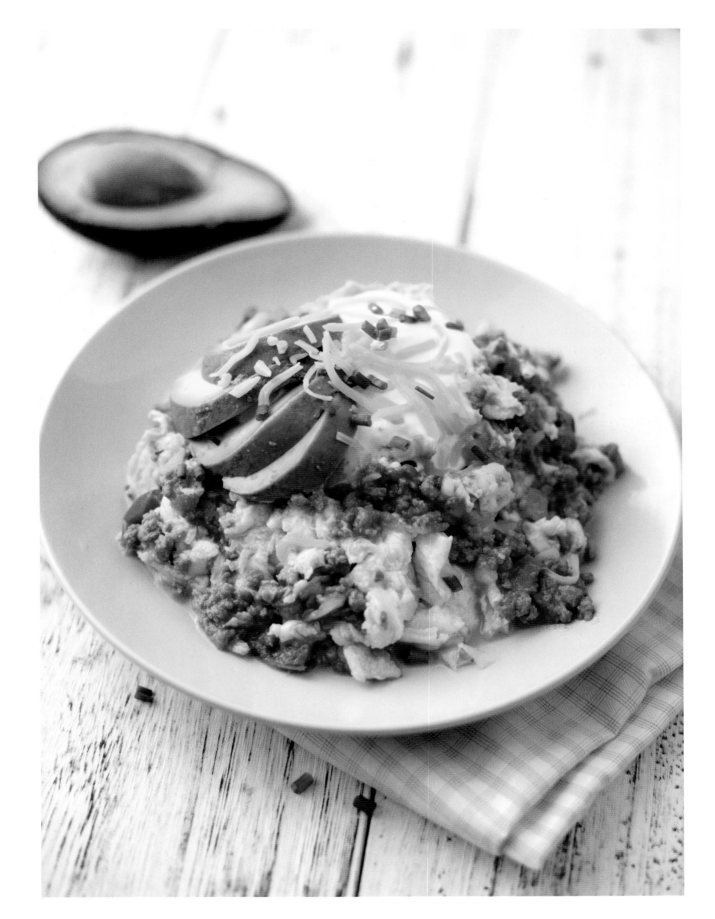

BISCUITS AND GRAVY

PREP TIME: 10 MINUTES (INCLUDING TIME TO MAKE BISCUITS)
COOK TIME: 15 MINUTES • YIELD: 2 SERVINGS

Growing up in South Carolina, we often enjoyed biscuits and gravy, one of the ultimate comfort foods! I created and tested this recipe with my dad by my side, just like the old days . . . but without all the carbs!

4 ounces bulk breakfast sausage

3 ounces cream cheese, softened

⅓ cup half-and-half

Salt and pepper

1 batch 60-Second Mug Biscuits (page 88), for serving

Chopped fresh parsley, for garnish (optional)

1   In a small saucepan over medium heat, brown the sausage, using a wooden spoon or spatula to break up the clumps of meat.

2   Add the cream cheese and stir until blended. Pour in the half-and-half and stir until well mixed.

3   Allow the gravy to reduce over medium heat until the desired consistency is reached, 3 to 5 minutes, then remove from the heat and season with salt and pepper to taste.

4   Serve the gravy over the biscuits. Garnish with parsley, if desired.

per serving:

CALORIES: 518 | FAT: 46 g | PROTEIN: 17.5 g | TOTAL CARBS: 8.5 g | NET CARBS: 6 g

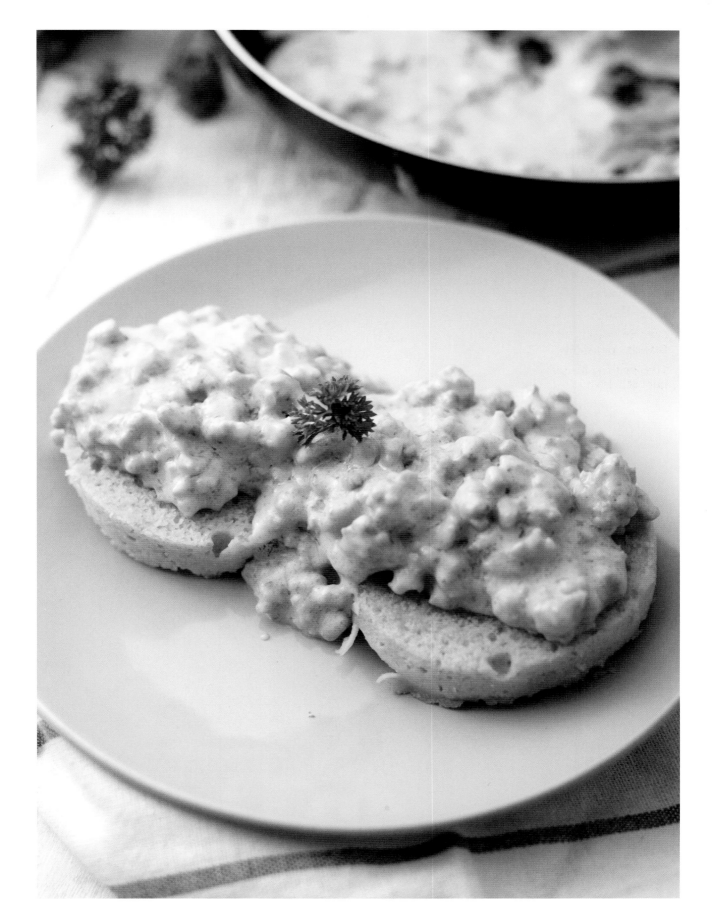

CHOCOLATE CHIP WAFFLE

PREP TIME: 5 MINUTES • COOK TIME: 5 MINUTES

YIELD: 1 LARGE WAFFLE (1 SERVING)

One of my favorite things about keto is that you can make almost any dish keto-friendly with a few simple swaps. Enter chocolate chip waffles! Enjoy this waffle topped with a pat of butter and some sugar-free syrup or Keto Whipped Cream (page 290).

⅓ cup blanched almond flour

½ tablespoon coconut flour

¼ teaspoon baking powder

2 large eggs

¼ teaspoon vanilla extract

4 drops liquid stevia

1 tablespoon stevia-sweetened chocolate chips (see notes)

For Topping (Optional)

Swerve confectioners'-style sweetener

Sugar-free syrup

Salted butter

notes: I use Lily's baking chips. These chocolate chips are dairy-free but are manufactured using equipment that may come into contact with dairy, so those with dairy allergies should be cautious.

This recipe can also be used to make chocolate chip pancakes if you don't have a waffle maker.

1 Preheat a waffle maker to medium-high heat.

2 Place all the ingredients except the chocolate chips in a large bowl and blend until smooth. Fold in the chocolate chips.

3 Spray the hot waffle maker with nonstick cooking spray.

4 Pour the batter into the hot waffle iron and cook for 3 to 5 minutes, until light golden brown.

5 Serve dusted with Swerve confectioners'-style sweetener and topped with sugar-free syrup and butter, if desired.

per waffle:

CALORIES: 398 | FAT: 31 g | PROTEIN: 23 g | TOTAL CARBS: 14 g | NET CARBS: 6.3 g

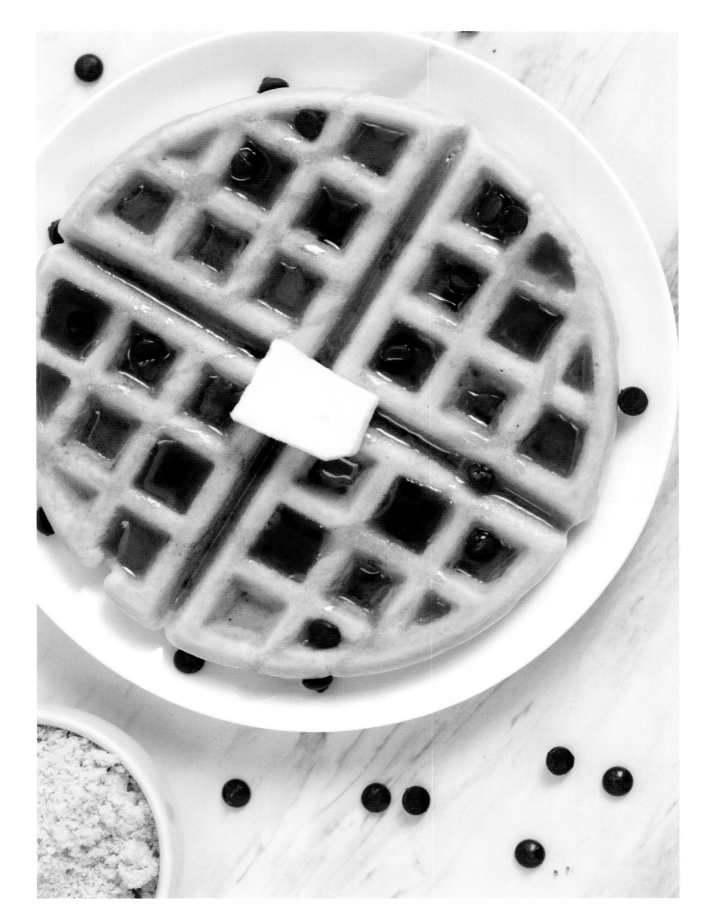

OLIVIA'S CREAM CHEESE PANCAKES

🕐 PREP TIME: 15 MINUTES • COOK TIME: 15 MINUTES • YIELD: 3 PANCAKES (1 SERVING)

Pancakes were by far my favorite breakfast food for the majority of my life. Thankfully, these delicious keto pancakes offer the same great taste, without the added sugar or stomachache. Enjoy them plain or add blueberries, stevia-sweetened chocolate chips, crispy bacon, or a little pumpkin with cinnamon for variety! My daughter, Olivia, and I make a double batch of these almost every weekend, and they taste great even with a little eggshell in them (but hey, I'm not pointing any fingers). This batter is a little thinner than traditional pancake batter, so make sure your pan is nice and hot before you pour in the batter.

2 medium eggs

2 ounces cream cheese

½ teaspoon vanilla extract

¼ cup blanched almond flour

1 teaspoon Swerve confectioners'-style sweetener

¼ teaspoon baking powder

Salted butter, for serving

Sugar-free syrup, for serving

notes: If you want a large batch of pancakes, this recipe can be doubled or tripled.

After cooking each batch, you can keep the pancakes warm by placing them in a pan in a preheated 200°F oven.

Extras can be stored in the freezer between sheets of parchment paper in a zip-top plastic bag.

1 Combine the eggs, cream cheese, vanilla, almond flour, sweetener, and baking powder in a blender and blend on medium-high speed until smooth. Use a fork to pop the large bubbles on the top of the batter.

2 Coat a medium-sized skillet with coconut oil spray or ghee and place over medium heat. Once hot, pour one-third of the batter into the pan. Flip the pancake when the sides are firm and bubbles appear evenly throughout, 1 to 3 minutes, then cook for another 1 to 3 minutes on the second side.

3 Repeat with the remaining batter to make a total of 3 pancakes.

4 Serve topped with butter and sugar-free syrup.

per serving:

CALORIES: 487 | FAT: 40 g | PROTEIN: 21 g | TOTAL CARBS: 12 g | NET CARBS: 6 g

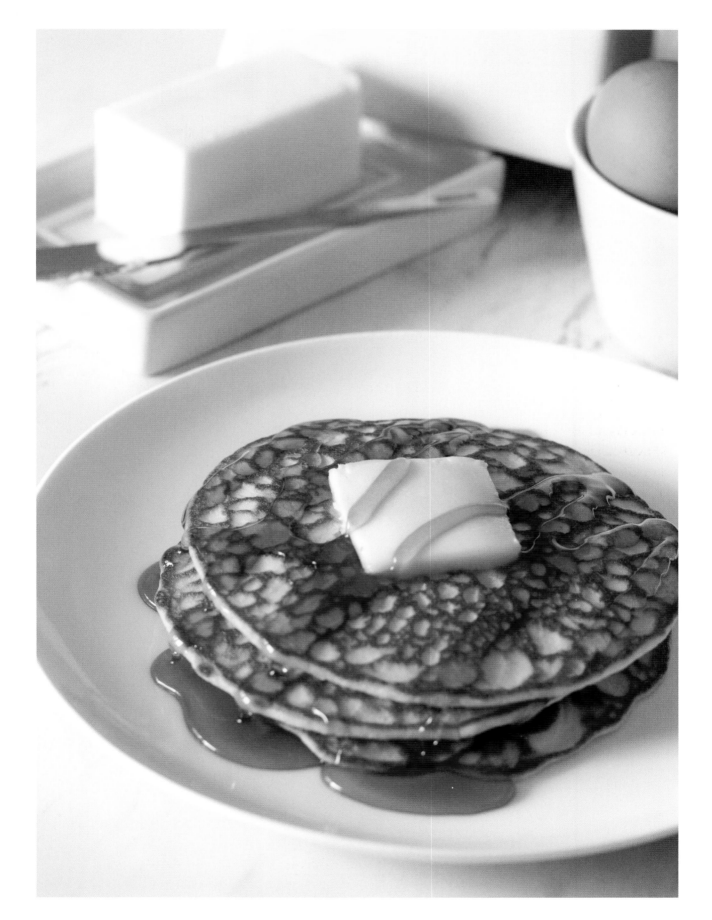

EASY EGG SCRAMBLE

PREP TIME: 10 MINUTES • COOK TIME: 15 MINUTES • YIELD: 2 SERVINGS

I discovered this delicious egg scramble in a cute little café in the heart of San Francisco. I enjoyed it so much that I re-created the dish when I got home! I'm a big fan of goat cheese, but if you aren't, feel free to substitute a cheese that you like.

1 tablespoon unsalted butter

1 cup sliced white mushrooms

4 large eggs

3 ounces goat cheese, crumbled (about ⅓ cup)

⅓ cup cooked chopped bacon

2 large fresh basil leaves, chopped

Salt and pepper

1 In a medium-sized skillet, melt the butter over medium-high heat. Add the mushrooms and sauté until tender, 4 to 5 minutes.

2 Add the eggs and scramble, stirring constantly, until almost fully cooked, 4 to 5 minutes.

3 Sprinkle the goat cheese, bacon, and basil over the eggs and mushrooms; toss a few times. Season to taste with salt and pepper and serve.

per serving:

CALORIES: 381 | FAT: 28 g | PROTEIN: 29.5 g | TOTAL CARBS: 2 g | NET CARBS: 1.5 g

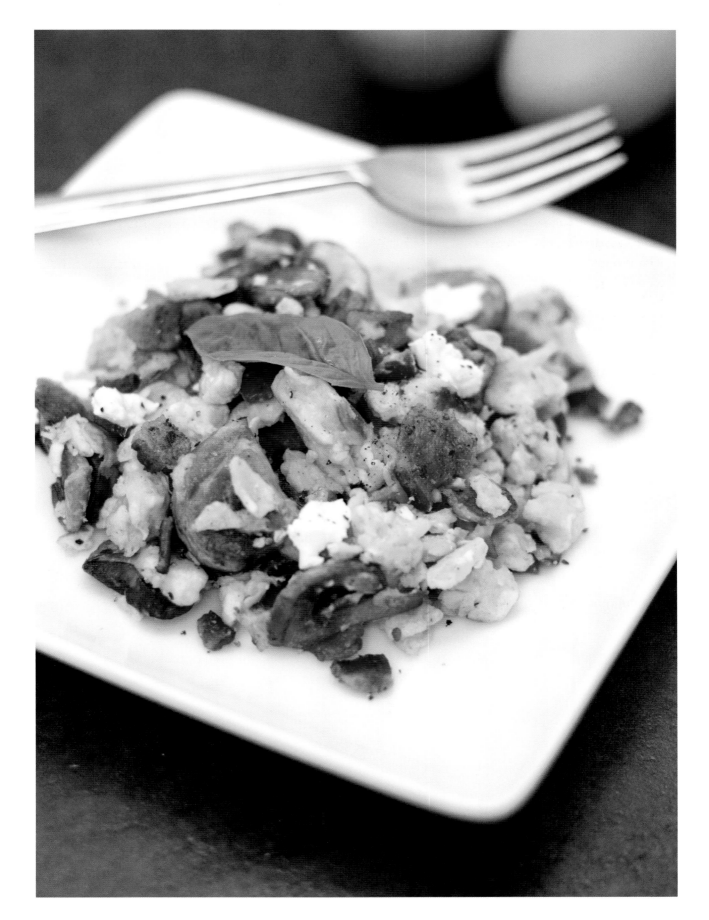

EGGS BENEDICT

PREP TIME: 15 MINUTES (NOT INCLUDING TIME TO MAKE BISCUITS OR HOLLANDAISE)
COOK TIME: 20 MINUTES • YIELD: 2 SERVINGS

This delicious breakfast is my go-to on weekends when I have a little extra time to play around in the kitchen. Eggs Benny can easily be made ketogenic by swapping the English muffins for my 60-Second Mug Biscuits, avocado slices, or even leftover Low-Carb Crab Cakes (page 222)!

1 batch 60-Second Mug Biscuits (page 88)

4 slices bacon, cooked and cut in half crosswise

½ avocado, sliced (optional)

4 large eggs

⅓ cup Simple Hollandaise (page 76), warm

Salt and pepper

Snipped fresh chives, for garnish (optional)

tip: Eggs Benedict is a great option for breakfast when dining out on keto. Often restaurants are happy to leave out the bread or even swap the bread for sliced avocado.

1 If desired, toast the biscuits.

2 Cook the bacon in a skillet over medium heat and set aside.

3 Bring a medium-sized pot of water to a simmer over medium-high heat. Do not let the water boil.

4 Crack an egg into a small bowl. Use a spoon to create a gentle whirlpool in the simmering water, then gently drop in the egg. Poach for 3 minutes. Gently remove the cooked egg with a slotted spoon and place on a paper towel–lined plate to absorb the excess water. Repeat with the remaining eggs.

5 Place 2 biscuits on each plate. Top each biscuit with 2 half-slices of bacon and avocado slices, if using. Top with a poached egg and drizzle the warm hollandaise over the top. Season with salt and pepper to taste. Garnish with chives, if desired.

per serving, without avocado:

CALORIES: 572 | FAT: 49.3 g | PROTEIN: 25.8 g | TOTAL CARBS: 8.3 g | NET CARBS: 4.6 g

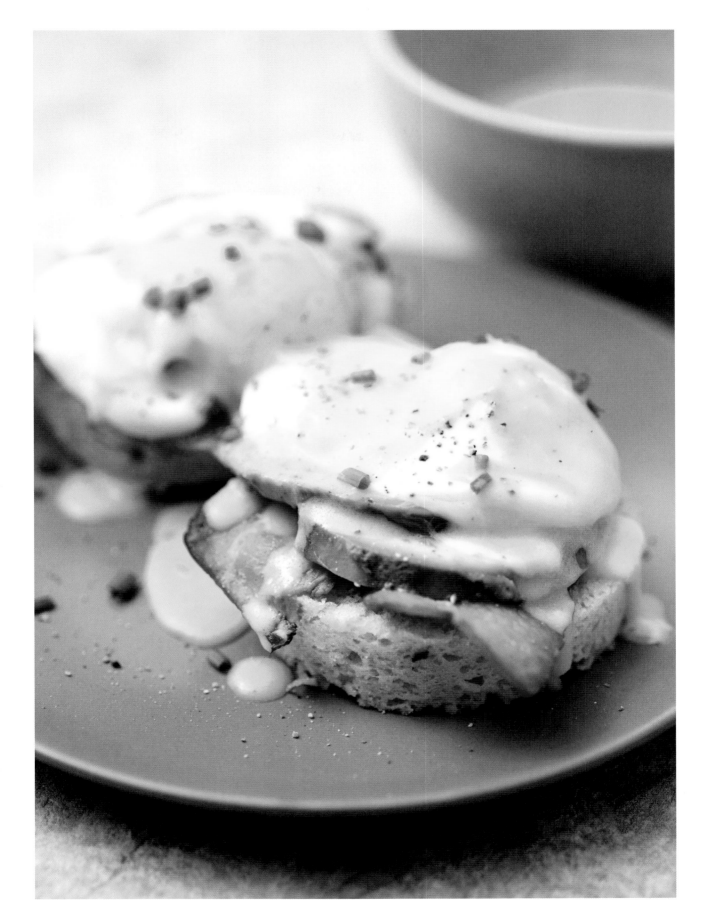

LOX AND CREAM CHEESE SLIDERS

PREP TIME: 15 MINUTES • YIELD: 20 SLIDERS (5 PER SERVING)

Looking for egg-free breakfast ideas? My friend Jessica and I developed this quick and easy recipe, perfect for busy weekday mornings! While I often eat these for breakfast, I have also served them as an appetizer at gatherings with family and friends.

1 English cucumber

3½ ounces whipped cream cheese

3 ounces wild lox, cut into bite-sized pieces

Fresh dill, for garnish (optional)

Capers, for garnish (optional)

1. Peel and slice the cucumber into ¼- to ⅜-inch-thick rounds.

2. Spread about 1 teaspoon of cream cheese on each cucumber slice. Top each slice with a bite-sized piece of lox. Insert a toothpick down the center to hold the sliders together.

3. Garnish with fresh dill and capers, if desired.

per serving:

CALORIES: 139 | FAT: 9.8 g | PROTEIN: 7.8 g | TOTAL CARBS: 3.7 g | NET CARBS: 3.2 g

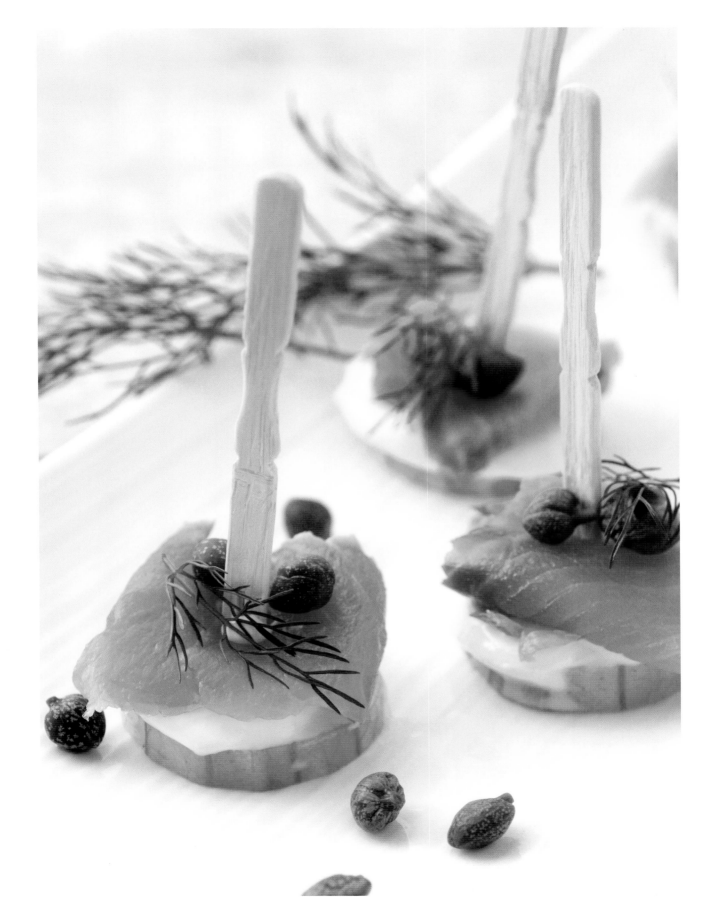

QUICK AND EASY
CAPICOLA EGG CUPS

PREP TIME: 5 MINUTES • COOK TIME: 14 MINUTES
YIELD: 6 EGG CUPS (2 PER SERVING)

Weekday mornings are pretty hectic in our house, and these egg cups are always there to save the day! I recommend prepping them on Sunday night to have them ready for the busy week ahead.

6 slices capicola (regular or spicy)

¾ cup shredded cheddar cheese or other cheese of choice (optional)

6 large eggs

Salt and pepper

Thinly sliced fresh basil, for garnish (optional)

notes: *You can use prepackaged or deli capicola, or substitute other meats, like ham or bacon.*

This recipe can easily be doubled or tripled for meal prep. Store the egg cups in airtight containers in the refrigerator for up to 4 days or in the freezer for up to 3 months.

1 Preheat the oven to 400°F. Spray 6 wells of a standard-size muffin pan with nonstick cooking spray.

2 Place a slice of capicola in each of the 6 greased wells, forming a bowl shape. If using cheese, sprinkle 2 tablespoons into each of the cups formed by the capicola.

3 Crack an egg into each cup and season with salt and pepper.

4 Bake for 12 to 14 minutes, until the egg whites are set. Serve hot, garnished with basil, if desired.

per serving, with cheese:

CALORIES: 260 | FAT: 19.6 g | PROTEIN: 23 g | TOTAL CARBS: 1.6 g | NET CARBS: 1.6 g

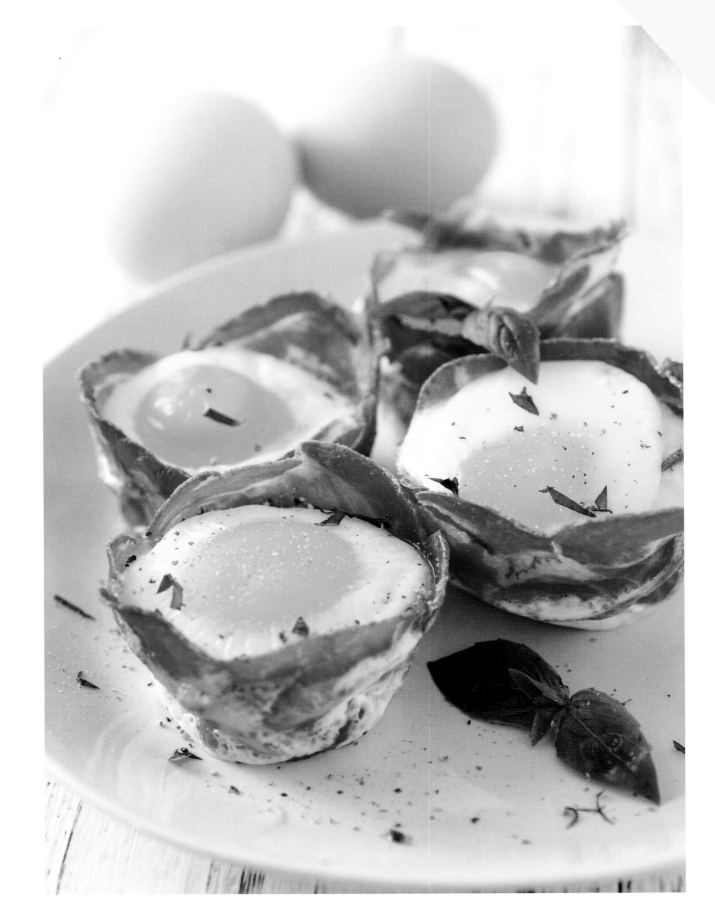

SAGE, EGG, AND CHEESE
KFAST BAKE

PREP TIME: 15 MINUTES • COOK TIME: 35 MINUTES • YIELD: 6 SERVINGS

This egg bake is my husband's favorite breakfast; I'm pretty sure he would eat it every day if he could! This simple and delicious dish is warm, filling, and ready in less than an hour!

1 tablespoon unsalted butter

⅓ cup chopped yellow onions

1 pound bulk breakfast sausage

8 large eggs

⅓ cup heavy whipping cream

1 clove garlic, pressed

1 teaspoon salt

½ teaspoon ground black pepper

1 cup shredded cheddar cheese

note: Feel free to play around with the ingredients in this recipe. For example, try spinach, mushrooms, or other meats, like cooked bacon crumbles.

1 Preheat the oven to 350°F. Lightly coat an 8-inch deep-dish pie dish or baking dish with coconut oil or nonstick cooking spray.

2 Heat the butter in a large skillet over medium heat. Add the onions and sauté until soft, 3 to 4 minutes.

3 Add the sausage and cook until evenly browned, 4 to 5 minutes. Drain and set aside.

4 In a large bowl, whisk the eggs, cream, garlic, salt, and pepper.

5 Spread the sausage evenly on the bottom of the prepared dish and top with the cheese. Pour the egg mixture over the cheese.

6 Bake for 35 minutes, until the eggs are set and the top is lightly golden brown.

7 Allow to cool for 3 to 5 minutes before serving. Leftovers can be covered and stored in the refrigerator for up to 4 days.

per serving:

CALORIES: 394 | FAT: 33 g | PROTEIN: 21.8 g | TOTAL CARBS: 2.6 g | NET CARBS: 2.6 g

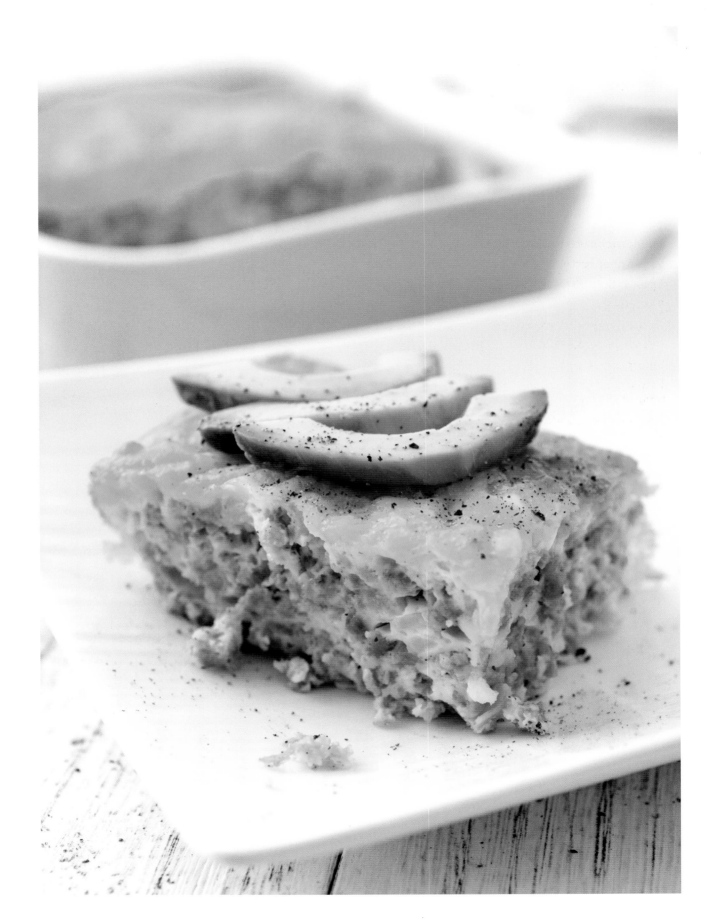

WAFFLE BREAKFAST SANDWICHES

⏱ 🥛 **PREP TIME: 10 MINUTES • COOK TIME: 20 MINUTES • YIELD: 2 SERVINGS**
OPTION

The perfect combination for a savory and delicious breakfast sandwich. Feel free to play around with the ingredients inside the waffle sandwich, like swapping out the bacon for sausage or ham!

Waffles

2 large eggs

⅓ cup blanched almond flour

½ tablespoon coconut flour

¼ teaspoon baking powder

Pinch of salt

¼ teaspoon vanilla extract

4 drops liquid stevia

Sandwich Fillings

4 slices bacon

2 large eggs

2 slices cheddar cheese or other cheese of choice (optional)

½ avocado, sliced

Salt and pepper

1. Preheat a waffle maker to medium-high heat.

2. Make the waffles: In a medium-sized mixing bowl, beat the eggs. Add the almond flour, coconut flour, baking powder, salt, vanilla, and stevia and mix until smooth.

3. Pour the batter into the preheated waffle maker and close the lid; cook for 3 to 5 minutes, until light golden brown and slightly crisp. Remove the cooked waffle and set aside.

4. Make the sandwich fillings: In a skillet over medium heat, fry the bacon until crispy. Remove the bacon and set aside, leaving the bacon fat in the skillet.

5. Crack the eggs into the skillet with the bacon fat (cooked over easy so that the yolks are runny).

6. After flipping the eggs, cover each with a slice of cheese, if using, and cover the pan with a lid to help melt the cheese.

7. To assemble the sandwiches, cut the waffle into quarters. Place a quarter waffle on each plate and top each with 2 slices of bacon and a cheese-topped egg. Top each stack with avocado slices and season with salt and pepper to taste. Top each sandwich with one of the remaining waffle quarters.

per serving, without cheese filling:

CALORIES: 393 | FAT: 31 g | PROTEIN: 23.5 g | TOTAL CARBS: 8.5 g | NET CARBS: 3.5 g

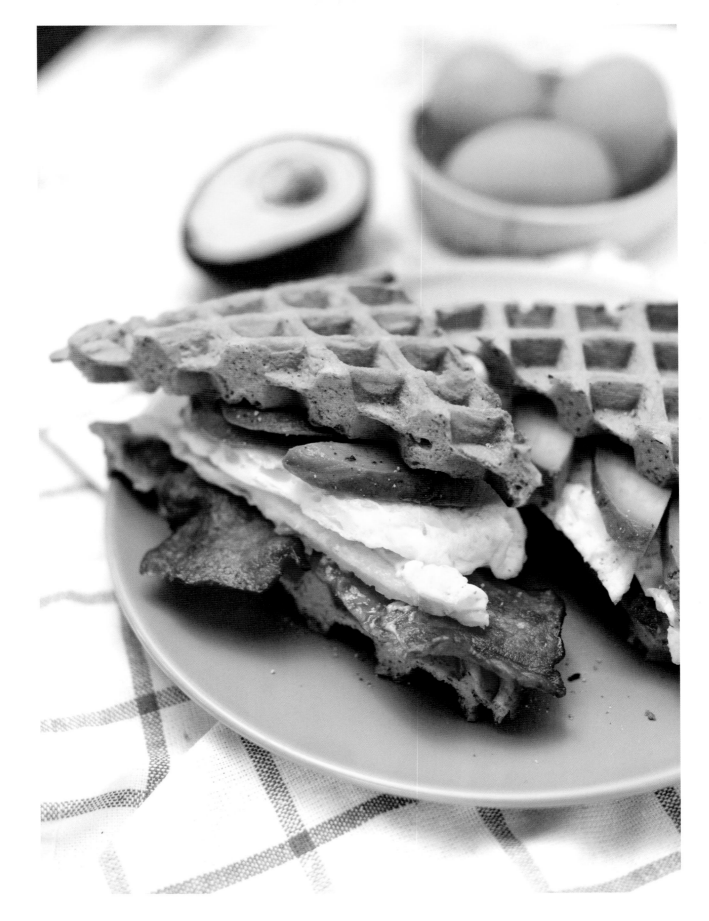

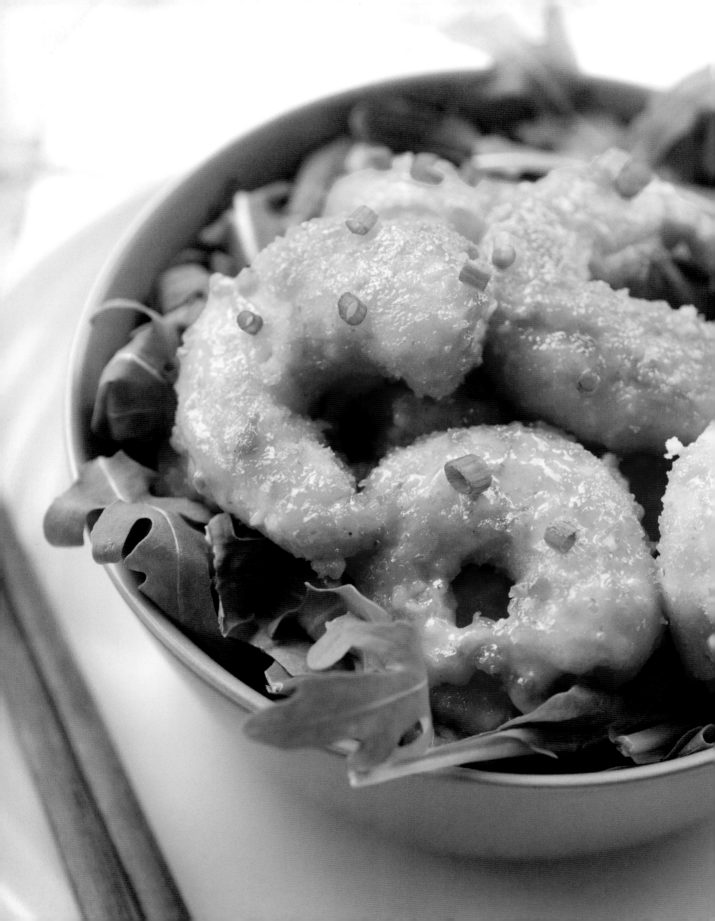

APPETIZERS AND SNACKS

BACON CHEDDAR JALAPEÑO POPPERS

PREP TIME: 15 MINUTES • COOK TIME: 20 MINUTES • YIELD: 12 POPPERS (4 PER SERVING)

These delicious poppers are my favorite appetizer—perfect for Sunday night football, cookouts, or gatherings! Just be sure to make a few batches if you're having company over, because they go quickly.

5 slices bacon (see tip)

6 jalapeño peppers

3 ounces cream cheese, softened

¼ cup shredded cheddar cheese

¼ teaspoon garlic powder

tip: As a shortcut, you can use packaged bacon bits/pieces (nitrate-free if possible) instead of frying your own bacon.

1   In a skillet over medium heat, fry the bacon until crispy. Set aside on a paper towel–lined plate to cool. When cool enough to handle, chop the bacon into bits.

2   Preheat the oven to 400°F. Line a rimmed baking sheet with parchment paper.

3   Slice the jalapeño peppers in half lengthwise. Use a spoon to scrape out the seeds and membranes. (If you prefer spicy food, feel free to incorporate the jalapeño seeds and membranes into the cheese sauce instead of discarding them.)

4   In a medium-sized bowl, use a fork to combine the cream cheese, cheddar cheese, garlic powder, and bacon bits. Spoon some of the mixture into each jalapeño half and set the peppers cheese side up on the lined baking sheet. Bake for 18 to 20 minutes, until the cheese is melted and slightly crisp on top.

per serving:

CALORIES: 203 | FAT: 16.3 g | PROTEIN: 9 g | TOTAL CARBS: 3.3 g | NET CARBS: 2.6 g

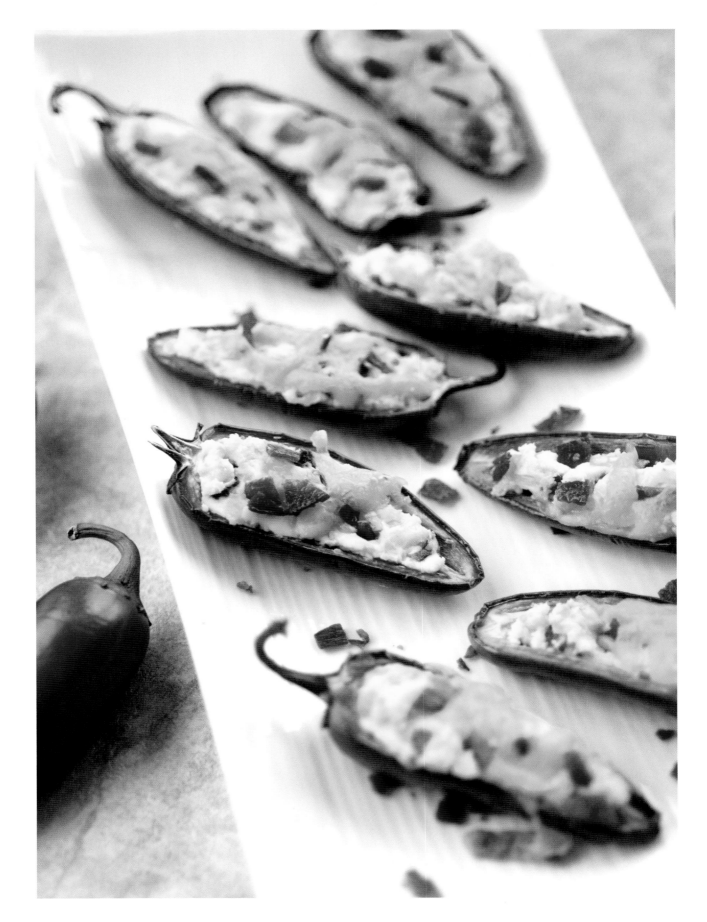

BAKED CRAB DIP

PREP TIME: 15 MINUTES • COOK TIME: 25 MINUTES • YIELD: 4 TO 6 SERVINGS

This rich, warm crab dip is the ultimate comfort-food appetizer! I love to pair it with Cheese Crisps (page 128), Keto Crackers (page 136), or fresh veggies, such as cucumber slices, celery sticks, bell pepper strips, or cherry or grape tomatoes.

4 ounces cream cheese, softened

½ cup shredded Parmesan cheese, plus ½ cup extra for topping (optional)

⅓ cup mayonnaise

¼ cup sour cream

1 tablespoon chopped fresh parsley

2 teaspoons fresh lemon juice

1½ teaspoons Sriracha sauce

½ teaspoon garlic powder

8 ounces fresh lump crabmeat

Salt and pepper

1 Preheat the oven to 375°F.

2 Combine all the ingredients except for the crabmeat in a mixing bowl and use a hand mixer to blend until smooth.

3 Put the crabmeat in a separate bowl, check for shells, and rinse with cold water, if needed. Pat dry or allow to rest in a strainer until most of the water has drained.

4 Add the crabmeat to the bowl with the cream cheese mixture and gently fold to combine. Taste for seasoning and add salt and pepper to taste, if needed. Pour into an 8-inch round or square baking dish and bake for 25 minutes, until the cheese has melted and the dip is warm throughout.

5 If desired, top the dip with another ½ cup of Parmesan cheese and broil for 2 to 3 minutes, until the cheese has melted and browned slightly.

per serving, with cheese topping, based on 6 servings:

CALORIES: 275 | FAT: 22.6 g | PROTEIN: 15.8 g | TOTAL CARBS: 1.3 g | NET CARBS: 1.3 g

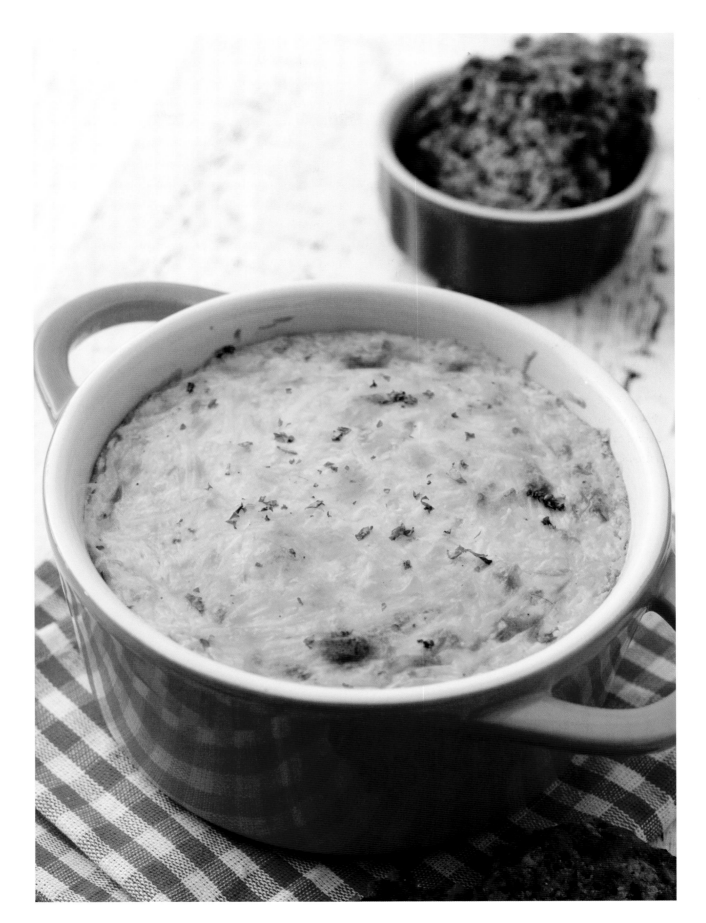

SWEET AND SPICY FRIED SHRIMP

⏱ 🚫 🥛 PREP TIME: 15 MINUTES • COOK TIME: 4 MINUTES • YIELD: 2 SERVINGS

This recipe is inspired by Bonefish Grill's Bang Bang Shrimp dish. It's the perfect combination of crunchy succulent shrimp with a slightly sweet and spicy sauce.

¼ cup coconut flour

¼ teaspoon garlic powder

¼ teaspoon salt

1 large egg

8 large shrimp, peeled and deveined, tails removed

¾ tablespoon coconut oil, for the pan

½ batch Mick's Spicy Aioli (page 78)

Arugula, for serving

Sliced green onions, for garnish (optional)

1. In a small bowl, mix together the coconut flour, garlic powder, and salt.

2. In a third small bowl, beat the egg.

3. Dip the shrimp into the beaten egg and then into the coconut flour mixture; press the mixture into both sides of the shrimp to coat.

4. In a medium-sized skillet over medium-high heat, heat the coconut oil. When hot, add the shrimp and fry for 2 to 4 minutes, flipping once, until the "breading" is golden brown on both sides.

5. Toss the shrimp in the spicy aioli. Serve over arugula and garnish with green onions, if desired.

per serving:

CALORIES: 272 | FAT: 19.5 g | PROTEIN: 14 g | TOTAL CARBS: 11.3 g | NET CARBS: 5.4 g

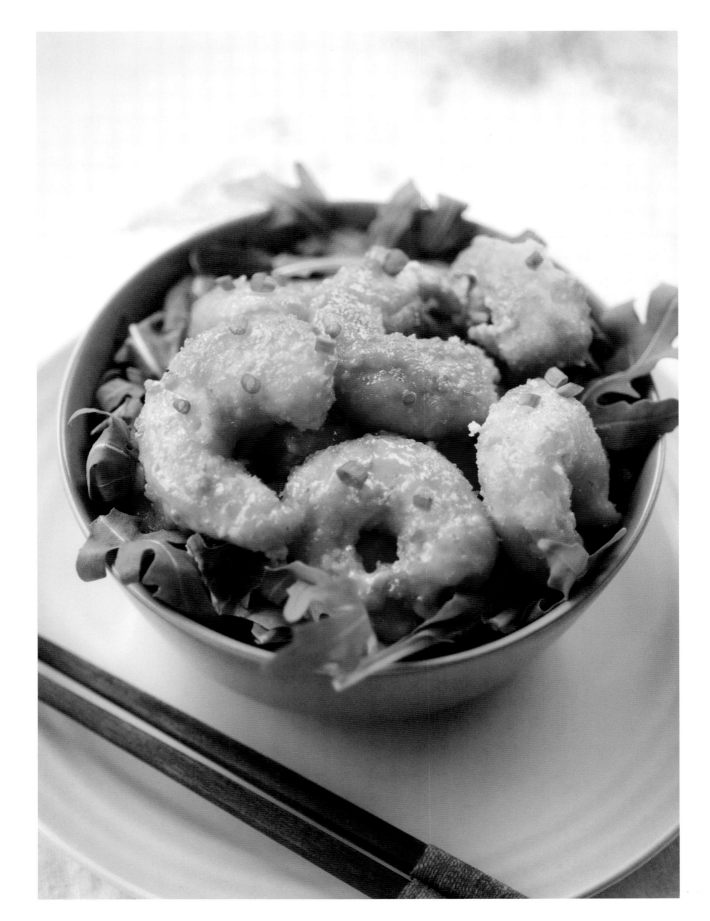

BUFFALO CHICKEN DIP

PREP TIME: 10 MINUTES • COOK TIME: 20 MINUTES • YIELD: 6 SERVINGS

Buffalo chicken dip is the ultimate game-day dip, but of course it can be enjoyed any day of the week. Pair it with celery sticks, pork rinds, or Keto Crackers (page 136) and enjoy!

3 slices bacon (see tip)

1½ cups shredded cooked chicken

1 (8-ounce) package cream cheese, softened

½ cup Buffalo sauce

½ cup ranch dressing (see note)

Chopped green onions, for garnish (optional)

tip: To save time and effort, you can use packaged bacon bits/pieces (nitrate-free if possible) instead of frying your own bacon, and purchase a rotisserie chicken from the supermarket.

note: Ingredients vary in different brands of ranch dressing. If you wish to make this recipe egg-free, please check ingredient labels closely and find a brand that meets your needs.

1 Preheat the oven to 375°F.

2 In a skillet over medium heat, fry the bacon until crispy. Set aside on a paper towel–lined plate to cool, then chop.

3 In a large bowl, combine the shredded chicken, cream cheese, Buffalo sauce, ranch dressing, and bacon; mix well. (If desired, reserve some of the bacon to sprinkle on top, as pictured.)

4 Transfer the chicken mixture to a shallow 1-quart baking dish and bake for 20 minutes, until warm throughout.

5 Garnish with chopped green onions, if desired.

per serving:

CALORIES: 286 | FAT: 24.6 g | PROTEIN: 11 g | TOTAL CARBS: 2.7 g | NET CARBS: 2.7 g

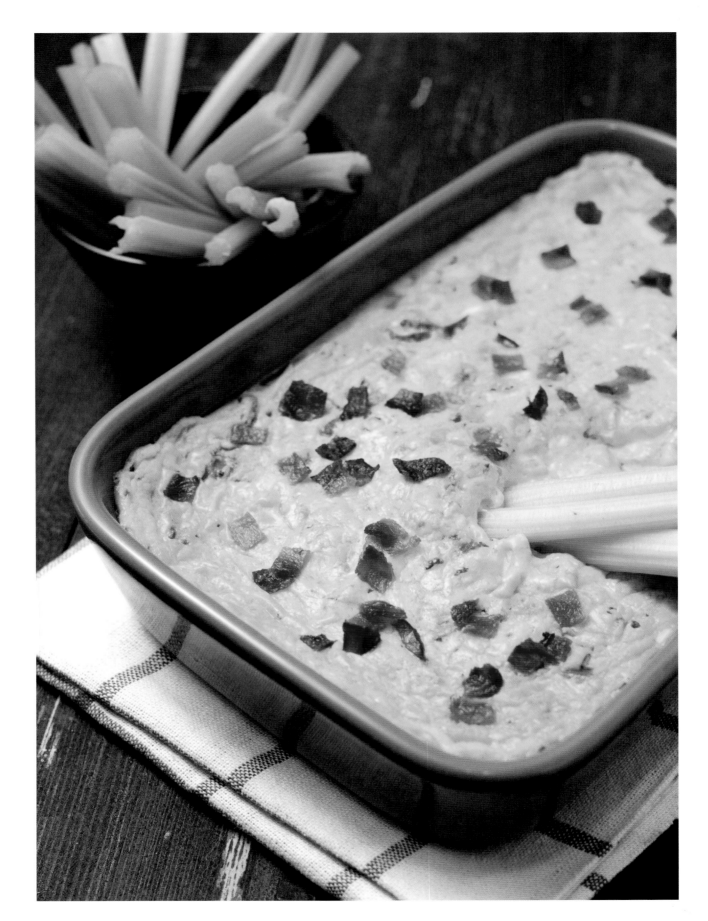

CAPRESE SKEWERS

PREP TIME: 15 MINUTES, PLUS 1 HOUR TO MARINATE • YIELD: 6 SERVINGS

Ciliegini are Italian fresh mozzarella cheese balls that are the size of small cherry tomatoes and packaged in water or a seasoning marinade. The tiny balls are perfect for salads, snacks, and a variety of appetizers, including this one. These caprese skewers are fresh, colorful, and great for picnics or cookouts!

8 ounces ciliegini mozzarella balls, drained and halved

9 grape tomatoes, halved

18 small to medium fresh basil leaves

Marinade

¼ cup extra-virgin olive oil

1 small to medium clove garlic, pressed or minced

1 tablespoon chopped fresh parsley

1 tablespoon dried ground oregano

1 tablespoon fresh lemon juice

Kosher salt and ground black pepper, to taste

tip: To save time, you can use premarinated ciliegini mozzarella balls instead of making your own marinade.

1 In a medium-sized bowl, combine the mozzarella balls with the marinade ingredients. Stir well and cover; place in the refrigerator to marinate for 1 hour.

2 To assemble, place a mozzarella ball, a basil leaf (folded in half lengthwise if needed), and a grape tomato half on a toothpick. (*Tip:* If you want the skewers to stand up on a plate, place the tomatoes cut side down.)

3 Serve right away or store in the refrigerator until ready to serve.

per serving:

CALORIES: 174 | FAT: 15.5 g | PROTEIN: 8 g | TOTAL CARBS: 2.2 g | NET CARBS: 2.2 g

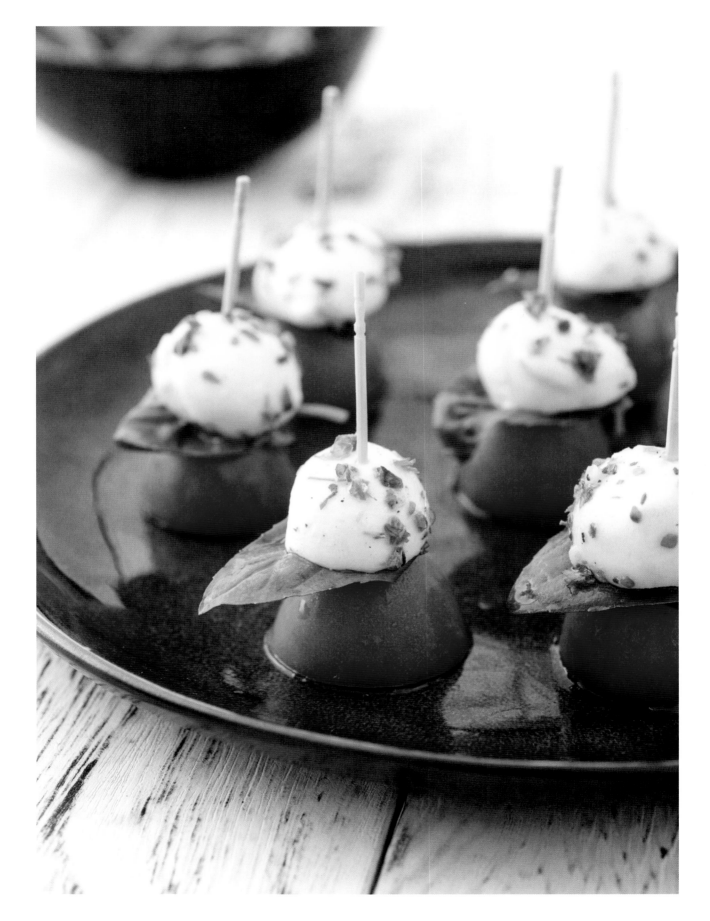

CHEESE AND CHARCUTERIE BOARD

🕧 ⊘ PREP TIME: 15 MINUTES • YIELD: 6 TO 8 SERVINGS

You can't go wrong with a meat and cheese board. This recipe will help you prepare the perfect platter for your next gathering!

4 ounces prosciutto, sliced

4 ounces Calabrese salami, sliced

4 ounces capicola, sliced

7 ounces Parrano Gouda cheese

7 ounces aged Manchego cheese

7 ounces Brie cheese

½ cup roasted almonds

½ cup mixed olives

12 cornichons (small, tart pickles)

1 sprig fresh rosemary or other herbs of choice, for garnish

note: Pairs perfectly with Keto Crackers (page 136).

Arrange the meats, cheeses, and almonds on a large wooden cutting board. Place the olives and pickles in separate bowls and set them on or alongside the cutting board. Garnish with a spring of rosemary or other fresh herbs of your choice.

per serving, based on 8 servings:

CALORIES: 445 | FAT: 35 g | PROTEIN: 31 g | TOTAL CARBS: 2.8 g | NET CARBS: 1.5 g

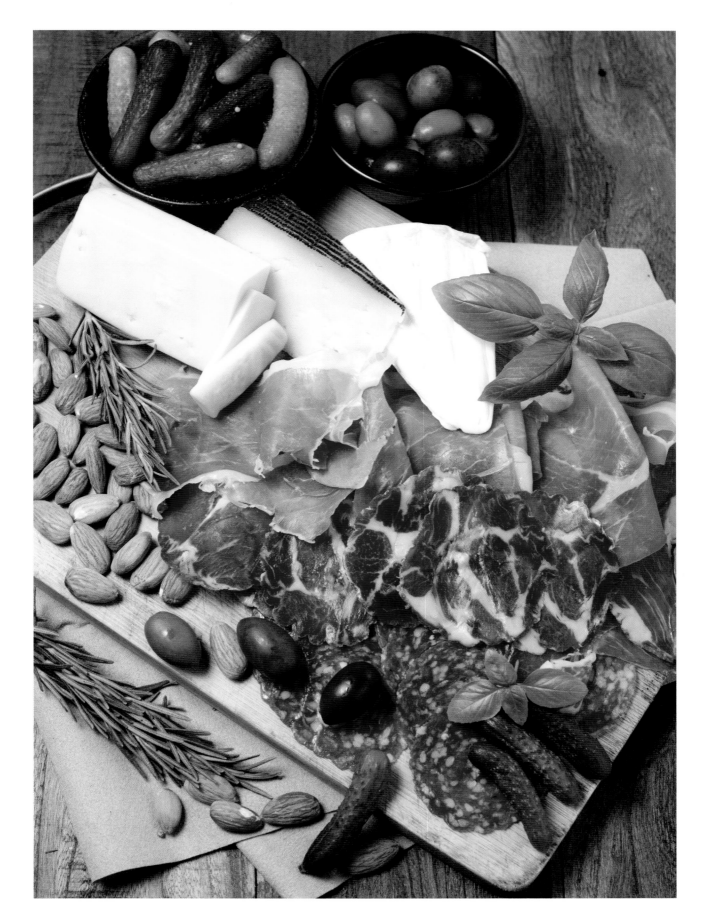

CHEESE CRISPS

⏱️(30) ⃠ ⃠   PREP TIME: 5 MINUTES • COOK TIME: 8 MINUTES • YIELD: 8 CRISPS (4 PER SERVING)

Who knew that crispy cheese could taste so good? Feel free to play around with the seasonings to create your own flavor combinations! Simply make your cheese piles and then add your flavoring ingredients. Try a variety of different spices, or even slices of pickled jalapeño!

½ cup shredded cheddar cheese

½ cup shredded Parmesan cheese

½ teaspoon dried basil

¼ teaspoon garlic powder

1   Preheat the oven to 400°F. Line a baking sheet with parchment paper.

2   In a medium-sized bowl, mix together all the ingredients.

3   Scoop up a heaping tablespoon of the mixture and place it on the parchment paper. Repeat, making a total of 8 small piles, spacing them 2 inches apart to prevent the cheese from running together.

4   Bake for 8 minutes, until golden brown. Let cool for 5 minutes before removing from the parchment paper.

per serving:

CALORIES: 195 | FAT: 13.4 g | PROTEIN: 14.5 g | TOTAL CARBS: 3 g | NET CARBS: 3 g

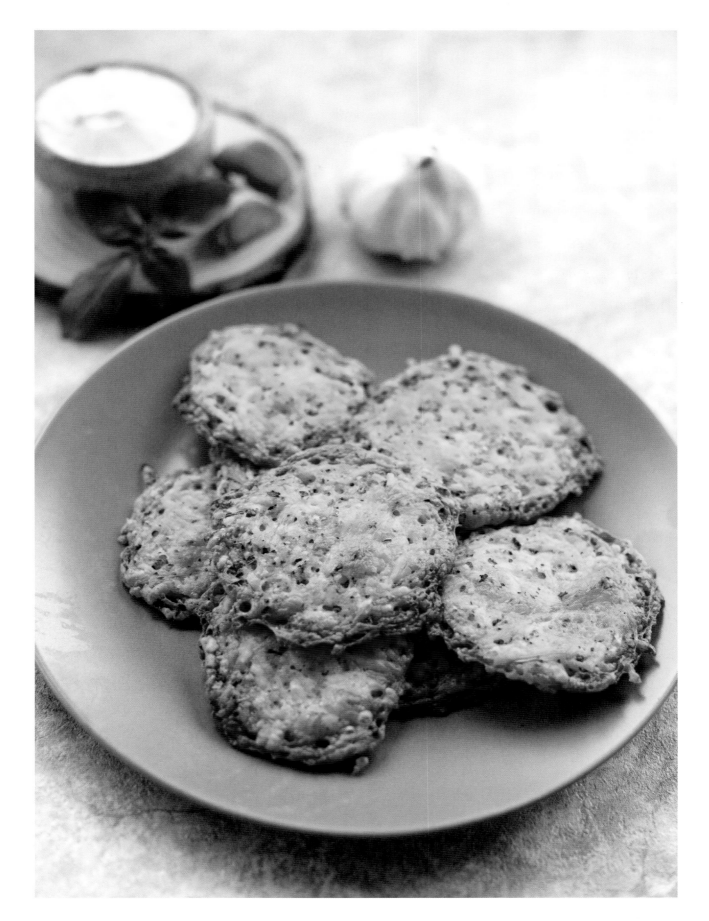

CALLIE'S CREAMY HERB DIP

 PREP TIME: 15 MINUTES, PLUS 30 MINUTES TO CHILL • COOK TIME: 5 MINUTES OR LESS
YIELD: 7 SERVINGS

This delicious dip pairs well with a variety of foods, such as sliced cucumbers, bell pepper strips (red, yellow, and green), celery sticks, cherry or grape tomatoes, sliced mushrooms, and broccoli or cauliflower florets. It's also great with chicken or even Keto Crackers (page 136). I created this recipe with one of my best friends, Callie.

1 (8-ounce) package cream cheese

½ cup half-and-half

¼ cup sour cream

3 tablespoons finely chopped fresh chives

2 tablespoons finely chopped onions

2 tablespoons finely chopped fresh parsley

½ teaspoon garlic powder

1 Place the cream cheese and half-and-half in a microwave-safe bowl and microwave on high for 1 minute; stir and repeat until the texture is smooth.

2 Add the remaining ingredients and stir to combine.

3 Place in the refrigerator to chill for at least 30 minutes before serving.

per serving:

CALORIES: 156 | FAT: 14 g | PROTEIN: 3.1 g | TOTAL CARBS: 2.4 g | NET CARBS: 2.4 g

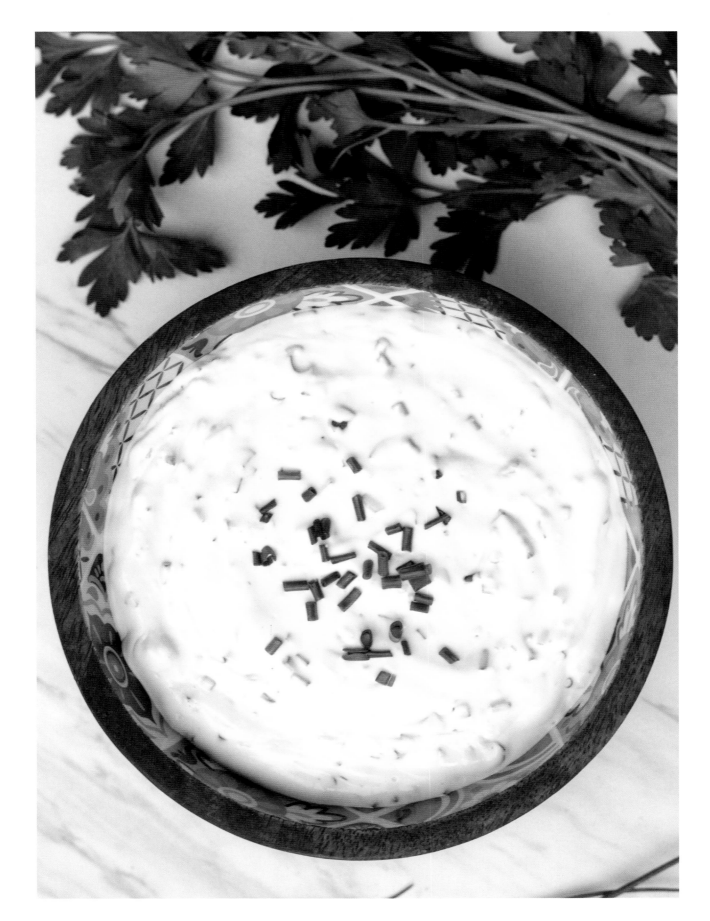

CRISPY FRIED PICKLES

PREP TIME: 5 MINUTES • COOK TIME: 5 MINUTES • YIELD: 2 SERVINGS

There's something about fried pickles that I absolutely love, but I find that people generally either love them or hate them. Which side are you on?

Avocado oil or coconut oil, for frying

3 tablespoons mayonnaise

¼ cup finely grated Parmesan cheese

3 tablespoons golden flaxseed meal

⅛ teaspoon garlic powder

12 dill pickle rounds

note: Pairs well with ranch dressing or Mick's Spicy Aioli (page 78).

1. Heat ¼ inch of oil in a small skillet over medium-high heat.

2. Place the mayonnaise in a bowl. In another bowl, mix together the Parmesan cheese, flaxseed meal, and garlic powder.

3. Place the pickle slices on a paper towel and cover with another paper towel to dry the tops.

4. Dip each pickle slice into the mayonnaise and then into the Parmesan and flaxseed "breading," making sure to coat the slices evenly.

5. When the temperature of the oil reaches 400°F, gently place the breaded pickles in the hot oil and fry until golden and crispy, 1 to 2 minutes per side. Place the fried pickles on a paper towel–lined plate to absorb the excess oil before serving.

per serving:

CALORIES: 376 | FAT: 37.5 g | PROTEIN: 7.5 g | TOTAL CARBS: 4.5 g | NET CARBS: 1 g

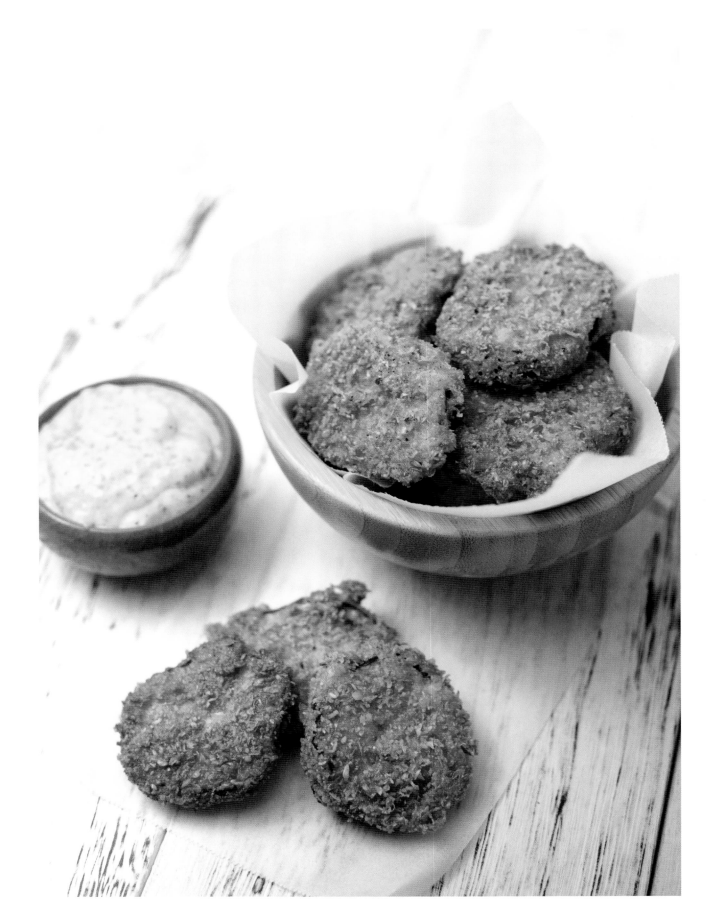

GUACAMOLE

⏱(30) ⊘ 🥑 🥛 OPTION PREP TIME: 15 MINUTES • YIELD: 4 SERVINGS

Fresh and simple guacamole, ready in just 15 minutes! Include the sour cream if you like a creamier guac.

2 ripe avocados

½ tomato, seeded and chopped

¼ cup minced red onions

2 tablespoons finely chopped fresh cilantro

1 tablespoon fresh lime juice

½ teaspoon minced garlic

½ teaspoon salt

1 tablespoon sour cream (optional)

note: Serve with pork rinds, celery, or Keto Crackers (page 136).

1 Slice the avocados in half lengthwise, remove the pits, and scoop the flesh into a medium-sized serving bowl. Mash the avocado flesh.

2 Stir in the tomato, onions, cilantro, lime juice, garlic, and salt. Fold in the sour cream, if using.

3 Serve right away or place in the refrigerator to chill until ready to serve.

per serving, with sour cream:

CALORIES: 133 | FAT: 11.8 g | PROTEIN: 1.5 g | TOTAL CARBS: 8 g | NET CARBS: 2.8 g

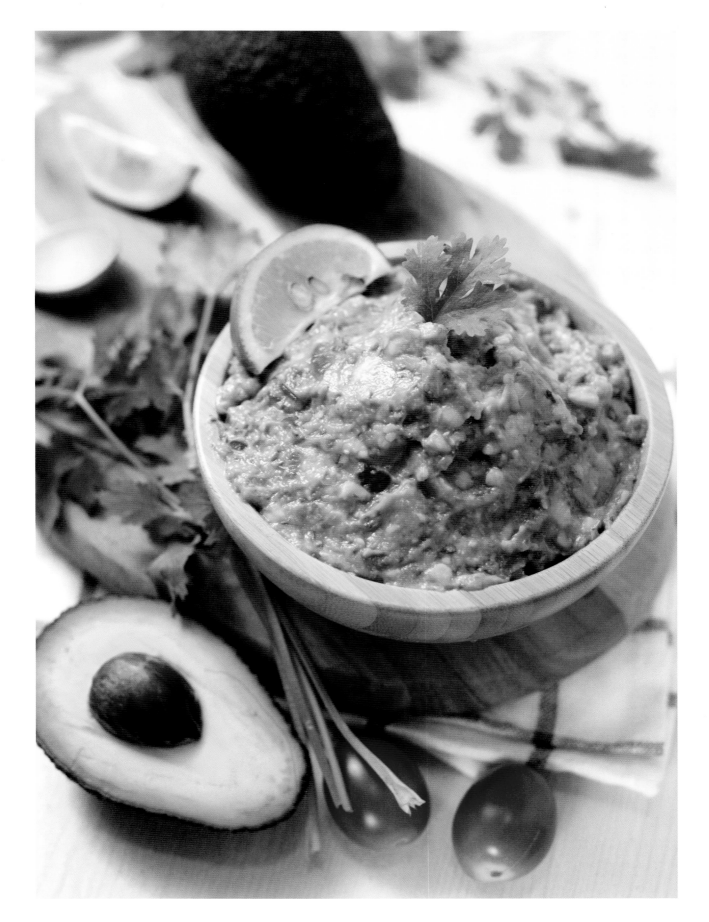

KETO CRACKERS—TWO WAYS

🕙 PREP TIME: 15 MINUTES • COOK TIME: 6 MINUTES • YIELD: 2 SERVINGS (ABOUT 20 PER SERVING)

Some things like cheese and dips just aren't the same without a crunchy scoop, so Mick and I set out to make a quick and easy keto cracker! The first is a more basic version, perfect for dipping, and the second is a cheddar cracker, which tastes similar to standard cheddar-flavored crackers. I often eat the cheese crackers on their own!

Simple Keto Crackers

½ cup shredded mozzarella cheese

⅓ cup blanched almond flour

⅛ teaspoon garlic powder

Dash of salt

1 large egg yolk

Keto Cheddar Cheese Crackers

½ cup shredded cheddar cheese

⅓ cup blanched almond flour

⅛ teaspoon garlic powder

Dash of salt

1 large egg yolk

1 Preheat the oven to 425°F.

2 In a microwave-safe bowl, combine the cheese, almond flour, garlic powder, and salt. Microwave for 30 seconds.

3 Use your hands to knead the dough until fully mixed. Add the egg yolk and knead until it's blended into the dough.

4 Lay a piece of parchment paper on a flat surface, place the dough on top, and place another piece of parchment on top of the dough. Press down and spread the dough (with your hands or a rolling pin) into a very thin, even rectangle.

5 Using a fork, gently poke holes in the dough to prevent it from bubbling while baking. (Don't skip this step!)

6 Use a knife to cut the dough into 1-inch squares.

7 Line a baking sheet with parchment paper and lay the squares on the parchment with a bit of space between them. Bake for 5 to 6 minutes, until golden brown.

8 For extra-crunchy crackers, flip them over and bake for an additional 2 to 4 minutes, watching closely to ensure that they don't burn!

per serving:

CALORIES: 234 | FAT: 20 g | PROTEIN: 12 g | TOTAL CARBS: 5 g | NET CARBS: 3 g

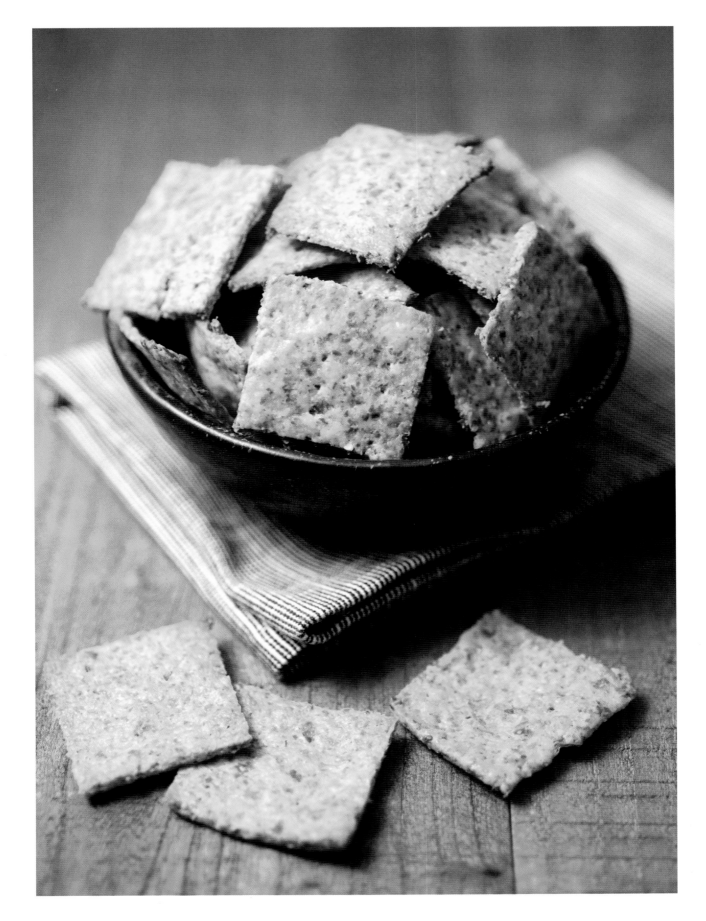

LIME BRUSSELS CHIPS

⏱️ 🚫 🍃 🧂 PREP TIME: 15 MINUTES • COOK TIME: 10 MINUTES • YIELD: 2 SERVINGS

I love Brussels sprouts in all forms, but these light and crispy chips are one of my very favorite preparations!

3 cups Brussels sprouts leaves (from 1½ to 2 pounds fresh Brussels sprouts)

Juice of ½ lime

2½ tablespoons avocado oil or melted coconut oil

Pink Himalayan salt

tip: *Trimming a little higher up than usual on the stem end of the Brussels sprouts helps the leaves come off easier.*

1 Preheat the oven to 400°F. Line a rimmed baking sheet with parchment paper.

2 Trim off the flat stem ends of the Brussels sprouts and separate the leaves. You should end up with 2 to 3 cups of leaves.

3 Place the separated leaves in a large bowl and add the lime juice.

4 Add the oil and season with salt to taste. Toss until the leaves are evenly coated.

5 Spread the leaves evenly on the prepared baking sheet and bake for 7 to 10 minutes, until lightly golden brown.

per serving:

CALORIES: 173 | FAT: 18 g | PROTEIN: 1.5 g | TOTAL CARBS: 4 g | NET CARBS: 2 g

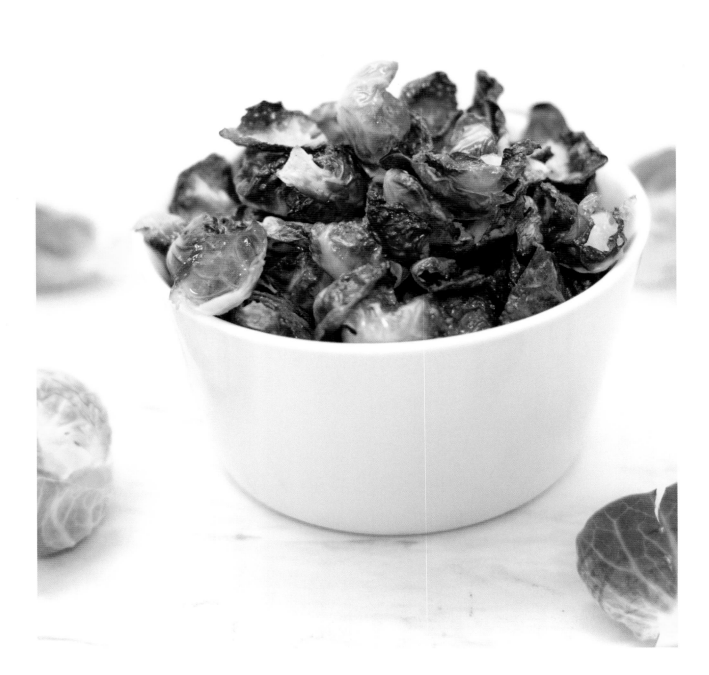

LOADED DEVILED EGGS

PREP TIME: 10 MINUTES • COOK TIME: 14 MINUTES • YIELD: 12 DEVILED EGGS (3 PER SERVING)

The only thing better than deviled eggs is deviled eggs with bacon, am I right? These loaded eggs are absolutely delicious, colorful, and perfect for parties.

6 large eggs

5 slices bacon

¼ cup mayonnaise

½ teaspoon prepared yellow mustard

¼ teaspoon garlic powder

Salt and pepper

⅓ cup shredded cheddar cheese, for topping

2 green onions, chopped, for topping

1 Place the eggs in a medium-sized saucepan and cover with cold water. Bring to a boil, then immediately remove the pan from the heat. Cover with a lid and allow the eggs to sit in the hot water for 12 to 14 minutes for firm yolks.

2 Meanwhile, fry the bacon in a skillet over medium heat. Set aside on a paper towel–lined plate to cool, then finely chop.

3 Carefully remove the eggs from the hot water and place in a bowl filled with ice water to halt the cooking. When the eggs are cool, peel them.

4 Cut the eggs in half lengthwise. Remove the yolks and place them in a medium-sized mixing bowl. Add the mayonnaise, mustard, garlic powder, two-thirds of the bacon, and salt and pepper to taste; mix well.

5 For easy filling, spoon the egg yolk mixture into a small zip-top plastic bag, seal, and cut off one corner of the bag. Gently squeeze the bag to pipe the yolk mixture into the egg white halves.

6 Top the filled egg white halves with the reserved bacon, cheddar cheese, and green onions. Eat right away or store in the refrigerator for up to 3 days.

per serving:

CALORIES: 290 | FAT: 25.8 g | PROTEIN: 14.3 g | TOTAL CARBS: 2 g | NET CARBS: 2 g

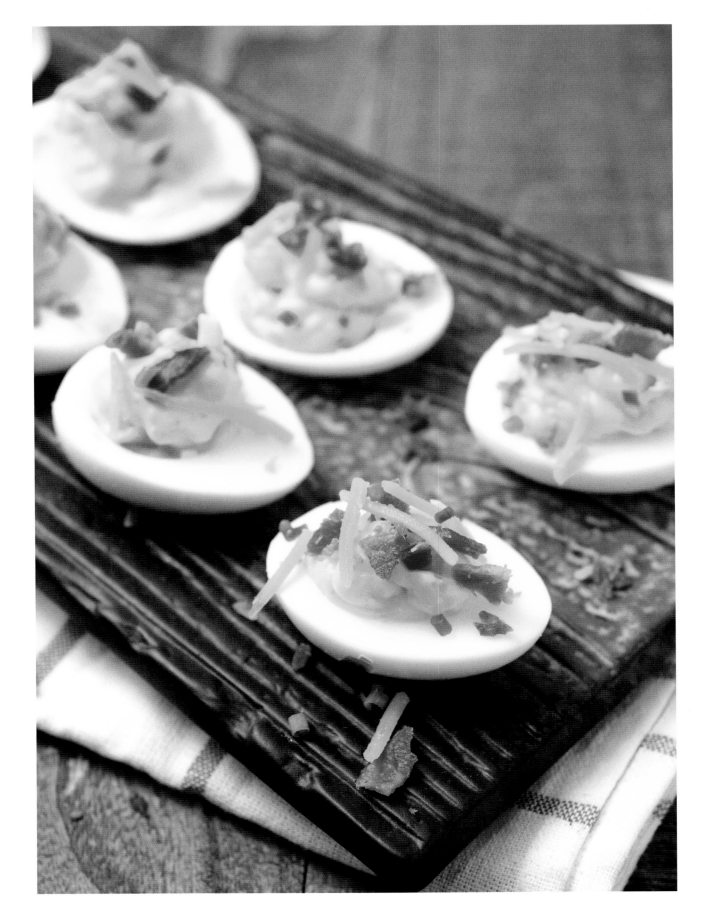

FRIED MOZZARELLA STICKS

PREP TIME: 10 MINUTES, PLUS 30 MINUTES TO FREEZE • COOK TIME: 4 MINUTES
YIELD: 10 STICKS (2 PER SERVING)

Mozzarella cheese sticks fried to golden perfection! Allowing enough time in the freezer is the key to making crispy low-carb fried mozzarella sticks, so be sure not to skip that important step.

1 large egg

¼ cup grated Parmesan cheese

¼ cup golden flaxseed meal

½ teaspoon Italian seasoning

¼ teaspoon garlic powder

Pinch of salt

5 mozzarella cheese sticks, cut in half crosswise to make 10 pieces

Avocado oil or coconut oil, for frying

Ranch dressing and/or no-sugar-added marinara sauce, warm, for serving

1 In a small bowl, beat the egg.

2 In another bowl, combine the Parmesan cheese, flaxseed meal, Italian seasoning, garlic powder, and salt; mix with a fork.

3 Dip each cheese stick into the beaten egg and then into the Parmesan cheese mixture. Press the Parmesan mixture into the cheese sticks to coat them evenly on all sides.

4 Place the breaded cheese sticks on a plate and place in the freezer for 30 to 45 minutes, until the Parmesan crust is firm and fully frozen.

5 In a small skillet, heat ½ inch of oil over medium-high heat. When the temperature of the oil reaches 400°F, add the cheese sticks and fry for 1 to 2 minutes, then flip and fry for 1 to 2 more minutes, until golden brown on both sides.

6 Serve with ranch dressing or marinara for dipping.

per serving:

CALORIES: 185 | FAT: 14.4 g | PROTEIN: 11.4 g | TOTAL CARBS: 3.4 g | NET CARBS: 2.2 g

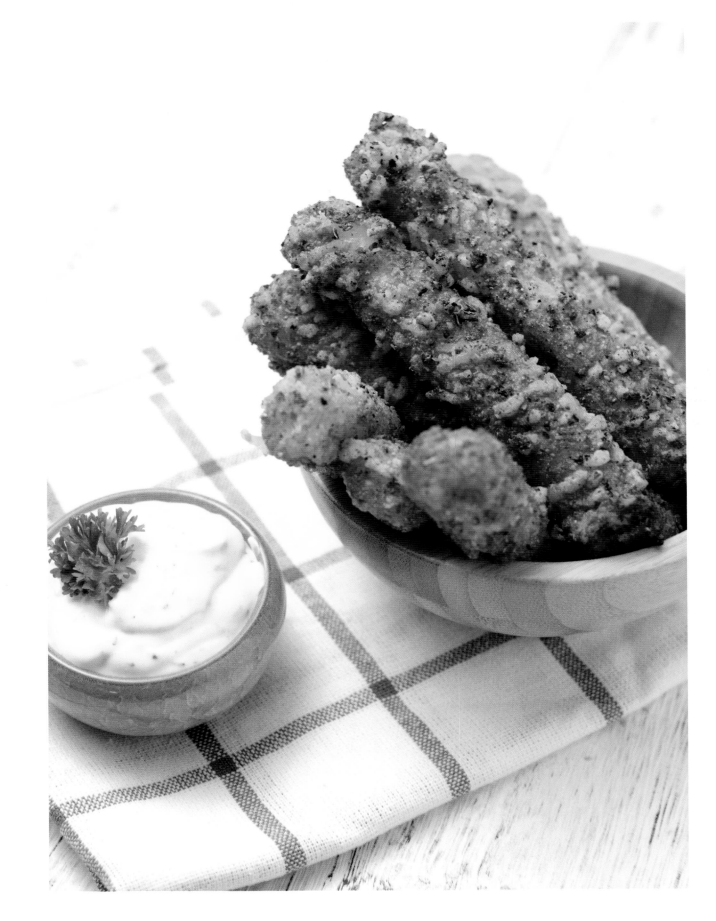

PROSCIUTTO–WRAPPED ASPARAGUS

PREP TIME: 5 MINUTES • COOK TIME: 12 MINUTES • YIELD: 6 SERVINGS

Prosciutto and asparagus are a perfect pairing. This delicious recipe works as an appetizer or a side dish.

18 asparagus spears, ends trimmed

2 tablespoons coconut oil, melted

6 slices prosciutto

1 teaspoon garlic powder

1 Preheat the oven to 400°F. Line a rimmed baking sheet with parchment paper.

2 Place the asparagus and coconut oil in a large zip-top plastic bag. Seal and toss until the asparagus is evenly coated.

3 Wrap a slice of prosciutto around 3 grouped asparagus spears. Repeat with the remaining prosciutto and asparagus, making a total of 6 bundles. Arrange the bundles in a single layer on the lined baking sheet. Sprinkle the garlic powder over the bundles.

4 Bake for 8 to 12 minutes, until the asparagus is tender.

per serving:

CALORIES: 122 | FAT: 10 g | PROTEIN: 7.5 g | TOTAL CARBS: 2.75 g | NET CARBS: 2 g

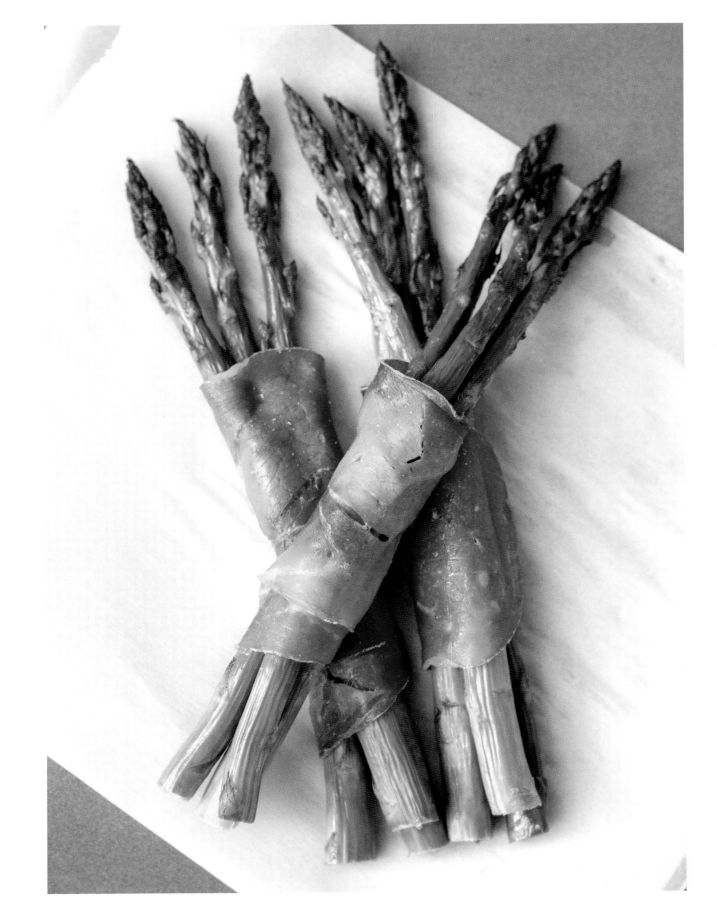

SPINACH AND ARTICHOKE–STUFFED MUSHROOMS

 PREP TIME: 15 MINUTES • COOK TIME: 20 MINUTES
YIELD: 15 STUFFED MUSHROOMS (5 PER SERVING)

Stuffed mushrooms baked until golden brown with a flavor-packed filling—yum!

15 cremini mushrooms or small white mushrooms

1 teaspoon unsalted butter

2 cloves garlic

3 cups fresh spinach, chopped

½ cup marinated artichoke hearts, drained and chopped

2 ounces cream cheese, softened

½ cup shredded Parmesan cheese, divided

Salt

tip: *You can use shredded mozzarella cheese in place of the fresh mozzarella if you prefer.*

1   Preheat the oven to 375°F. Line a 13 by 9-inch baking dish with aluminum foil or parchment paper.

2   Wash and destem the mushrooms. Set the caps aside and chop the stems.

3   Melt the butter in a medium-sized skillet over medium-high heat. Add the mushroom stems and garlic and sauté until soft, 3 to 5 minutes.

4   Add the spinach, artichoke hearts, cream cheese, ¼ cup of the Parmesan cheese, and salt to taste; stir until the spinach is soft and the filling is well blended.

5   Place the mushroom caps on the lined baking sheet and spoon the filling into the caps. Sprinkle the remaining ¼ cup of Parmesan cheese over the stuffed mushrooms.

6   Bake for 18 to 20 minutes, until the mushrooms are tender.

per serving:

CALORIES: 170 | FAT: 11.7 g | PROTEIN: 10 g | TOTAL CARBS: 6 g | NET CARBS: 4 g

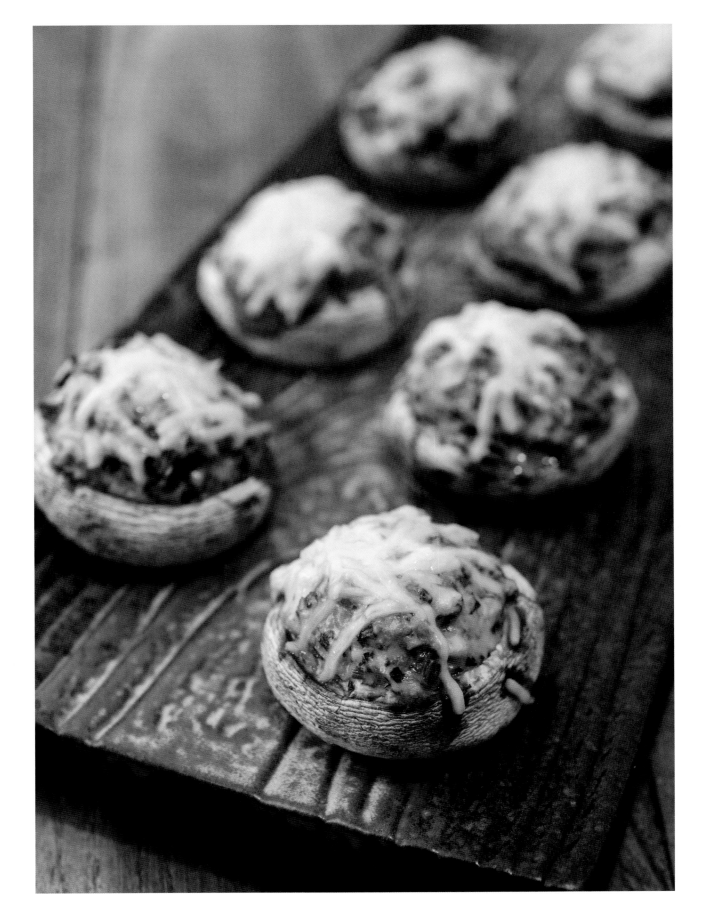

SALSA SHRIMP–STUFFED AVOCADOS

🕧 ⊘ ◍ PREP TIME: 10 MINUTES • COOK TIME: 15 MINUTES • YIELD: 4 SERVINGS

Down the street from my house there is a small Mexican restaurant that serves stuffed avocados. As soon as I tasted them, I knew I needed to re-create the recipe at home! These delicious stuffed avocados are perfect as an appetizer or a small meal.

2 avocados, halved and pitted

12 large precooked shrimp, peeled and deveined

3 tablespoons salsa

¼ cup shredded Mexican cheese blend

Finely chopped fresh cilantro, for garnish (optional)

Sour cream, for garnish (optional)

1 Preheat the oven to 350°F. Line a rimmed baking sheet with parchment paper.

2 Rinse the shrimp and halve lengthwise. Place in a bowl and top with the salsa. Stir to coat the shrimp evenly with the salsa.

3 Place the avocado halves cut side up on the lined baking sheet. Fill each half with salsa-coated shrimp and top with the cheese.

4 Bake for 15 minutes, until the cheese is melted.

5 Serve garnished with cilantro and/or topped with sour cream, if desired.

per serving:

CALORIES: 185 | FAT: 13.3 g | PROTEIN: 11.3 g | TOTAL CARBS: 7.3 g | NET CARBS: 6 g

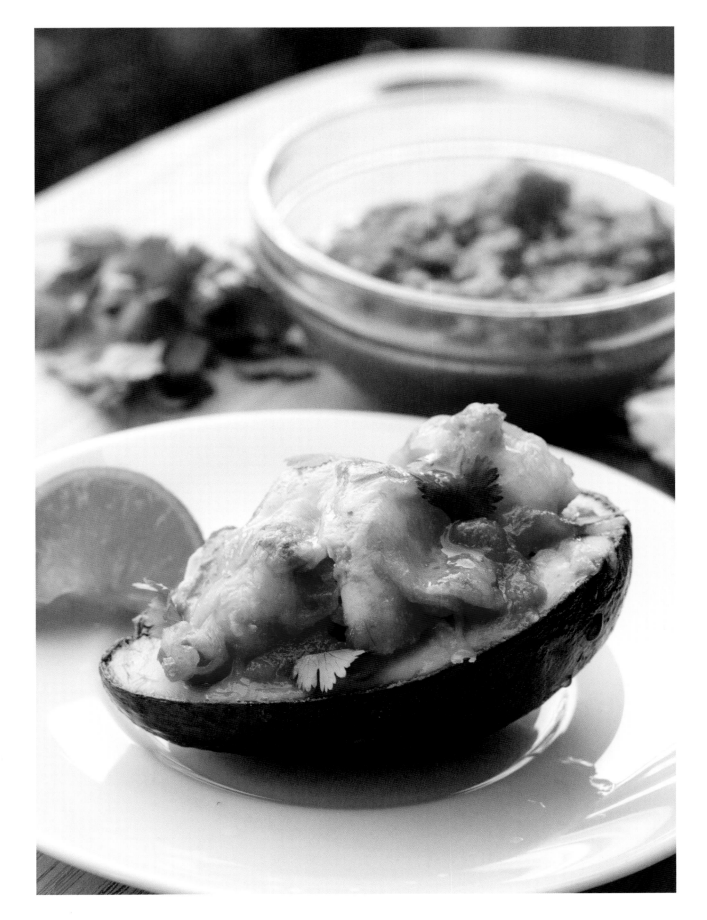

PORTOBELLO MARGHERITA PIZZAS

PREP TIME: 5 MINUTES • COOK TIME: 18 MINUTES • YIELD: 4 SERVINGS

The great taste of pizza without the carb-heavy crust! These mini portobello pizzas are fresh, delicious, and ready in under 30 minutes.

4 medium portobello mushroom caps, destemmed

Dash of salt

¼ cup no-sugar-added marinara sauce

4 tomato slices

4 ounces fresh mozzarella, cut into 4 slices

4 teaspoons extra-virgin olive oil or avocado oil

2 small cloves or 1 large clove garlic, minced

1 tablespoon chopped fresh basil and/or whole leaves, for garnish

1 Preheat the oven to 375°F. Place a wire rack in a rimmed baking sheet (this will keep the mushrooms from sitting in the liquid they release while cooking and getting soggy bottoms as a result).

2 Set the mushroom caps on top of the wire rack. Place 1 tablespoon of marinara and a slice of tomato in each cap, then a mozzarella slice. Drizzle with olive oil, then top with the minced garlic.

3 Bake for 15 to 18 minutes, until the cheese is melted and the mushrooms are tender.

4 Remove from the oven and top with the basil before serving.

per serving:

CALORIES: 141 | FAT: 10 g | PROTEIN: 8.3 g | TOTAL CARBS: 5.8 g | NET CARBS: 4.5 g

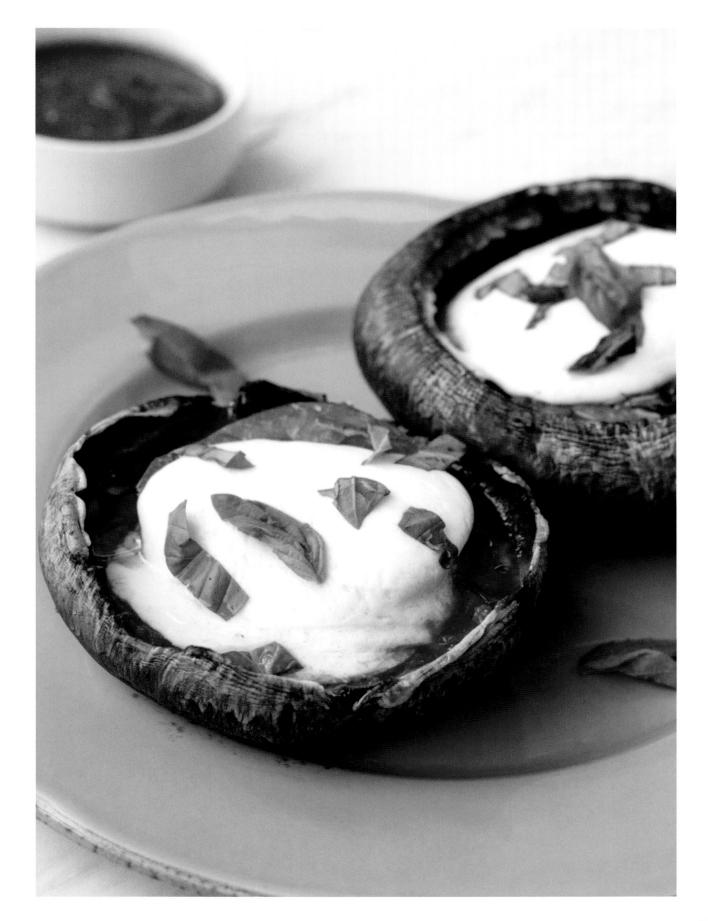

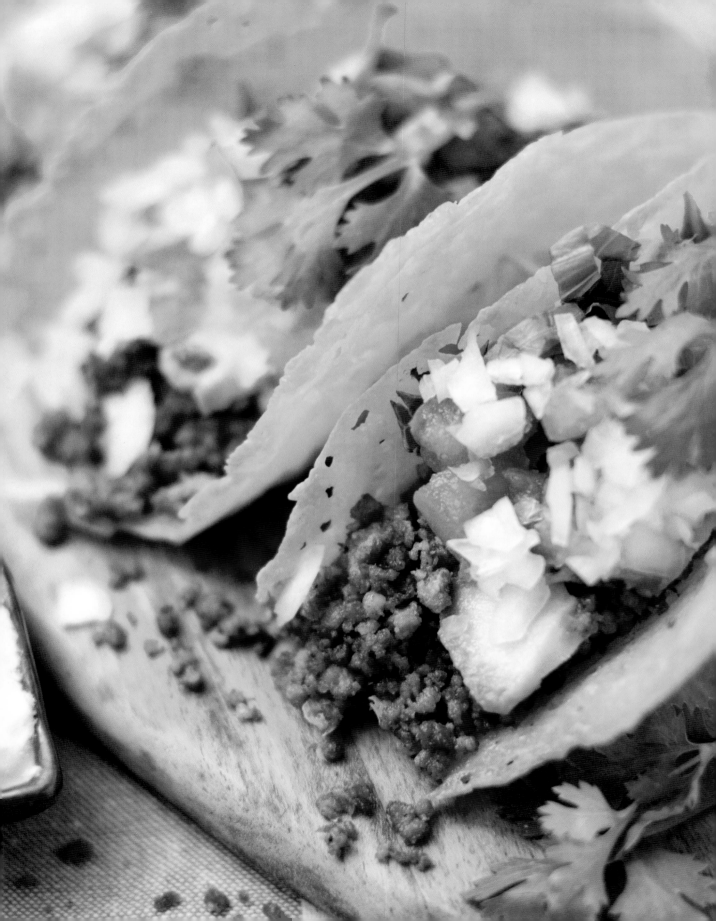

BEEF AND PORK

BLTA LETTUCE WRAPS

PREP TIME: 15 MINUTES • COOK TIME: 5 MINUTES • YIELD: 4 WRAPS (2 PER SERVING)

Vine-ripened tomato, crispy bacon, creamy avocado, and tangy mayo come together to create the perfect spin on a classic sandwich! Sorry, bread, you aren't invited to the party.

6 slices bacon

3 tablespoons mayonnaise

4 butter lettuce leaves

½ avocado

2 slices tomato, halved

Salt and pepper

1   In a large skillet over medium heat, fry the bacon until crispy, about 5 minutes. Set aside on a paper towel–lined plate to cool. When cool enough to handle, cut each strip in half crosswise.

2   Squeeze a line of mayonnaise onto each of the lettuce leaves. Top each leaf with a half-slice of tomato, 3 half-slices of bacon, and a slice of avocado. Season to taste with salt and pepper and enjoy!

per serving:

CALORIES: 387 | FAT: 34 g | PROTEIN: 14.5 g | TOTAL CARBS: 4.5 g | NET CARBS: 2 g

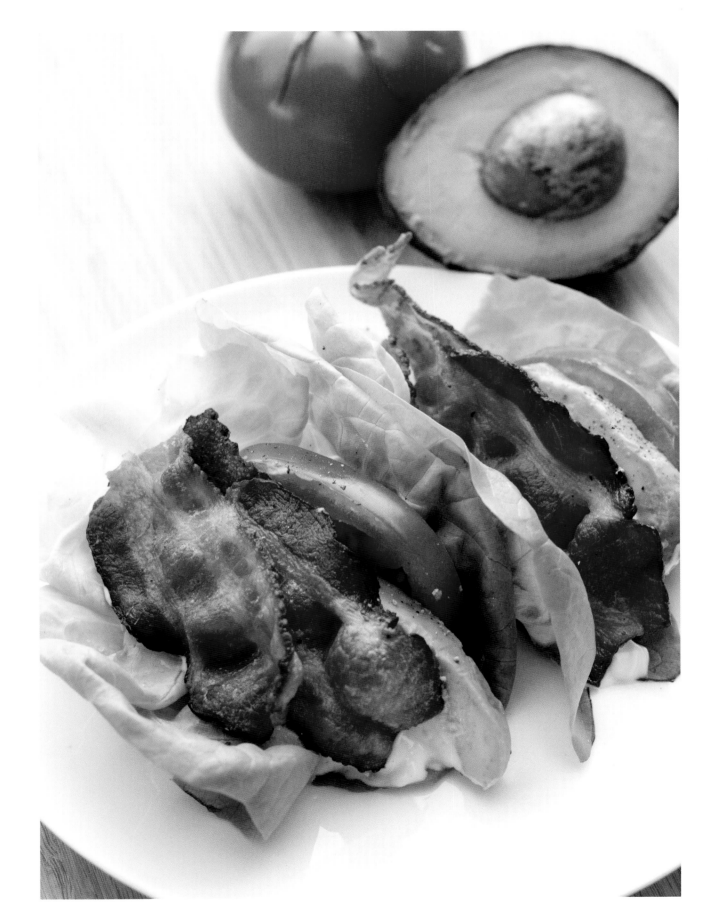

KETO CHILI

⊘ ⊘ 🥛 PREP TIME: 20 MINUTES • COOK TIME: 5 TO 8 HOURS • YIELD: 6 SERVINGS
   OPTION

One day I had a craving for chili, but I couldn't find any simple low-carb chili recipes, so I decided to create my own. This keto chili is absolutely delicious, and I promise you won't miss the beans! Leftovers can be used for Chili Cheese Dogs (page 160) or Chili Egg Scramble (page 94).

1 pound ground beef

1 pound bulk sausage, mild or hot

1 green bell pepper, diced

½ medium yellow onion, chopped

3 to 4 cloves garlic, minced, or 1 tablespoon garlic powder

1 (14½-ounce) can diced tomatoes (with juices)

1 (6-ounce) can tomato paste (see note)

1 tablespoon chili powder

1½ teaspoons ground cumin

⅓ cup water

Topping Suggestions

Shredded cheddar cheese

Sliced green onions

Sour cream

Sliced jalapeños

note: When buying tomato paste, check the labels and find the lowest-carb option available. The macros for this recipe may vary slightly depending on the brand of tomato paste you use.

1. In a large pot, brown the ground beef and sausage, using a wooden spoon to break up the clumps. Drain the meat, reserving half of the drippings.

2. Transfer the drained meat to a slow cooker. Add the reserved drippings, bell pepper, onion, garlic, tomatoes with juices, tomato paste, chili powder, cumin, and water and mix well.

3. Place the lid on the slow cooker and cook on low for 6 to 8 hours or on high for 5 hours, until the veggies are soft.

4. Serve topped with shredded cheese, green onions, sour cream, and/or sliced jalapeños, if desired.

per serving:

CALORIES: 387 | FAT: 24.6 g | PROTEIN: 33.5 g | TOTAL CARBS: 11.4 g | NET CARBS: 7.9 g

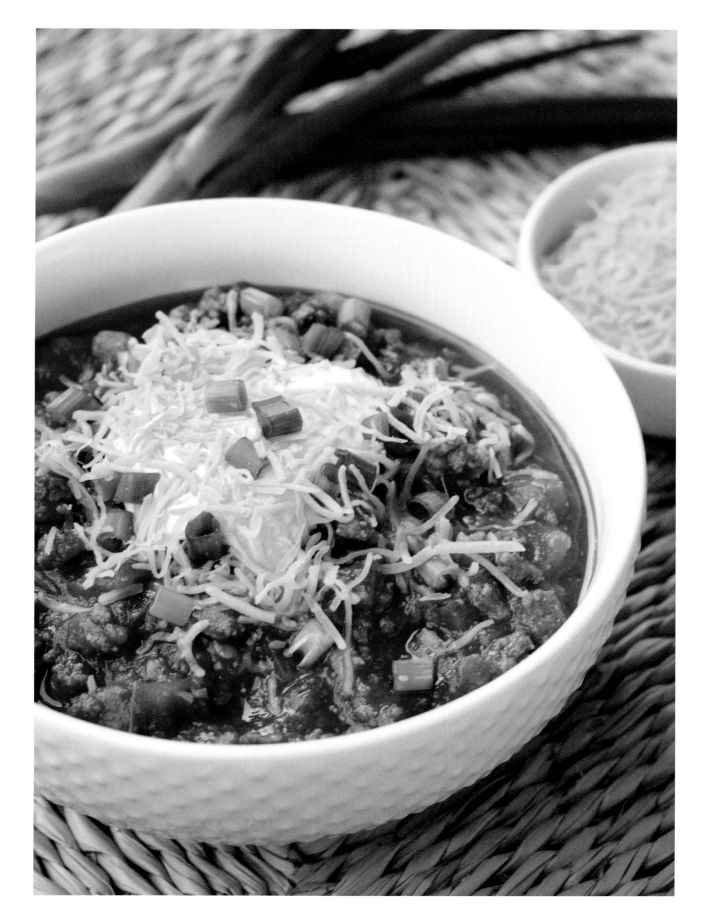

CHEESE SHELL TACOS

⏱ ⊘ ⊘ PREP TIME: 5 MINUTES • COOK TIME: 20 MINUTES • YIELD: 6 TACOS (2 PER SERVING)

Although I love a good taco salad, sometimes you just want the crunch of a taco shell. This easy recipe provides every bit of that crunch you crave, without all the carbs! These shells are fun to make and can even be prepared in the microwave if you don't feel like heating up the oven; see tips below.

Cheese Shells
(makes 6 large shells)

2 cups shredded cheddar cheese

Taco Filling

½ pound ground beef

1 tablespoon sugar-free taco seasoning, homemade (page 82) or store-bought

¼ cup water

Topping Suggestions

2 cups shredded lettuce

1 medium tomato, diced

1 avocado, sliced

¾ cup sour cream

⅓ cup chopped yellow onions

Fresh cilantro, for garnish (optional)

1 Preheat the oven to 375°F. Line 2 baking sheets with parchment paper.

2 Arrange the shredded cheese into 6 piles on the parchment-lined baking sheet, leaving several inches between piles so the shells don't run together. Bake for 7 to 10 minutes, until the edges start to brown and the cheese is no longer runny.

3 Meanwhile, prop up a wooden spoon or two kabob skewers, spaced 1 inch apart, with two cups or cans.

4 Remove the melted cheese rounds from the oven and, while the cheese is still flexible, use a spatula to transfer the cheese and drape over a wooden spoon handle or skewers. Prop up the wooden spoon or skewers with 2 cups or cans. The shell will harden as it cools. Repeat this process with the remaining shells.

5 In a medium-sized skillet, brown the ground beef, then drain the fat. Add the taco seasoning and water. Stir well, bring to a simmer, and allow to reduce for 3 to 5 minutes. Remove from the heat.

6 Fill each cheese shell with meat and the toppings of your choice. Garnish with cilantro, if desired.

tips: These cheese shells are also great filled with eggs, bacon or sausage, and avocado for breakfast tacos!

The shells can be prepared individually in the microwave. Place ⅓ cup of shredded cheese on a piece of parchment paper and microwave on high for 1 minute, then follow Step 3. Repeat with the remaining cheese.

per serving, without toppings:

CALORIES: 389 | FAT: 29.7 g | PROTEIN: 28 g | TOTAL CARBS: 3.2 g | NET CARBS: 2.6 g

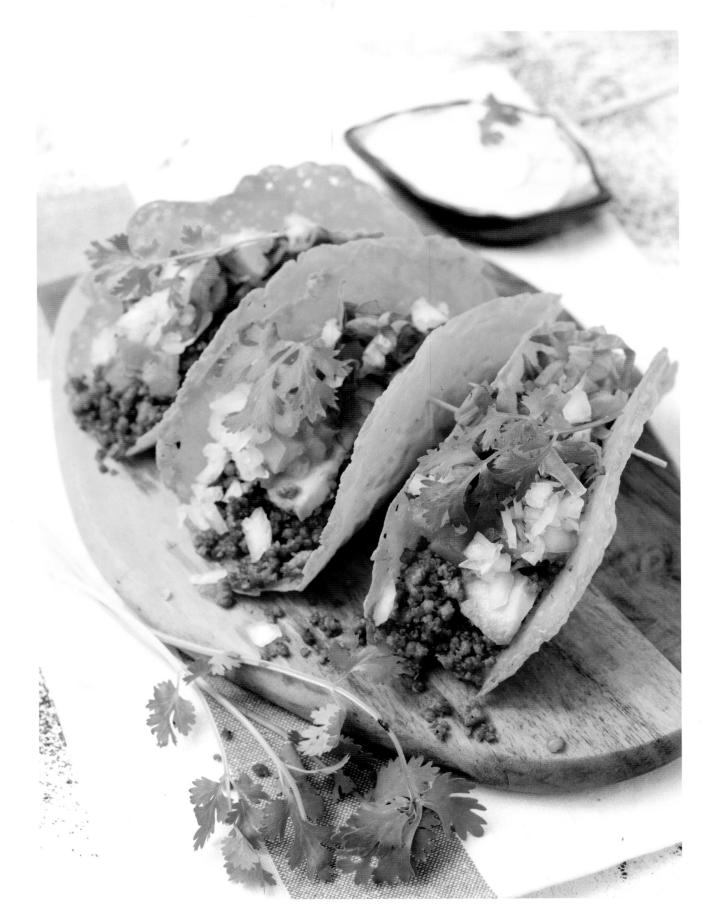

CHILI CHEESE DOGS

PREP TIME: 10 MINUTES (IF USING LEFTOVER CHILI) • COOK TIME: 10 MINUTES
YIELD: 2 SERVINGS

Chili cheese dogs are a classic, and a quick and easy meal to make with leftover Keto Chili!

4 nitrate-free hot dogs

1 cup Keto Chili (page 156), warm

½ cup shredded cheddar cheese

¼ cup diced yellow onions

¼ cup pickled jalapeño slices (optional)

Low-carb hot sauce, to taste (optional)

1   Grill or boil the hot dogs until warmed through.

2   Cut the hot dogs into segments and divide among 2 serving plates. Top each hot dog with half of the warm chili, half of the shredded cheese, and half of the diced onions. If you like extra heat, top the chili cheese dogs with jalapeño slices or your favorite low-carb hot sauce.

per serving:

CALORIES: 610 | FAT: 47 g | PROTEIN: 34.5 g | TOTAL CARBS: 11.2 g | NET CARBS: 6.4 g

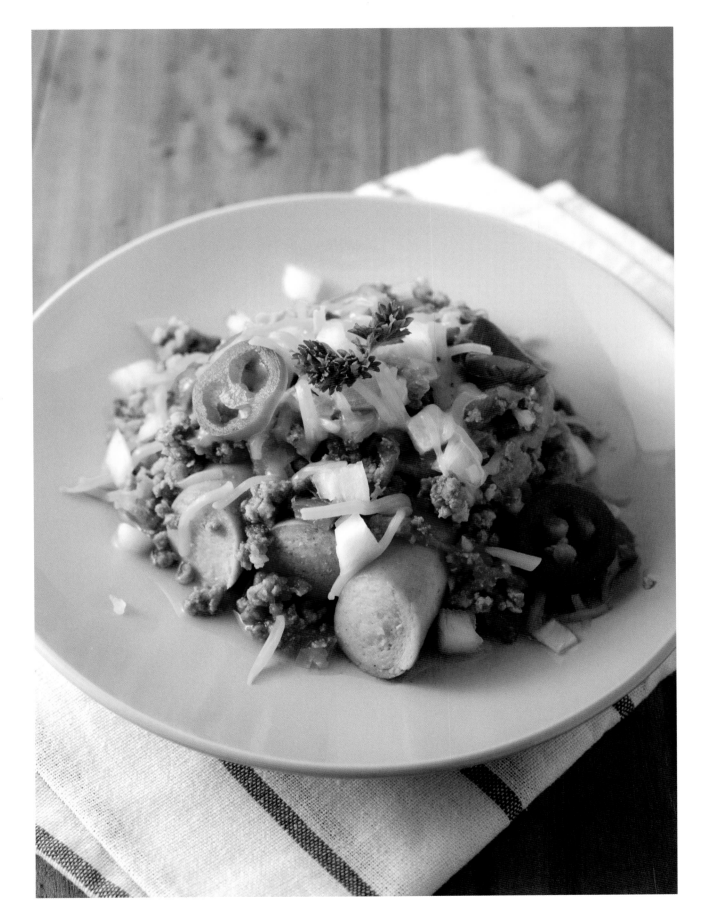

FAJITA KABOBS

PREP TIME: 15 MINUTES, PLUS 30 MINUTES TO MARINATE • COOK TIME: 10 MINUTES
YIELD: 6 KABOBS (2 PER SERVING)

These fajita kabobs are easy to prepare and are great for a quick and flavorful dinner!

Kabobs

1 pound boneless sirloin steak, cut into 1-inch cubes

1 green bell pepper

1 red bell pepper

½ red onion

Marinade

1 tablespoon chili powder

1½ teaspoons paprika

1 teaspoon ground cumin

½ teaspoon garlic powder

½ teaspoon salt

2 tablespoons avocado oil

Juice of 1 lime

Sliced jalapeños, for garnish (optional)

Special Equipment

- 6 wood or metal skewers (soak wood skewers in water for 30 minutes before grilling to prevent them from catching fire on the grill)

1 Place the cubed steak in a large zip-top plastic bag and set aside.

2 In a small bowl, combine the spices and salt for the marinade and mix with a fork. Add the avocado oil and lime juice, mix well, and pour over the steak in the bag. Remove the air from the bag and seal. From the outside of the bag, shift the steak around to evenly coat all the pieces in the marinade, then place in the refrigerator for 30 to 45 minutes.

3 Preheat a grill to medium-high heat.

4 Remove the seeds and membranes from the bell peppers, then cut the peppers into 1- to 2-inch chunks.

5 Peel and slice the onion into 1- to 2-inch pieces (no more than 2 or 3 onion layers per piece).

6 Place the marinated steak, peppers, and onions on the skewers, alternating between the three ingredients.

7 Grill the kabobs for 7 to 10 minutes, turning as needed, until browned. Serve garnished with sliced jalapeños, if desired.

tips: If you prefer medium-rare beef, the cook times for the meat and vegetables will differ. In this case, make all-meat and all-veggie kabobs. Put all the kabobs on the grill at the same time, but pull the meat off the grill after about 4 minutes; continue to cook the vegetables until done, 7 to 10 minutes total.

These kabobs pair well with Guacamole (page 134), Cilantro Lime Cauliflower Rice (page 243), sour cream, salsa, and shredded cheese.

per serving:

CALORIES: 429 | FAT: 29 g | PROTEIN: 32 g | TOTAL CARBS: 8.5 g | NET CARBS: 5.5 g

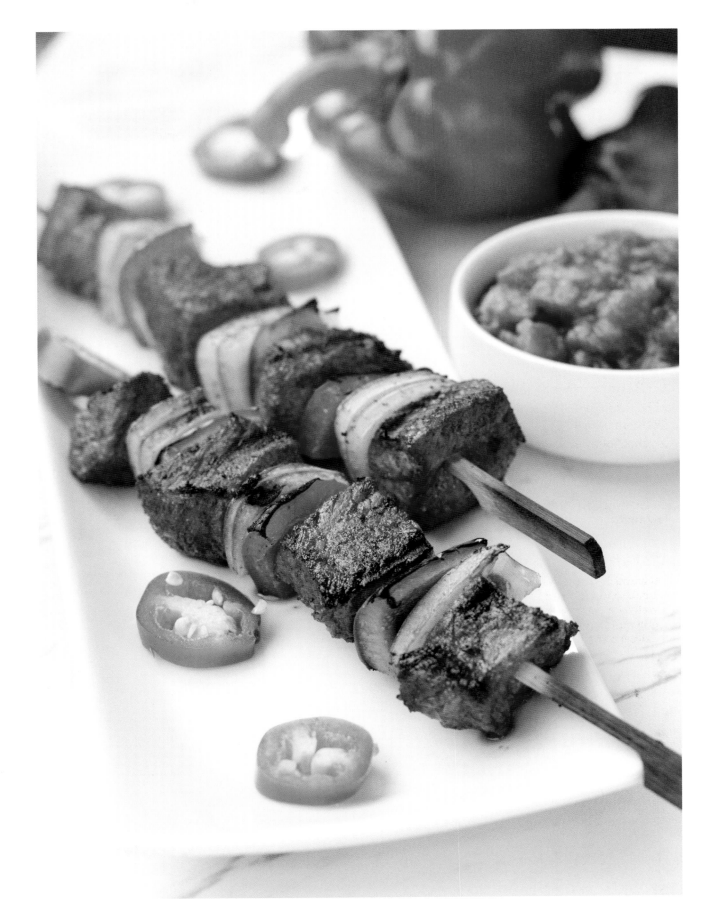

FILET MIGNONS WITH GORGONZOLA SAUCE

 PREP TIME: 15 MINUTES, PLUS 30 MINUTES TO MARINATE • COOK TIME: 20 MINUTES
YIELD: 4 SERVINGS

There's nothing like a perfectly cooked filet mignon. Even if you aren't generally a big fan of blue cheese (like me), you will love this sauce. If you are looking for an alternative, you can simply top this steak with butter to add more fat and delicious flavor.

4 (5-ounce) filet mignons

Kosher salt and pepper

2 teaspoons avocado oil

Gorgonzola Sauce

2 tablespoons unsalted butter

1 clove garlic, minced

⅓ cup crumbled Gorgonzola cheese

¼ cup finely grated Parmesan cheese

¼ cup heavy whipping cream

1 teaspoon onion powder

Salt and pepper, to taste

note: Pairs well with asparagus.

1 Remove the steaks from the refrigerator and season them generously with kosher salt and pepper. Allow to sit at room temperature for 30 minutes.

2 Preheat the oven to 450°F.

3 Pour the avocado oil into a large oven-safe skillet over high heat. When hot, add the steaks and sear for 3 to 4 minutes on each side.

4 Transfer the skillet to the oven and cook for 4 to 6 minutes for medium-rare steaks, or cook longer if you like your steaks more well-done.

5 Place the steaks on a plate and allow to rest for 5 minutes before slicing.

6 While the steaks are resting, make the sauce: In a small saucepan over low heat, combine the butter and garlic. When the butter is melted, add the remaining sauce ingredients. Stir to combine, then raise the heat to medium-high. Allow the sauce to simmer and reduce for 3 to 5 minutes, stirring often, until the desired consistency is achieved. Pour the sauce over the filets and serve.

per serving:

CALORIES: 446 | FAT: 31 g | PROTEIN: 36.5 g | TOTAL CARBS: 1 g | NET CARBS: 1 g

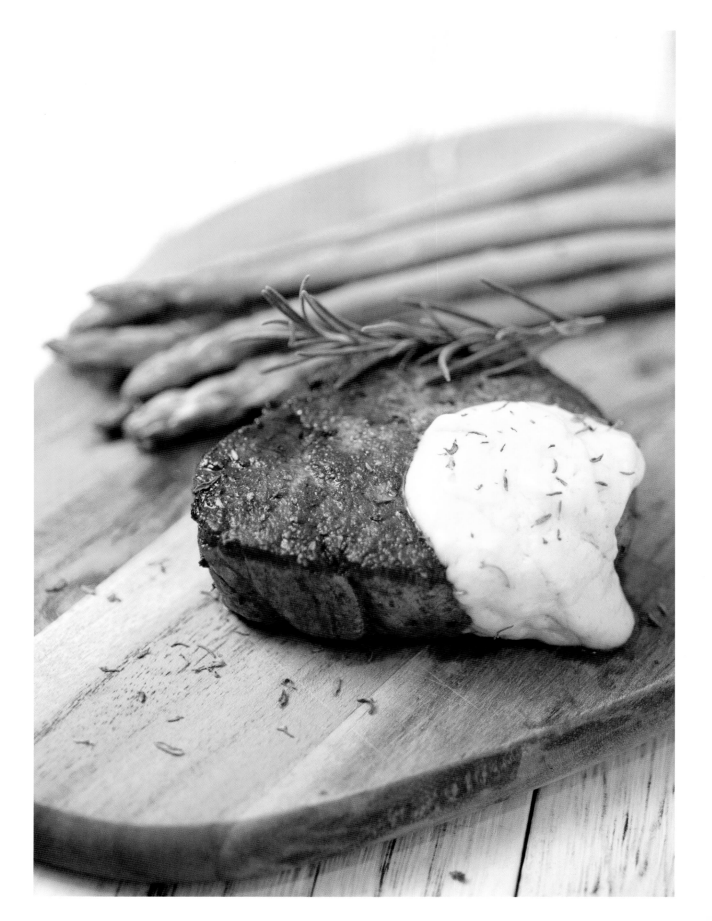

GARLIC BUTTER–BASTED RIB-EYE

PREP TIME: 10 MINUTES • COOK TIME: 10 MINUTES • YIELD: 2 SERVINGS

Rosemary and butter unite for the most epic and flavorful steak!

2 (6-ounce) or 1 (12-ounce) boneless rib-eye steak (about 1 inch thick)

2 teaspoons kosher salt

Pepper

2 tablespoons unsalted butter

2 teaspoons avocado oil

2 cloves garlic, smashed with the side of a knife

2 sprigs fresh rosemary

1 Remove the steaks from the refrigerator and season on both sides with the kosher salt and a generous amount of pepper. Allow to sit at room temperature for 30 minutes.

2 Heat the oil in a large cast-iron skillet or grill pan over medium-high heat. Place the steaks in the skillet and sear for 5 to 7 minutes, until a nice crust forms on one side. Turn the steaks over and top with the butter and rosemary sprigs, letting the butter melt over the steaks. Add the smashed garlic to the skillet and continue to cook, basting the steaks with the melted butter, for another 5 to 7 minutes for medium-rare steaks, or cook longer if you like your steaks more well-done.

3 Remove the steaks from the heat, cover loosely with aluminum foil, and allow to rest for 5 minutes before serving.

per serving:

CALORIES: 477 | FAT: 40 g | PROTEIN: 30 g | TOTAL CARBS: 0.5 g | NET CARBS: 0.5 g

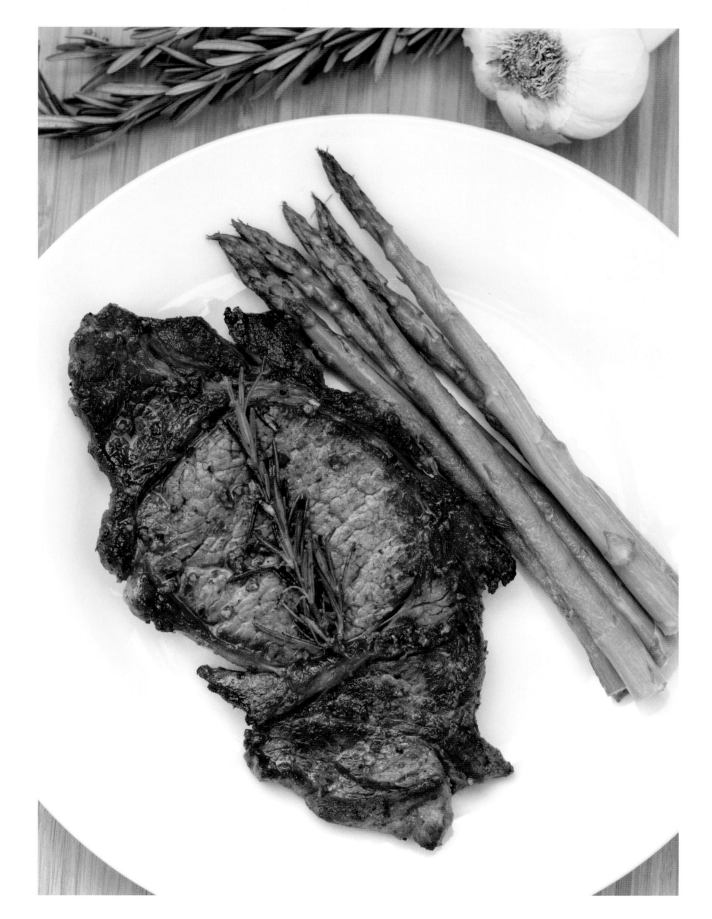

LEMON GARLIC PORK TENDERLOIN

PREP TIME: 15 MINUTES, PLUS 1 HOUR TO MARINATE • COOK TIME: 1 HOUR
YIELD: 4 SERVINGS

Pork tenderloin is one of my favorite cuts of meat because you can season it however you wish, toss it in the oven, and basically forget it while it cooks. I'm all about a low-maintenance meal!

Marinade

¼ cup extra-virgin olive oil

Zest and juice of ½ lemon

1½ tablespoons chopped fresh rosemary

1 tablespoon onion powder

2 cloves garlic, peeled

Salt and pepper, to taste

1½ pounds pork tenderloin

1. Combine the marinade ingredients in a small bowl and whisk to combine.

2. Place the pork in a large zip-top plastic bag and pour the marinade over it. Squeeze most of the air out of the bag and seal. Allow to marinate in the refrigerator for at least 1 hour.

3. About 20 minutes before cooking, remove the pork from the refrigerator and place the bag on the counter to allow the meat to come to room temperature.

4. Preheat the oven to 375°F. Line a baking dish with parchment paper.

5. Place the pork on the lined baking dish and cook for 50 to 60 minutes, until the internal temperature of the meat reaches 145°F. Allow to rest for 5 minutes before slicing and serving.

per serving:

CALORIES: 285 | FAT: 17 g | PROTEIN: 33.3 g | TOTAL CARBS: 3.3 g | NET CARBS: 3 g

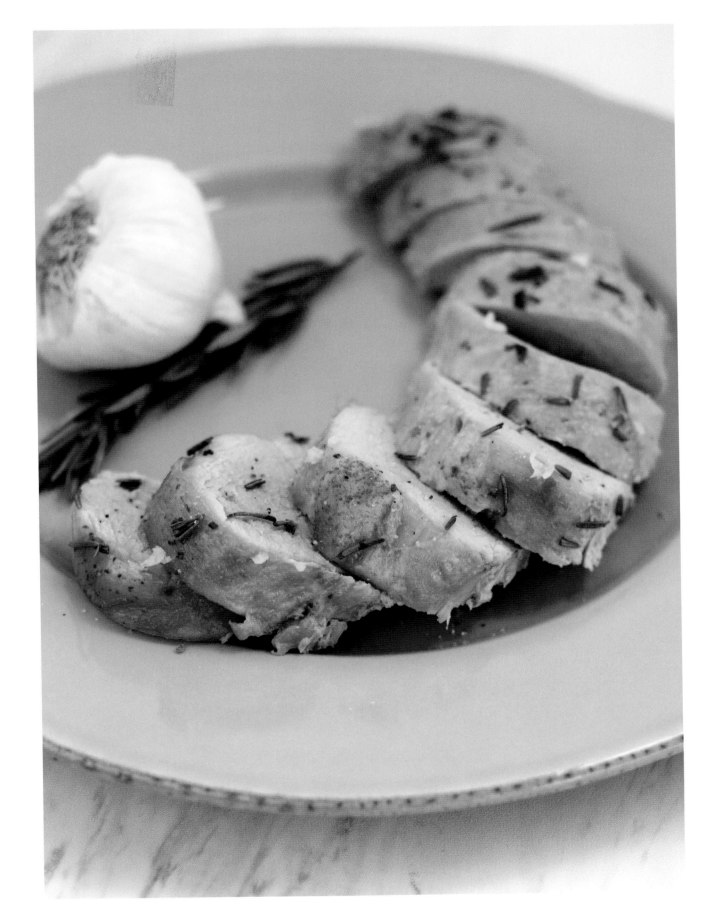

GOAT CHEESE, ROSEMARY, AND MUSHROOM STUFFED PORK CHOPS

⌀ ◍   PREP TIME: 15 MINUTES • COOK TIME: 40 MINUTES • YIELD: 2 SERVINGS

Have I mentioned how much I love goat cheese? These stuffed pork chops are absolutely delicious. If you double or triple the recipe, it's a great way to wow your family and friends at dinner!

1 slice bacon

½ cup chopped white mushrooms

2 ounces goat cheese, crumbled

1 teaspoon chopped fresh rosemary

1 large clove garlic, pressed

2 (12-ounce) bone-in pork chops (about 1 inch thick)

Salt and pepper

1 tablespoon avocado oil or ghee

1   Preheat the oven to 350°F.

2   Pan-fry the bacon in a small skillet over medium heat. Set aside on a paper towel–lined plate to cool. When cool enough to handle, chop and put in a small bowl.

3   To the bowl with the bacon, add the mushrooms, goat cheese, rosemary, and garlic and gently stir until evenly mixed.

4   Cut a large slit in the side of each pork chop to make a pocket for the filling. Be sure not to pierce the back or sides of the chop so that the filling won't spill out.

5   Stuff the pork chops with the mushroom filling, then press closed. (Optional: Secure the chops closed with a toothpick.) Season the stuffed chops generously with salt and pepper.

6   Heat the avocado oil in a large cast-iron or other oven-safe skillet over medium-high heat. Add the stuffed chops and sear until golden brown, 2 to 3 minutes per side.

7   Transfer the skillet to the oven and cook for 25 to 30 minutes, until the internal temperature of the chops reaches 145°F.

8   Allow the pork chops to rest for 3 to 5 minutes before serving.

per serving:

CALORIES: 483 | FAT: 33.5 g | PROTEIN: 43 g | TOTAL CARBS: 1.5 g | NET CARBS: 1.5 g

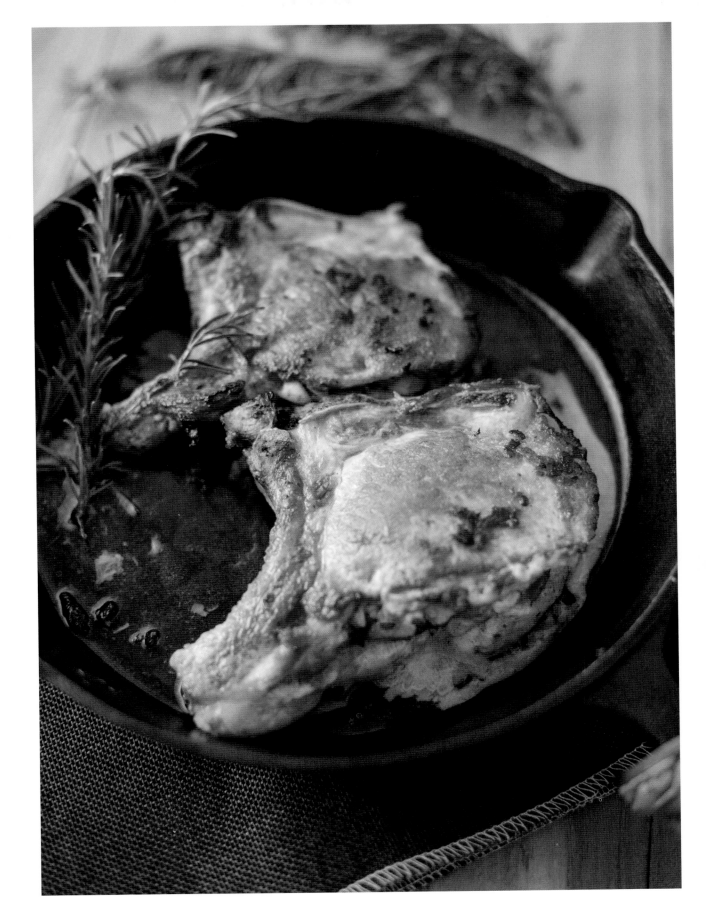

GYRO LETTUCE WRAPS

PREP TIME: 10 MINUTES • COOK TIME: 20 TO 25 MINUTES • YIELD: 8 WRAPS (2 PER SERVING)

This low-carb spin on a classic gyro gives you all the flavor you'd expect, but without any unnecessary carbs!

Meatballs

½ pound ground beef

½ pound ground lamb

1 large egg

¼ cup finely chopped yellow onions

1 tablespoon minced garlic

1 teaspoon ground cumin

½ teaspoon dried ground oregano

½ teaspoon salt

½ teaspoon ground black pepper

⅓ cup crumbled feta cheese

For Serving

8 butter lettuce leaves or other lettuce wraps of choice

1 large tomato, sliced

¼ red onion, thinly sliced

½ batch Tzatziki Sauce (page 84)

note: The meatballs can also be served on their own as an appetizer, with Tzatziki Sauce.

1. Preheat the oven to 400°F and line a rimmed baking sheet with parchment paper.

2. In a large bowl, combine all the meatball ingredients except for the feta cheese and use your hands to incorporate. Carefully fold in the feta.

3. Form the mixture into sixteen 1-inch meatballs and place on the lined baking sheet, spaced at least 1 inch apart.

4. Bake the meatballs for 20 to 25 minutes, until the outsides are browned and the internal temperature reaches 160°F.

5. Let cool for 5 minutes, then cut each meatball into 3 slices.

6. To assemble the wraps, divide the meatball slices evenly among the lettuce leaves. Top with tomato and red onion slices and tzatziki sauce.

per serving:

CALORIES: 396 | FAT: 27.3 g | PROTEIN: 29 g | TOTAL CARBS: 8.1 g | NET CARBS: 6 g

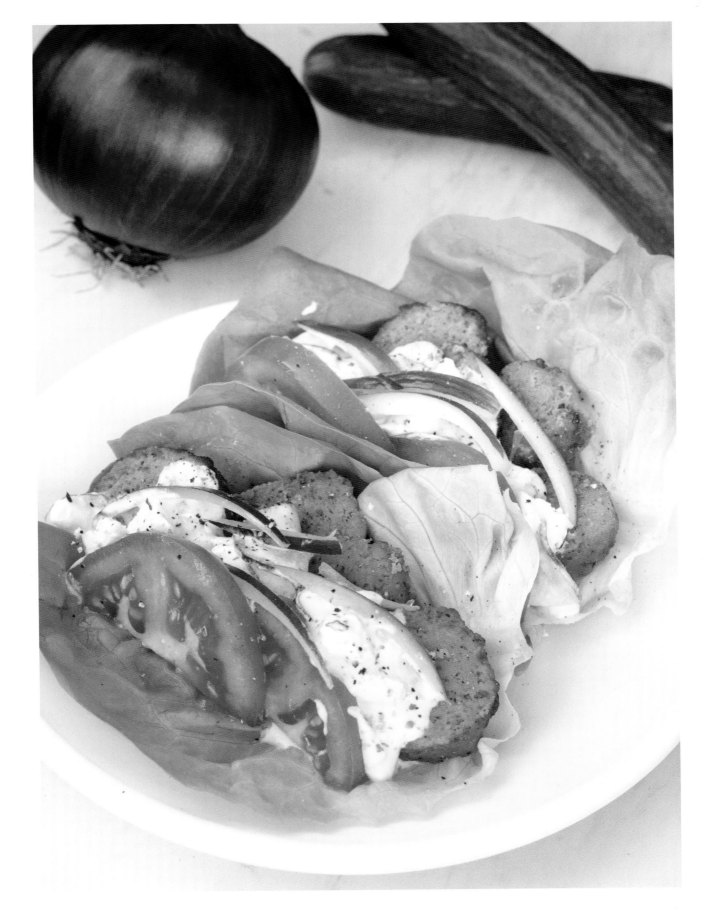

BUNLESS PHILLY CHEESESTEAKS

PREP TIME: 15 MINUTES • COOK TIME: 10 MINUTES • YIELD: 2 SERVINGS

Crunched for time? This easy meal is ready in a little over 15 minutes, and it's packed full of flavor and cheesesteak goodness. Serve as is or over shredded lettuce!

1 tablespoon unsalted butter

1 cup white mushrooms, halved

½ cup chopped onions

⅓ cup chopped green bell peppers

¼ teaspoon garlic powder

8 ounces rare roast beef slices

2 slices provolone cheese

Salt and pepper

note: To make this recipe dairy-free, use ghee instead of butter and omit the cheese.

1   In a medium-sized saucepan over medium heat, melt the butter. Add the mushrooms, onions, bell peppers, and garlic powder and cook until the veggies are soft, 4 to 5 minutes.

2   Cut the roast beef into 1-inch squares.

3   Add the roast beef to the saucepan and toss with the vegetables for 1 minute, until heated through.

4   Reduce the heat to low and top the roast beef and veggie mixture with the provolone cheese. Cover the pan with a lid for 2 to 3 minutes to allow the cheese to melt. Season with salt and pepper to taste, then serve.

per serving:

CALORIES: 305 | FAT: 16 g | PROTEIN: 33 g | TOTAL CARBS: 6 g | NET CARBS: 4.5 g

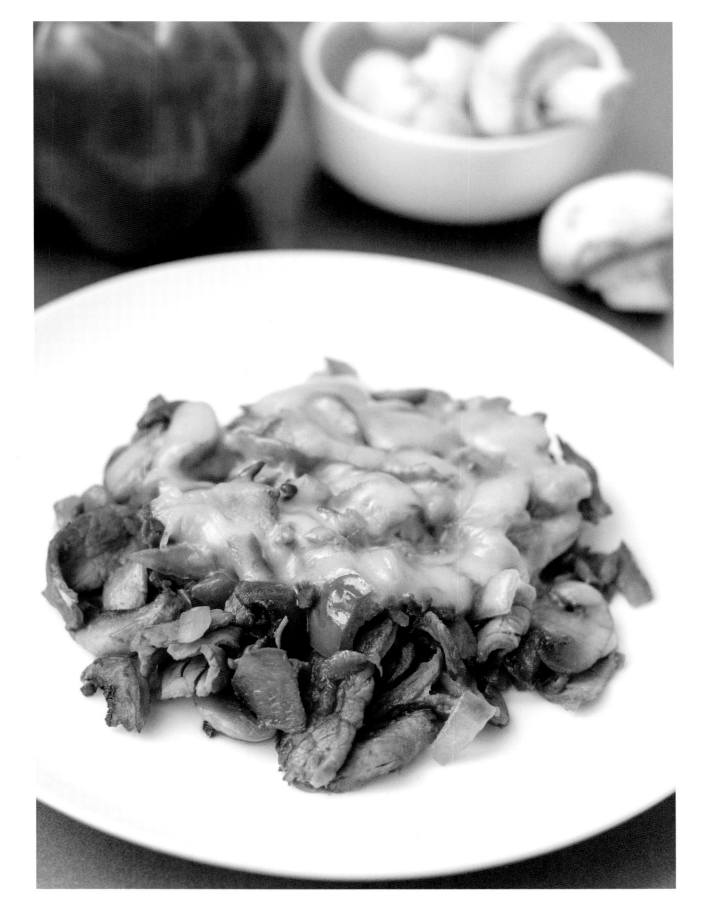

SLOW COOKER CARNITAS

PREP TIME: 15 MINUTES • COOK TIME: 8 TO 10 HOURS • YIELD: 15 SERVINGS

This is a delicious and easy slow cooker meal that you can set up in the morning and come home to in the evening.

Carnitas

2 medium onions, chopped, divided

1½ cups chicken broth

Juice of 1 lime

1 (4½-pound) bone-in pork shoulder, or 1 (3-pound) boneless pork shoulder

½ cup chopped fresh cilantro

Salt and pepper

Dry Rub

1 tablespoon garlic powder

2 teaspoons chili powder

2 teaspoons ground cumin

2 teaspoons salt

For Serving

1 to 2 heads butter lettuce, leaves separated

1 avocado, peeled, pitted, and sliced

Chopped fresh cilantro

Diced red onions

1 lime, cut into wedges

1 In a slow cooker, combine half of the chopped onions, the chicken broth, and the lime juice.

2 Rinse the pork shoulder with cold water and pat dry.

3 In a bowl, combine the dry rub ingredients. Rub the mixture over the entire pork shoulder.

4 Place the seasoned pork shoulder in the slow cooker on top of the onion mixture. Top with the remaining onions and the cilantro. Cover and cook on low for 8 to 10 hours, until the pork is fully cooked and shreds easily.

5 Remove the pork from the slow cooker, leaving the juices in the slow cooker. Shred the meat and return it to the pot with the juices; season to taste with salt and pepper, if needed. Cover and place on the keep warm setting for 30 minutes.

6 Preheat the oven to 400°F. Place the shredded pork on a rimmed baking sheet and bake for 15 to 20 minutes until crisp.

7 Serve in butter lettuce leaves topped with avocado slices, chopped cilantro, and diced red onions, with the lime wedges on the side.

per serving:

CALORIES: 376 | FAT: 24 g | PROTEIN: 31.5 g | TOTAL CARBS: 2.4 g | NET CARBS: 2 g

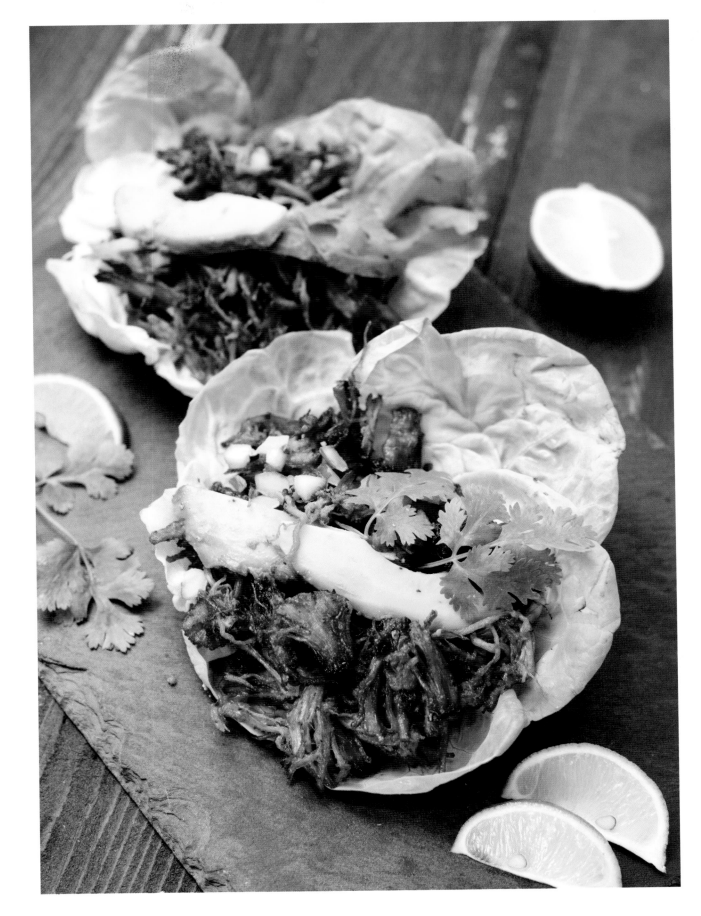

SUNNY-SIDE-UP BURGERS

PREP TIME: 10 MINUTES • COOK TIME: 15 MINUTES • YIELD: 4 SERVINGS

Bunless burgers are a common choice for keto-ers on the go and at home. Adding a fried egg and some sliced avocado gives these burgers additional fat and flavor to complete your meal!

1 pound ground beef

2 teaspoons garlic powder

Salt and pepper

4 slices cheddar cheese

1 tablespoon unsalted butter

4 large eggs

1 medium avocado, sliced

1 small tomato, cut into 4 slices

½ small yellow onion, sliced

4 butter lettuce leaves, for serving (optional)

note: Optional toppings include mayonnaise, mustard, pickles, jalapeño slices, and/or crispy bacon.

1 Preheat a grill or grill pan to medium-high heat.

2 In a bowl, combine the ground beef and garlic powder. Season generously with salt and pepper and mix well. Use your hands to form the mixture into four ½-inch patties.

3 Grill the patties for 3 to 4 minutes on each side for medium-done burgers, flipping once. After flipping the patties, top each patty with a slice of cheese and allow to melt while the other side cooks.

4 In a skillet over medium heat, melt the butter. Crack the eggs into the pan and fry until cooked to your liking. (I recommend sunny side up or over easy.)

5 Place the burgers on a plate and top each burger with a slice of tomato, onion slices, avocado slices, and a fried egg. Season to taste with salt and pepper. Eat as is or enjoy wrapped in a butter lettuce leaf.

per serving:

CALORIES: 459 | FAT: 33.8 g | PROTEIN: 34 g | TOTAL CARBS: 5 g | NET CARBS: 2.3 g

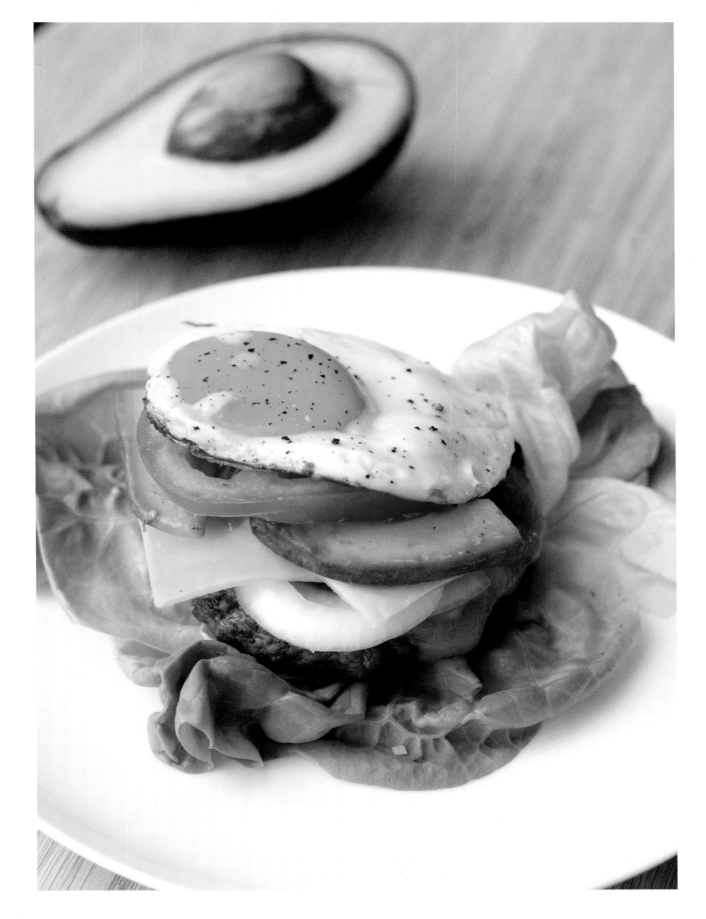

QUICK AND EASY PERSONAL PIZZA

🕒 PREP TIME: 5 MINUTES • COOK TIME: 15 MINUTES • YIELD: 1 SERVING

My husband, Mick, loves pizza, so I set out to create a crust that is both easy to make and delicious. We went through several rounds of recipe testing (which Mick never seemed to complain about) and eventually landed on this delicious low-carb recipe. Personal pizzas ready in under 20 minutes, perfect for those busy weeknights!

Crust

⅓ cup shredded mozzarella cheese

¼ cup blanched almond flour

⅛ teaspoon garlic powder

Pinch of salt

1 large egg yolk

Toppings

1½ tablespoons no-sugar-added pizza sauce

¼ cup shredded mozzarella cheese

5 slices pepperoni

¼ teaspoon Italian seasoning

note: Feel free to create your own pizza toppings or season the crust with different spices! Fresh basil also complements this recipe really nicely.

1. Place an oven rack in the top position. Preheat the oven to 425°F.

2. Make the crust: In a microwave-safe bowl, combine the mozzarella cheese, almond flour, garlic powder, and salt and stir until well blended. Microwave for 25 seconds.

3. Knead the dough with your hands for a few seconds. Add the egg yolk while the dough is still warm. Knead until combined and roll into a ball. Form a disk as if you were making a hamburger patty. Place the dough on a parchment-lined baking sheet and use your hands to press into a circle 5 to 6 inches in diameter and about ¼ inch thick (or use a rolling pin). If the dough cools too much to form properly, place it back in the microwave for 10 seconds.

4. Use a fork to poke holes in several places throughout the crust before baking. Bake on the top rack for 8 to 10 minutes, until the crust is golden brown.

5. Remove the crust from the oven and flip it over. Top the flatter side with the pizza sauce and sprinkle with half of the cheese. Next, add the pepperoni slices, then sprinkle with the remaining cheese. Bake for another 3 to 4 minutes, until the cheese is melted.

6. Sprinkle the pizza with Italian seasoning before serving.

per serving:

CALORIES: 479 | FAT: 39 g | PROTEIN: 25 g | TOTAL CARBS: 11 g | NET CARBS: 7.8 g

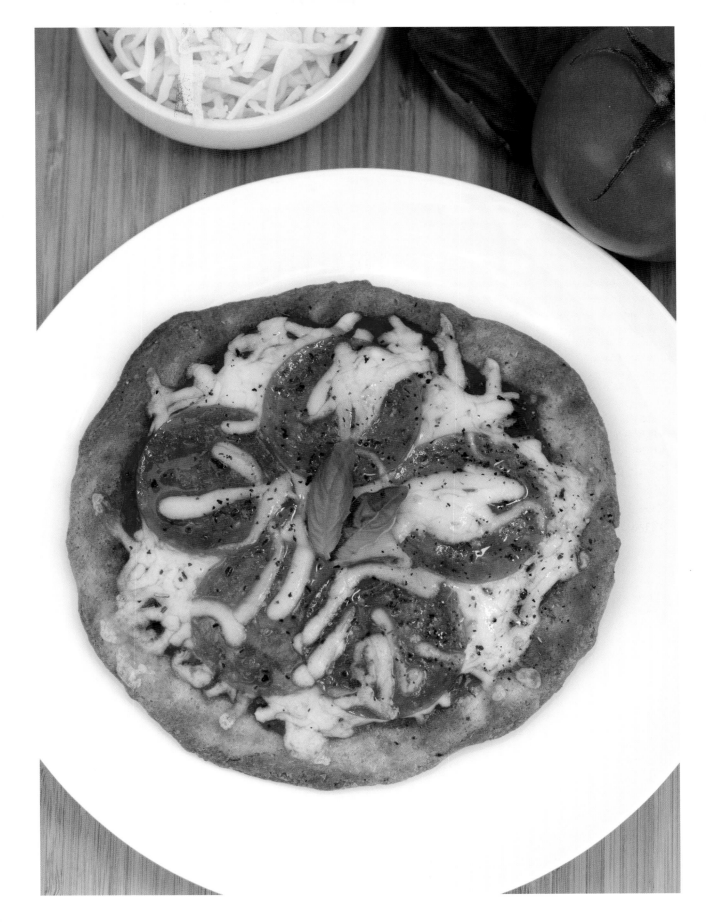

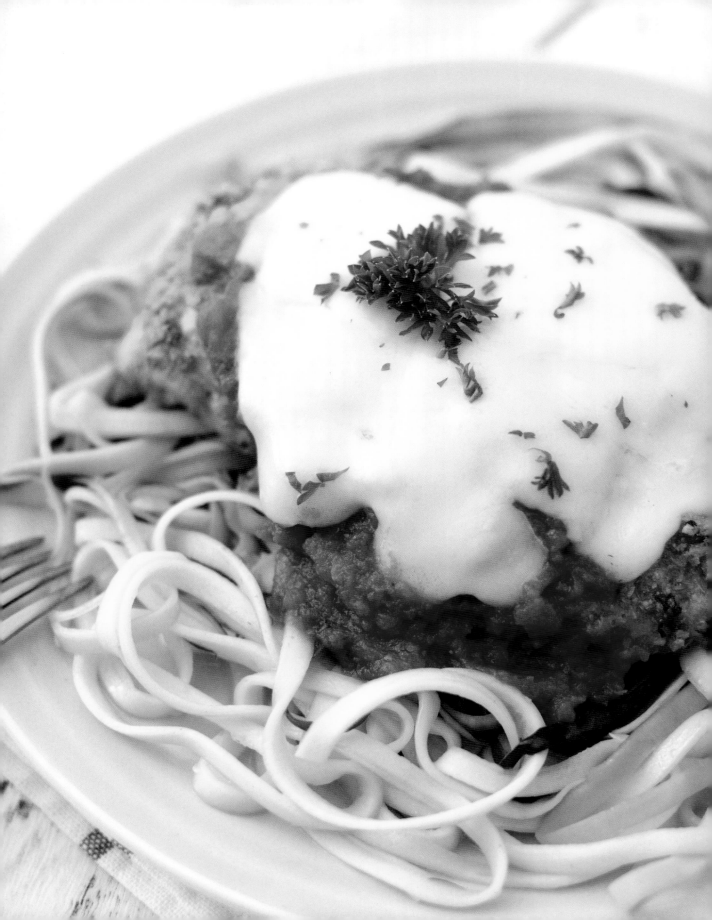

CHICKEN

BACON AND RANCH CHICKEN SALAD

(30) • PREP TIME: 10 MINUTES • COOK TIME: 10 MINUTES • YIELD: 3 SERVINGS

OPTION

When I'm in a rush for lunch, I often make homemade chicken salad. Your typical chicken salad can easily be made with mayo, celery, onion, and a little seasoning, but when you're hungry for a little variety, this version is delish!

5 slices bacon

1½ cups cubed cooked chicken (about 12 ounces; see notes)

⅓ cup mayonnaise

3 tablespoons ranch dressing (see notes)

½ stalk celery, chopped (optional)

Salt and pepper

6 butter lettuce leaves, for serving

Chopped fresh parsley, for garnish (optional)

1 In a skillet over medium heat, fry the bacon until crispy. Set aside on a paper towel–lined plate to cool.

2 Place the cooked chicken in a medium-sized mixing bowl. Add the mayonnaise, ranch dressing, and celery, if using.

3 Chop the bacon and add to the chicken mixture.

4 Fold all the ingredients with a spoon until the chicken is evenly coated. Season with salt and pepper to taste.

5 Divide the chicken salad evenly among the lettuce leaves. Garnish with chopped parsley, if desired.

notes: I use leftover Simply Roasted Chicken (page 204) or a precooked rotisserie chicken.

Ingredients vary in different brands of ranch dressing. If you wish to make this recipe dairy-free, please check ingredient labels closely and find a brand that meets your needs.

If you prefer, you can spoon this chicken salad into avocado halves instead of lettuce leaves.

per serving:

CALORIES: 397 | FAT: 35.3 g | PROTEIN: 18 g | TOTAL CARBS: 1.3 g | NET CARBS: 1 g

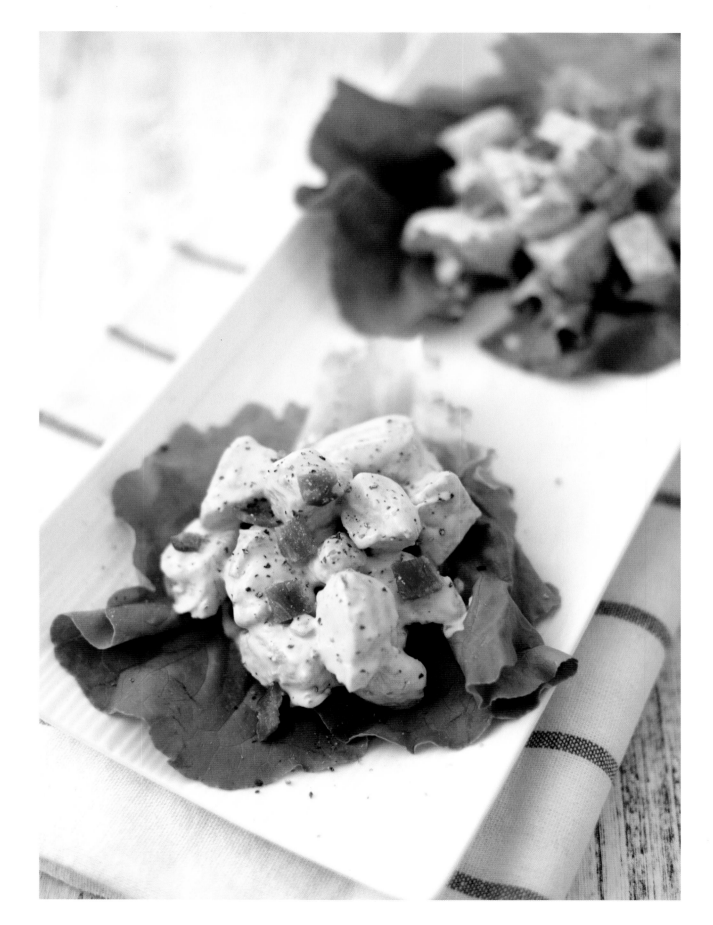

BACON-WRAPPED CHEESY CHICKEN

⊘ ⊘   PREP TIME: 15 MINUTES • COOK TIME: 35 MINUTES • YIELD: 4 SERVINGS

OPTION

This recipe is a keto-friendly spin on a famous Outback Steakhouse dish called Alice Springs Chicken that I used to love. The crisp bacon, mushrooms, honey mustard, and melted cheese blend together for a most delicious keto meal!

2 boneless, skinless chicken breast halves (about 1½ pounds)

Salt and pepper

2 tablespoons Keto Honey Mustard (page 73) or ranch dressing (see note), plus extra for serving

1 cup white mushrooms, sliced

¾ cup shredded cheddar cheese

8 slices thin-sliced or regular bacon, cut in half crosswise

Chopped fresh parsley, for garnish (optional)

note: Ingredients vary in different brands of ranch dressing. If you wish to make this recipe egg-free, please check ingredient labels closely and find a brand that meets your needs.

1. Preheat the oven to 375°F. Line a shallow baking pan with parchment paper.

2. Cut each chicken breast in half horizontally to make four fillets that are about ½ inch thick at the wider end. Season the chicken with salt and pepper.

3. Place the chicken in a bowl and top with the honey mustard or ranch dressing; toss to coat.

4. Place the coated chicken fillets in the lined baking pan, spaced 1 inch apart. Top each fillet with ¼ cup of the mushrooms, then sprinkle 3 tablespoons of the cheddar cheese on top of the mushrooms.

5. Drape each chicken stack with 4 half-slices of bacon, fully covering the surface of the chicken.

6. Bake for 25 to 30 minutes, until the internal temperature of the chicken reaches 165°F, then set the oven to broil for 5 minutes to crisp the bacon. Garnish with parsley before serving, if desired. Serve with honey mustard or ranch.

per serving:

CALORIES: 357 | FAT: 19 g | PROTEIN: 47 g | TOTAL CARBS: 1.8 g | NET CARBS: 1.2 g

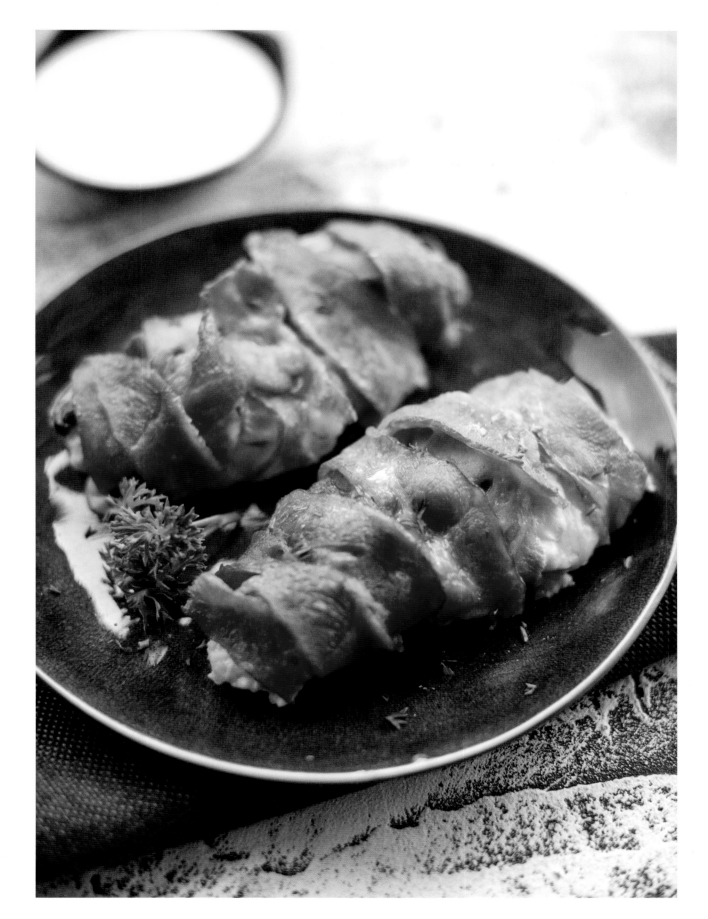

CHICKEN CAESAR SALAD

🕐 🥬 PREP TIME: 15 MINUTES • YIELD: 2 SERVINGS

This salad is a re-creation of one of my favorite salads from a local burger joint near my house called Jack's Prime. This is the first restaurant I ever went to that put avocado in Caesar salad, and anytime you add avocado to anything (well, almost anything), I'm a fan!

1 (9-ounce) bag hearts of romaine, or 9 ounces prewashed and prechopped romaine lettuce

6 ounces cooked rotisserie chicken breast, chopped

6 cherry tomatoes, halved

⅓ cup Quick and Easy Caesar Dressing (page 74)

1 avocado, sliced or cubed

¼ cup shaved Parmesan cheese

Ground black pepper

note: If you're in a hurry and need to buy premade Caesar dressing, be sure to check the labels! Most Caesar dressings are keto-friendly, but it's best to check the macros and ingredients of different brands.

1. Rinse and pat dry the romaine, then chop (or use prewashed and chopped hearts of romaine).

2. In a large mixing bowl, combine the romaine, chopped chicken, tomatoes, and dressing, then toss well. Top with the avocado, shaved Parmesan cheese, and a sprinkle of fresh ground pepper.

per serving:

CALORIES: 594 | FAT: 48 g | PROTEIN: 30 g | TOTAL CARBS: 13 g | NET CARBS: 4.5 g

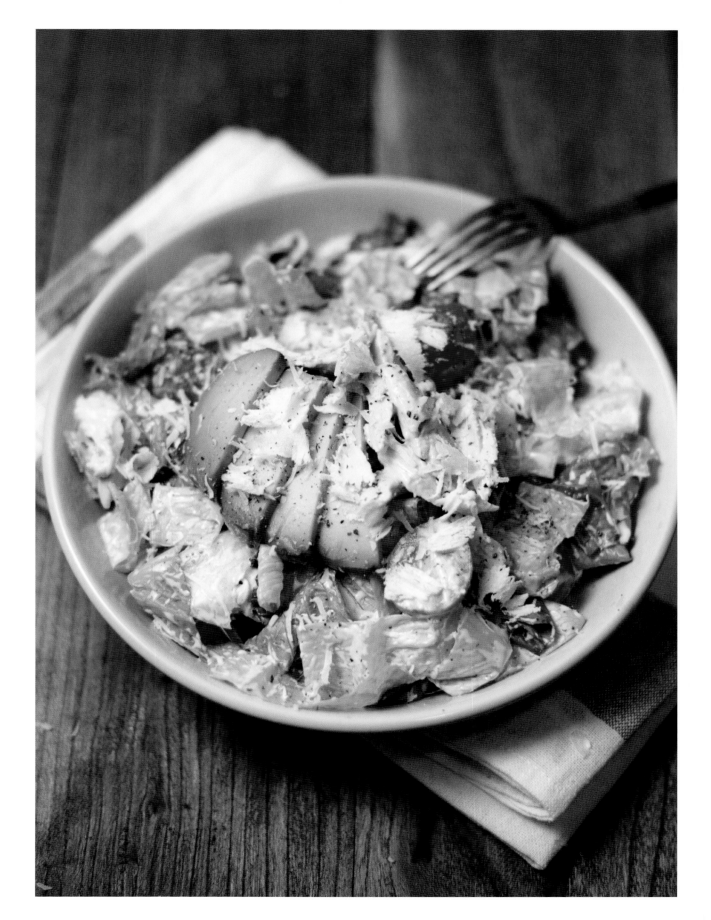

CHICKEN AND BROCCOLI ALFREDO BOWLS

⏱ ⊘ ⊗ PREP TIME: 15 MINUTES • COOK TIME: 15 MINUTES • YIELD: 4 SERVINGS

Chicken Alfredo is creamy, full of flavor, and did I mention quick and easy to make at home? It is a great option when dining out as well. When ordering chicken Alfredo at an Italian restaurant, simply substitute broccoli for the pasta.

1 tablespoon unsalted butter

½ cup chopped yellow onions

1 clove garlic, pressed

8 ounces white mushrooms, sliced

1 pound boneless, skinless chicken breasts or thighs, cooked and cubed (I use a prepared rotisserie chicken)

2 cups broccoli florets, steamed

1 cup Alfredo sauce, homemade (page 68) or store-bought

½ cup shaved Parmesan cheese

2 teaspoons chopped fresh parsley, or 1 teaspoon dried parsley (optional)

1 Melt the butter in a large skillet over medium heat. Add the onions, garlic, and mushrooms and cook until the onions are translucent and the mushrooms are cooked.

2 Add the chicken, steamed broccoli, and Alfredo sauce. Stir and simmer for 2 to 3 minutes.

3 Divide among 4 bowls and serve topped with the shaved Parmesan. Garnish with parsley, if desired.

per serving:

CALORIES: 422 | FAT: 26.2 g | PROTEIN: 31 g | TOTAL CARBS: 9 g | NET CARBS: 7 g

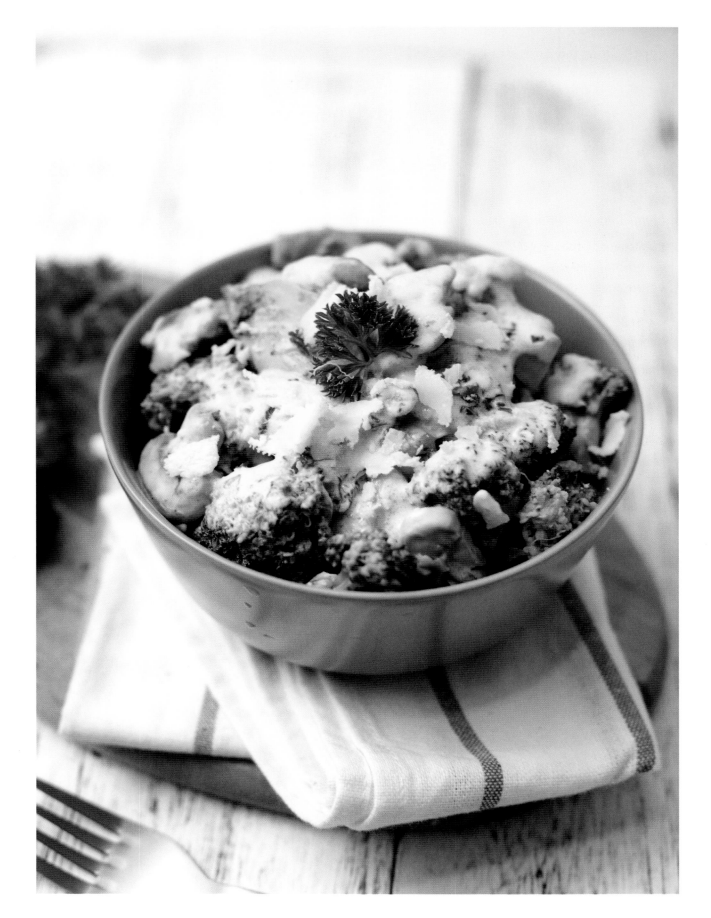

CHICKEN CORDON BLEU

PREP TIME: 15 MINUTES • COOK TIME: 40 MINUTES • YIELD: 6 SERVINGS

Did you know that crushed pork rinds can be used as a grain-free breading for a variety of foods? In this delicious and easy chicken dish, I've combined pork rinds and cheese for the perfect "breading"!

3 large boneless, skinless chicken breast halves (about 1½ pounds)

6 slices Swiss cheese

6 slices ham

¼ cup (½ stick) unsalted butter, melted

Chopped fresh parsley, for garnish (optional)

Breading

1 ounce plain pork rinds (6 to 8 large pork rinds)

⅔ cup finely grated Parmesan cheese

1 teaspoon garlic powder

¼ teaspoon salt

⅛ teaspoon ground black pepper

Special Equipment

• Toothpicks

1 Preheat the oven to 350°F. Line a medium-sized baking dish with parchment paper.

2 Cut the chicken breasts in half lengthwise. Place on a cutting board and cover with a piece of parchment paper. Use a kitchen mallet to pound the chicken to a thickness of ½ inch.

3 Top each chicken breast with one slice each of Swiss cheese and ham. Roll each breast so that the cheese and ham are locked inside the chicken. Secure with a toothpick to prevent the chicken from unrolling.

4 Make the breading: In a zip-top plastic bag, combine the pork rinds, Parmesan cheese, garlic powder, salt, and pepper. Crush and shake until the mixture resembles breadcrumbs. Transfer the "breading" to a bowl and set aside.

5 Place the butter in a microwave-safe bowl and microwave until melted.

6 Dip the chicken rolls, one at a time, into the butter and coat evenly. Place the butter-coated chicken rolls in the breading bowl and coat evenly. Place the breaded chicken rolls in the prepared baking dish.

7 Bake for 40 minutes, or until the internal temperature of the chicken reaches 165°F.

8 Place the chicken on a plate and spoon the drippings from the baking dish over the top before serving. Garnish with parsley, if desired.

per serving:

CALORIES: 373 | FAT: 22.8 g | PROTEIN: 39 g | TOTAL CARBS: 2.3 g | NET CARBS: 2.3 g

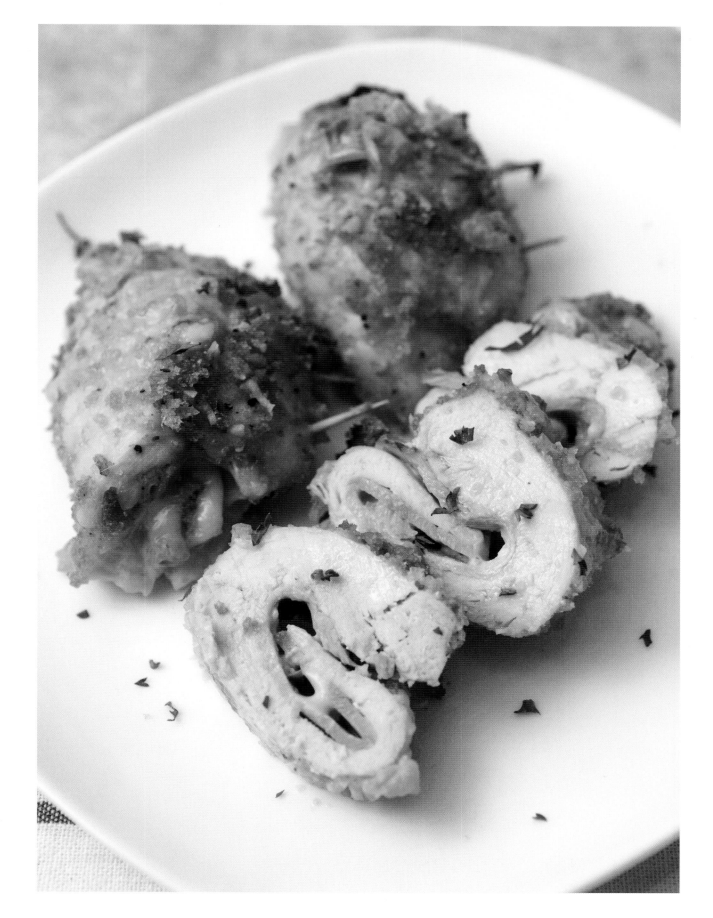

CHICKEN PARMESAN

PREP TIME: 10 MINUTES • COOK TIME: 30 MINUTES • YIELD: 2 SERVINGS

Chicken Parmesan is one of the ultimate Italian comfort foods! This simple recipe is ready in under an hour. It pairs perfectly with Zoodles for a low-carb Italian feast!

2 (6-ounce) chicken breast halves

⅓ cup mayonnaise

⅓ cup golden flaxseed meal

2 tablespoons chopped fresh parsley, plus extra for garnish

½ teaspoon garlic powder

½ teaspoon Italian seasoning

½ cup no-sugar-added marinara sauce, warm

½ cup shredded mozzarella cheese

1 batch Zoodles (page 254), for serving

1   Preheat the oven to 350°F. Line a shallow baking dish with parchment paper.

2   Pound the chicken to a thickness of ½ inch.

3   In a medium-sized mixing bowl, combine the chicken and mayonnaise and toss to coat evenly.

4   In a separate bowl, mix together the flaxseed meal, parsley, garlic powder, and Italian seasoning.

5   Place the mayonnaise-coated chicken in the flaxseed mixture, pressing the mixture onto the chicken to evenly coat all sides.

6   Place the coated chicken breasts in the prepared baking dish. Bake for 20 to 25 minutes, until the juices run clear and the internal temperature of the chicken reaches 165°F.

7   Top each breast with ¼ cup of the warm marinara and ¼ cup of the mozzarella cheese and return to the oven for 3 to 5 minutes, until the sauce is warm and the cheese is melted. Garnish with parsley and serve over zoodles.

per serving:

CALORIES: 675 | FAT: 51 g | PROTEIN: 47.5 g | TOTAL CARBS: 13 g | NET CARBS: 7.5 g

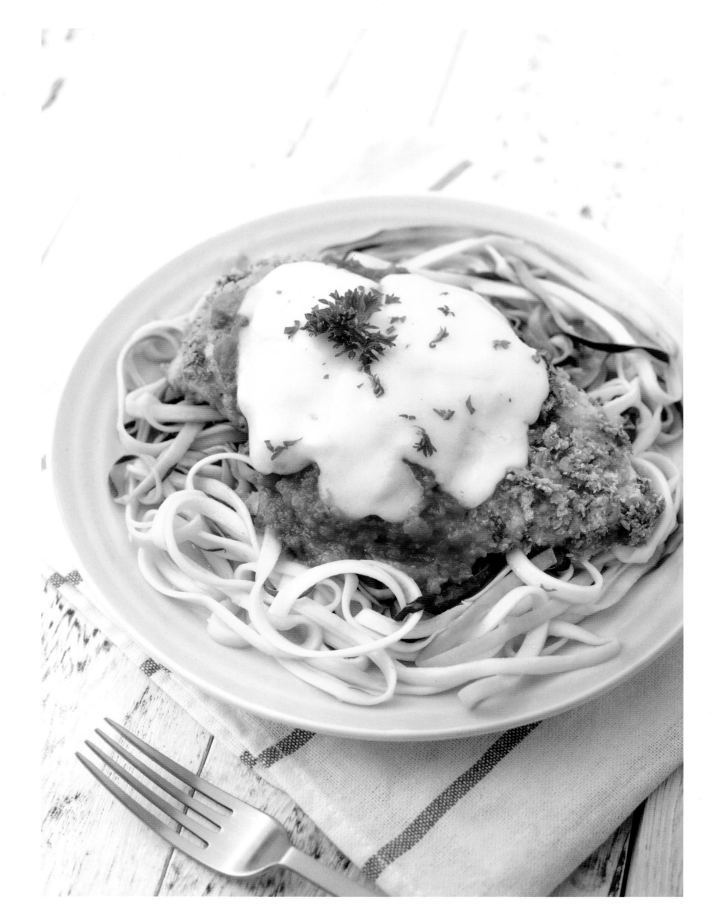

CREAMY PESTO CHICKEN

PREP TIME: 15 MINUTES • COOK TIME: 20 MINUTES • YIELD: 4 SERVINGS

Alfredo and pesto team up for a creamy and cheesy sauce with a big hit of flavor!

2 tablespoons avocado oil

½ cup diced onions

2 cloves garlic, minced

1½ pounds boneless, skinless chicken breasts, cubed

1 (5-ounce) bag fresh spinach, chopped

1 cup Alfredo sauce, homemade (page 68) or store-bought

3 tablespoons pesto, homemade (page 70) or store-bought

Salt and pepper

½ cup shaved Parmesan cheese

tip: Serve this chicken on its own in a bowl or serve over Zoodles (page 254) or steamed broccoli.

1 Heat the avocado oil in a large, deep skillet over medium-high heat. Add the onions and garlic and cook for about 1 minute, until fragrant.

2 Add the chicken and cook for 8 to 10 minutes, tossing as needed, until the internal temperature of the chicken reaches 165°F and the juices run clear.

3 Add the spinach and stir to combine. Cook for 2 to 3 minutes, until wilted, then pour in the Alfredo sauce and pesto. Stir until everything is well blended and the sauces are warmed.

4 Plate, season with salt and pepper to taste, and sprinkle with the shaved Parmesan.

per serving:

CALORIES: 564 | FAT: 36.4 g | PROTEIN: 48 g | TOTAL CARBS: 6.6 g | NET CARBS: 5.5 g

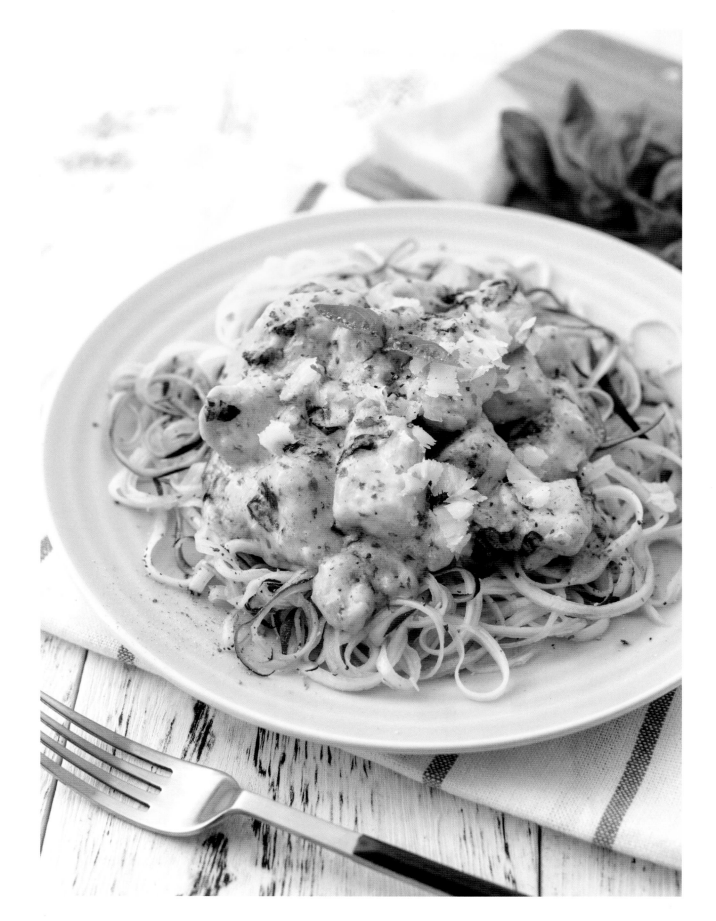

GRILLED CHICKEN AND BACON RANCH KABOBS

 PREP TIME: 15 MINUTES, PLUS 30 MINUTES TO MARINATE • COOK TIME: 15 TO 20 MINUTES
YIELD: 6 KABOBS (2 PER SERVING)

These easy-to-make kabobs are seriously the ultimate, full of a variety of flavors and textures!

Marinade

⅓ cup ranch dressing

½ teaspoon Italian seasoning

¼ teaspoon garlic powder

Kabobs

1¼ pounds boneless, skinless chicken breasts, cubed (24 cubes total)

6 slices bacon

12 small white mushrooms, halved (optional)

Special Equipment

- 6 wood or metal skewers (soak wood skewers in water for 30 minutes before grilling to prevent them from catching fire on the grill)

1 Make the marinade: In a medium-sized bowl, mix together the ranch dressing, Italian seasoning, and garlic powder.

2 Add the chicken to the bowl with the marinade and stir to coat. Cover and refrigerate for 30 minutes.

3 Preheat a grill to medium-high heat.

4 Thread the end of a slice of bacon onto a skewer. Add one piece of chicken and one mushroom half (if using) to the skewer, then loop the bacon around and thread it onto the skewer again. Add another piece of chicken and another mushroom, then thread the bacon onto the skewer again, creating an "S" pattern covering each level of chicken and mushroom with bacon. Repeat until each skewer has 4 pieces of chicken and 4 mushroom halves.

5 Grill the skewers for 15 to 20 minutes, until the internal temperature of the chicken reaches 165°F and the juices run clear, and the bacon is cooked.

per serving:

CALORIES: 421 | FAT: 22.5 g | PROTEIN: 46 g | TOTAL CARBS: 3 g | NET CARBS: 2.6 g

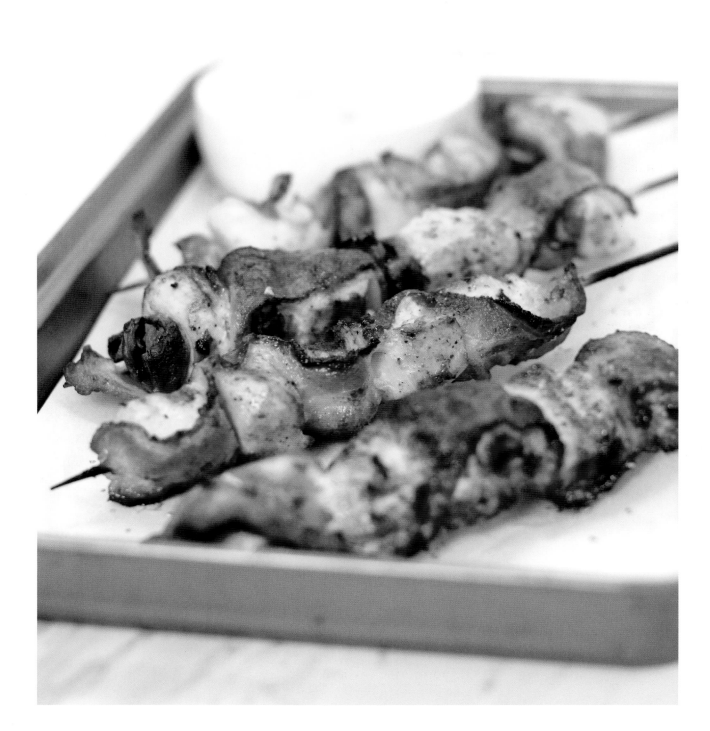

RED CURRY CHICKEN

PREP TIME: 10 MINUTES (NOT INCLUDING TIME TO MAKE RICE)
COOK TIME: 20 MINUTES • YIELD: 3 SERVINGS

If I had to pick one type of cuisine to eat for the rest of my life, it would likely be Thai food. My dad and I used to go for red curry (and Tom Kha Gai, a coconut and chicken soup) almost every week. Even though we live 3,000 miles apart now, this dish always reminds me of those special times together.

2 teaspoons avocado oil

1 pound boneless, skinless chicken thighs

1 green bell pepper, sliced

1 red bell pepper, sliced

1 (13½-ounce) can full-fat coconut milk

2 tablespoons fish sauce (optional)

2 tablespoons red curry paste

1½ teaspoons Swerve confectioners'-style sweetener or other keto sweetener of choice

8 to 10 fresh basil leaves, sliced, plus additional leaves for garnish (optional)

1 batch Basic Cauliflower Rice (page 242), for serving (optional)

1   Heat the oil in a large skillet over medium heat. When hot, add the chicken and bell peppers and cook until the peppers are soft and the internal temperature of the chicken reaches 165°F and the juices run clear. Remove from the pan and set aside.

2   In the same skillet over medium heat, combine the coconut milk, fish sauce (if using), curry paste, and sweetener; stir well to combine and simmer for 4 to 5 minutes to reduce.

3   Chop the chicken into bite-sized pieces. Once the sauce has reduced, add the cooked chicken and peppers and fresh basil leaves. Stir and simmer for 2 to 3 minutes, until the basil is soft.

4   Serve over cauliflower rice, if desired. Garnish with fresh basil, if desired.

per serving, not including rice:

CALORIES: 425 | FAT: 27.3 g | PROTEIN: 32 g | TOTAL CARBS: 12.5 g | NET CARBS: 6.6 g

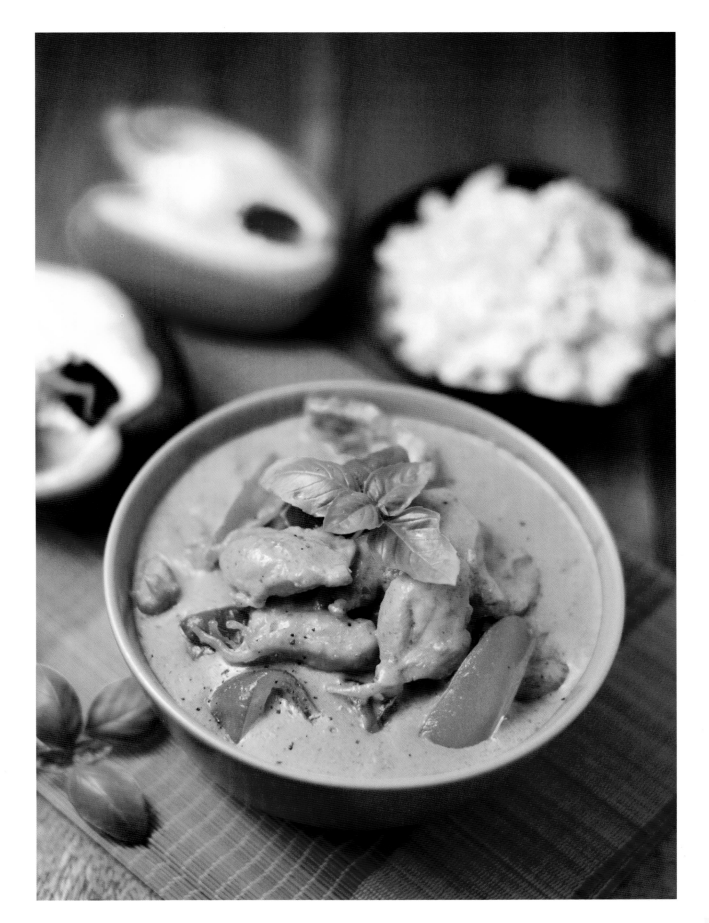

BREADED CHICKEN TENDERS

PREP TIME: 5 MINUTES • COOK TIME: 25 MINUTES • YIELD: 3 SERVINGS

Breaded chicken strips are a popular choice for people of all ages; my little girl requests them often! These simple chicken tenders are low in carbs but deliver great taste. They can be enjoyed as is, dipped in a variety of low-carb sauces, or added to salads or lettuce wraps!

¼ cup golden flaxseed meal

1 tablespoon fresh parsley, chopped

½ teaspoon garlic powder

1 pound boneless, skinless chicken breasts or tenders

⅓ cup mayonnaise

Keto Honey Mustard (page 73) or ranch dressing, for dipping

1 Preheat the oven to 350°F. Line a shallow baking dish with parchment paper.

2 Place the flaxseed meal, parsley, and garlic powder in a medium-sized bowl and mix with a fork.

3 If using chicken breasts, slice the breasts lengthwise into 1½-inch-thick strips. Place the strips, or tenders, in another medium-sized bowl with the mayonnaise and toss to coat evenly.

4 Dip the coated chicken strips one at a time into the flaxseed meal mixture, pressing the mixture onto the chicken to coat all sides.

5 Place the breaded chicken tenders on the lined baking dish and bake for 25 minutes, until the internal temperature of the chicken reaches 165°F.

6 Serve with honey mustard or ranch for dipping.

per serving:

CALORIES: 366 | FAT: 26 g | PROTEIN: 32 g | TOTAL CARBS: 3 g | NET CARBS: 0.5 g

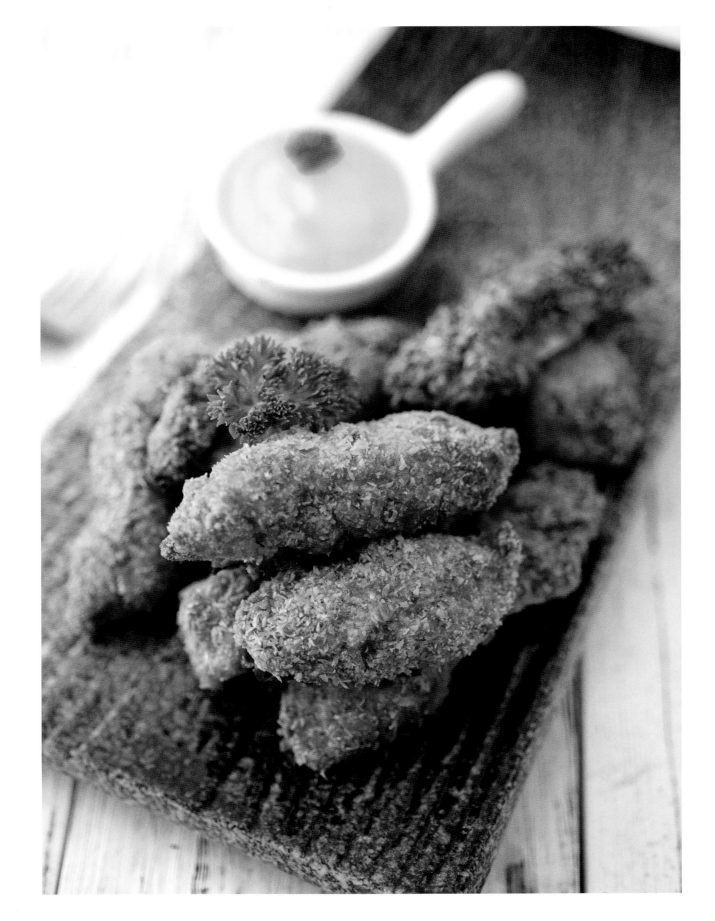

SIMPLY ROASTED CHICKEN

PREP TIME: 15 MINUTES • COOK TIME: 1 HOUR 30 MINUTES • YIELD: 5 SERVINGS

This delicious and moist roasted chicken will have you second-guessing all those past drives to the store for rotisserie chicken.

1 (3- to 4-pound) whole chicken

½ yellow onion, halved

2 large cloves garlic, halved

2 to 3 sprigs fresh rosemary

½ cup (1 stick) unsalted butter

1 lemon, quartered

2 tablespoons extra-virgin olive oil

2 teaspoons garlic powder

Salt and pepper

Special Equipment

- Butcher's twine

note: Leftovers can easily be made into Bacon and Ranch Chicken Salad (page 184).

1 Preheat the oven to 350°F. Line a roasting pan or deep baking dish with parchment paper.

2 Remove and discard the giblet bag from inside of the chicken and rinse the chicken with cold water. Pat dry and place in the lined baking dish.

3 Stuff the chicken cavity with the onion, garlic, rosemary, butter, and 3 of the lemon quarters. Tuck the wing tips under the breast and tie the legs together with butcher's twine.

4 Drizzle the olive oil over the entire chicken and rub it into the skin. Season the outside of the chicken with the garlic powder, generous amounts of salt and pepper, and the juice from the remaining lemon quarter.

5 Bake for 1 hour 30 minutes, or until the internal temperature of the chicken reaches 165°F. Once fully cooked, baste the chicken with the melted butter and pan drippings, then allow to rest for 10 minutes before slicing and serving.

per serving:

CALORIES: 320 | FAT: 18.9 g | PROTEIN: 36 g | TOTAL CARBS: 1.8 g | NET CARBS: 1.4 g

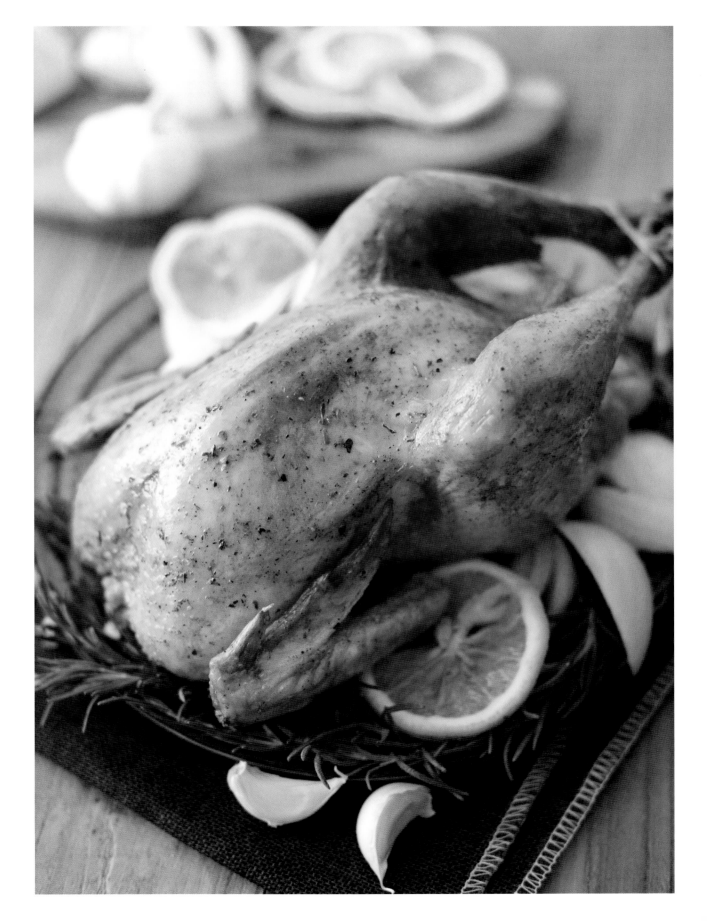

TINA'S SLOW COOKER SALSA CHICKEN LETTUCE WRAPS

PREP TIME: 10 MINUTES • COOK TIME: 4 TO 10 HOURS • YIELD: 7 SERVINGS

Slow cooker meals are great, especially for people who have busy schedules—which means pretty much all of us! When selecting a salsa for this recipe, be sure to read the labels and watch for added sugars; my favorite salsas are found in the refrigerated section of the grocery store. I created this recipe with one of my best friends, Tina.

2½ pounds boneless, skinless chicken breasts

2 cups salsa (see note)

6 ounces cream cheese, softened

Hot sauce (optional)

12 butter lettuce leaves, for serving

Topping Suggestions

Shredded Mexican-style cheese

1 avocado, sliced just before serving

note: Check several brands of salsa to find one that is low in carbs.

1 Place the chicken and salsa in a slow cooker and stir to coat the chicken evenly with the salsa. Cover and cook on low for 6 to 10 hours or on high for 4 to 6 hours, until the chicken is white throughout and the juices run clear.

2 Remove half of the liquid from the slow cooker and set aside. Add the softened cream cheese and hot sauce, if using, to the slow cooker and stir with a fork, shredding the chicken as you mix in the cream cheese. If desired, add some of the reserved liquid to moisten the chicken to your liking.

3 Scoop the chicken into the lettuce leaves, then top with shredded cheese and sliced avocado.

per serving:

CALORIES: 280 | FAT: 11 g | PROTEIN: 32.4 g | TOTAL CARBS: 5.4 g | NET CARBS: 5.4 g

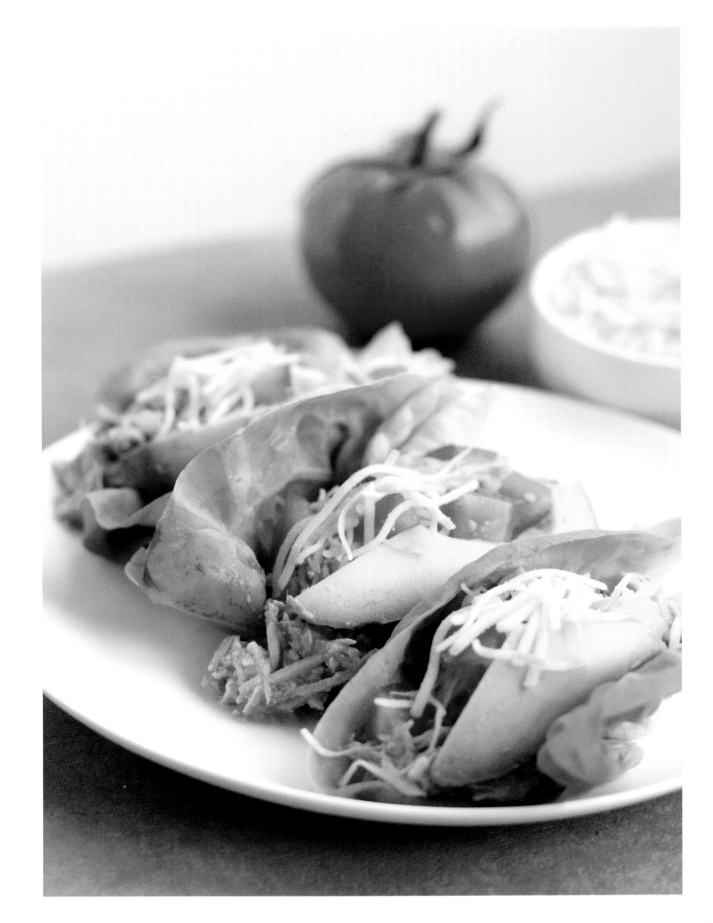

TUSCAN CHICKEN

PREP TIME: 10 MINUTES • COOK TIME: 25 MINUTES • YIELD: 4 SERVINGS

Although sun-dried tomatoes need to be used in moderation on a ketogenic diet due to their higher carb count, a little goes a long way in this dish! This is one of the most popular recipes on my blog, ketokarma.com, and it's a favorite in our home.

4 (6-ounce) boneless, skinless chicken breast halves

1 teaspoon olive oil

Salt and pepper

4 ounces goat cheese, sliced into 4 (1-ounce) rounds

Tuscan Sauce

8 tablespoons (1 stick) unsalted butter, divided

¼ cup minced yellow onions

3 cloves garlic, minced

¼ cup fresh lemon juice

¼ cup dry white wine

4 sun-dried tomato halves, sliced (about 1¼ ounces)

6 to 8 fresh basil leaves, chopped

note *Pairs well with Mashed Cauliflower (Fauxtatoes) (page 246) or Zoodles (page 254).*

1. Preheat a grill to medium-high heat.

2. Coat each chicken breast lightly with the olive oil and season with salt and pepper.

3. Grill the chicken, flipping once, until the internal temperature reaches 165°F, 15 to 25 minutes, depending on the thickness of each breast.

4. When the chicken is almost finished cooking, top each breast with a round of goat cheese, close the grill lid, and allow the cheese to soften, 2 to 3 minutes.

5. Make the sauce: In a medium-sized saucepan over medium heat, melt 1 tablespoon of the butter. Add the onions and garlic and sauté until soft and translucent. Add the lemon juice and wine, stir, and simmer until the sauce is reduced by almost half, 4 to 5 minutes.

6. Cube the remaining 7 tablespoons of butter and add to the sauce, one cube at a time, stirring to allow each cube to melt before adding the next.

7. Add the sun-dried tomatoes, lower the heat to medium-low, and simmer for 2 to 3 minutes to reduce the sauce.

8. Add the basil, toss to combine, and remove from the heat.

9. Remove the chicken from the grill, plate, and spoon the Tuscan sauce over each breast.

per serving:

CALORIES: 511 | FAT: 37 g | PROTEIN: 41.5 g | TOTAL CARBS: 5.5 g | NET CARBS: 5.25 g

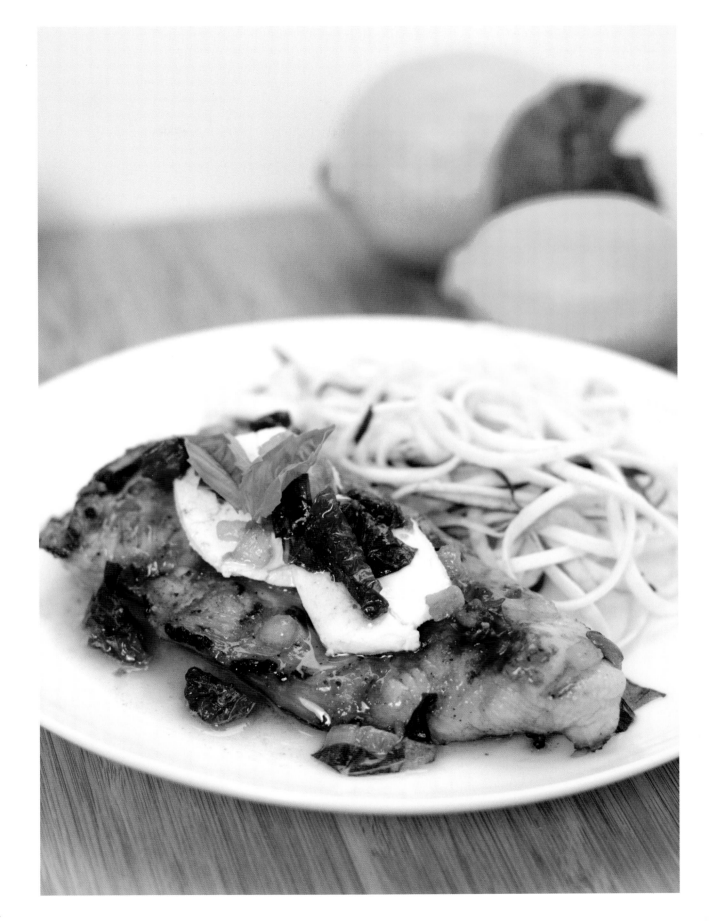

GRILLED PARMESAN GARLIC WINGS

⊘ 🍃 PREP TIME: 2 MINUTES • COOK TIME: 25 MINUTES • YIELD: 2 SERVINGS

I love chicken wings, from traditional Buffalo wings served with crunchy celery and ranch dressing to this grilled Italian-themed version. Feel free to switch up the seasonings in the sauce or just go for a basic Buffalo sauce. Be sure to check the labels, but most store-bought Buffalo sauces are pretty low in carbs.

1 to 1¼ pounds chicken wings

1 tablespoon avocado oil

Salt and pepper

Sauce

3 tablespoons unsalted butter, melted

¼ cup finely grated Parmesan cheese

½ teaspoon Italian seasoning

½ teaspoon fresh lemon juice

1 small clove garlic, minced

Shredded Parmesan cheese, for garnish (optional)

Thinly sliced green onions, for garnish (optional)

2 tablespoons chopped fresh parsley, for garnish (optional)

Lemon wedges, for serving (optional)

1 Preheat a grill to medium-high heat.

2 In a large mixing bowl, toss the wings with the avocado oil, then season lightly with salt and pepper.

3 Grill the wings until the internal temperature reaches 165°F (20 to 25 minutes, depending on your grill).

4 Meanwhile, make the wing sauce: In a medium-sized bowl, combine the melted butter, Parmesan cheese, Italian seasoning, lemon juice, garlic, and salt to taste.

5 As soon as you remove the wings from the grill, toss them in the sauce and and divide between 2 plates. If desired, garnish with shredded Parmesan cheese, sliced green onions, and chopped parsley, and serve with lemon wedges.

tip: If you don't have a grill, these wings can be baked in the oven. Preheat the oven to 425°F and line a rimmed baking sheet with foil or a wire rack. After completing Step 2, place the wings on the pan and bake for 30 minutes, then turn them over and bake for another 10 to 15 minutes, until the skin is crispy and the internal temperature reaches 165°F. Follow Steps 4 and 5 to complete the recipe.

per serving:

CALORIES: 738 | FAT: 61 g | PROTEIN: 47 g | TOTAL CARBS: 1 g | NET CARBS: 1 g

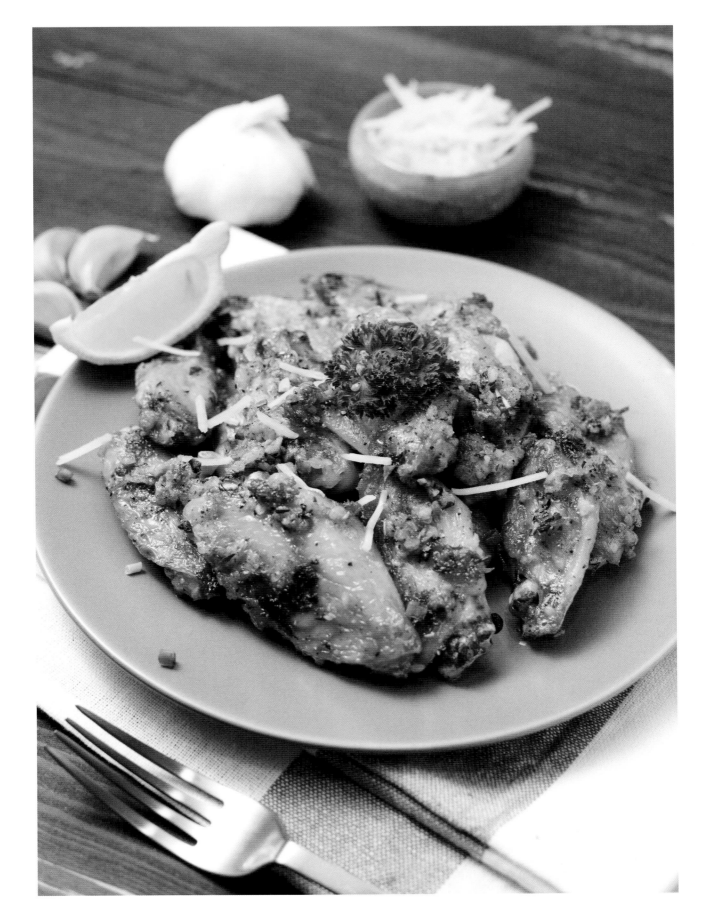

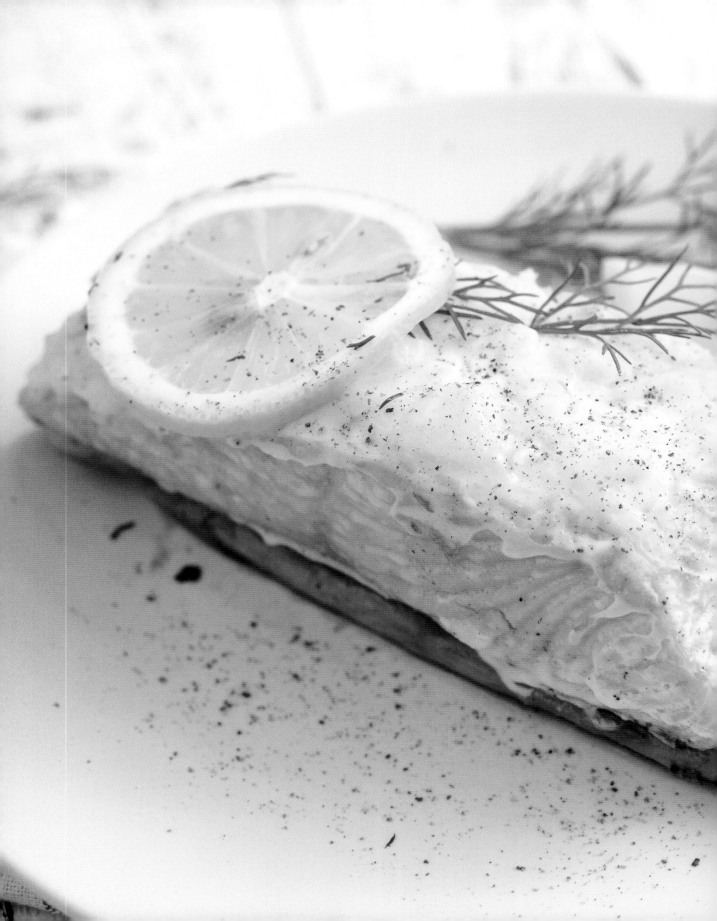

SEAFOOD

AHI TUNA POKE BOWLS WITH SPICY MAYONNAISE

⏱ 🍃 PREP TIME: 10 MINUTES • YIELD: 4 SERVINGS

Before I started keto, sushi was one of my favorite foods. While the majority of sushi rolls aren't keto-friendly, you can make a few simple modifications when dining out or preparing sushi at home to make your preferred choices lower in carbs. For starters, you can simply prepare or order sashimi, which is slices of sushi-grade raw fish. When dining out, I often ask the sushi chef to make my rolls with a cucumber wrap and without rice or sugary sauces. Last but not least, you can prepare or order a poke bowl, skip the rice, and top it with the low-carb sauce of your choice. In the recipe, I use a delicious and easy Sriracha mayonnaise.

1 pound sushi-grade ahi tuna, cut into cubes

Spicy Mayonnaise

¼ cup mayonnaise

1 to 2 tablespoons Sriracha sauce (use 1 tablespoon if you want it less spicy)

2 avocados, cut into medium dice

¼ cup sliced green onions

1 tablespoon black and/or white sesame seeds

4 cups spring greens salad mix, or 1 batch Basic Cauliflower Rice (page 242), for serving (optional)

1 Place the tuna in a medium-sized mixing bowl and set aside.

2 Make the Spicy Mayonnaise: In a small mixing bowl, combine the mayonnaise and Sriracha sauce, then mix well.

3 Pour the Spicy Mayonnaise over the tuna and gently stir to coat. Add the cubed avocados, green onions, and sesame seeds and gently stir to combine. Serve as is or over a bed of spring greens or cauliflower rice.

per serving, with spring greens and 1 tablespoon Sriracha:

CALORIES: 358 | FAT: 23 g | PROTEIN: 28 g | TOTAL CARBS: 7.8 g | NET CARBS: 2.5 g

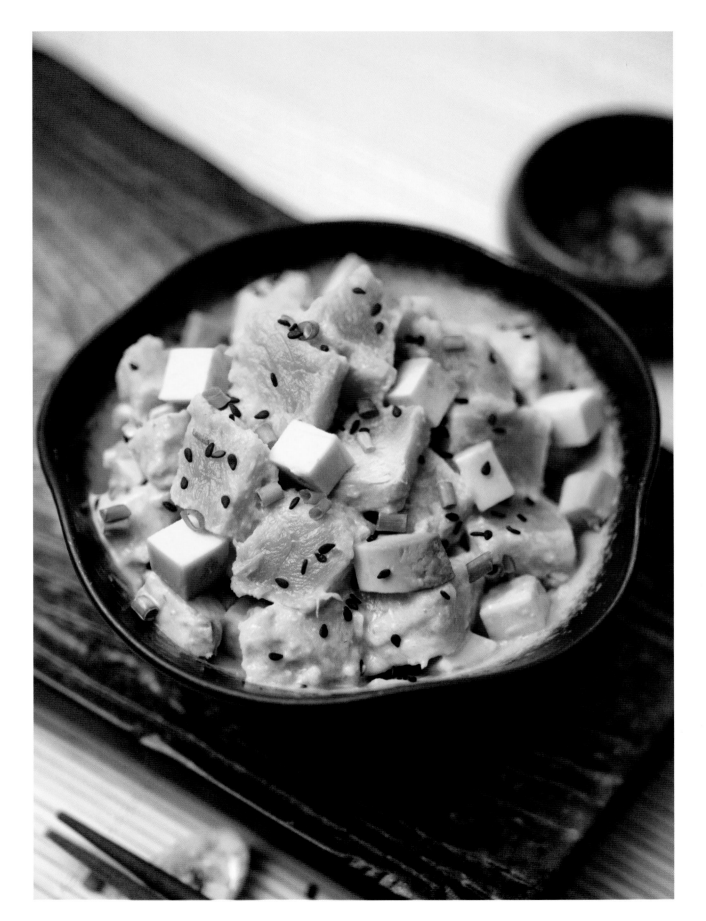

MACADAMIA NUT–CRUSTED TILAPIA

⏱ ⊘ ▯ PREP TIME: 5 MINUTES • COOK TIME: 15 MINUTES • YIELD: 2 SERVINGS

The perfect combination of flaky tilapia and a crunchy macadamia nut crust. Can we all just stop right here and take a trip to Maui?

2 (4-ounce) tilapia fillets

½ cup unsalted macadamia nuts

1 tablespoon chopped fresh parsley

1 tablespoon fresh lemon juice

2 teaspoons coconut oil

¼ teaspoon garlic powder

Lemon wedges, for serving

note: Pairs well with asparagus.

1 Preheat the oven to 400°F. Line a rimmed baking sheet with parchment paper.

2 Rinse the tilapia with cold water, pat dry with a paper towel, and place on the lined baking sheet.

3 Place the macadamia nuts, parsley, and lemon juice in a food processor and pulse/chop until the mixture is slightly chunkier than breadcrumb consistency. Be sure not to overblend, or you will end up with nut butter.

4 Top each fillet with 1 teaspoon of the coconut oil and then macadamia nut mixture, pressing it into the fish. Bake for 10 to 15 minutes, until the top is crisp and slightly golden brown. Serve with lemon wedges on the side.

per serving:

CALORIES: 383 | FAT: 32.5 g | PROTEIN: 22.5 g | TOTAL CARBS: 5.5 g | NET CARBS: 2.5 g

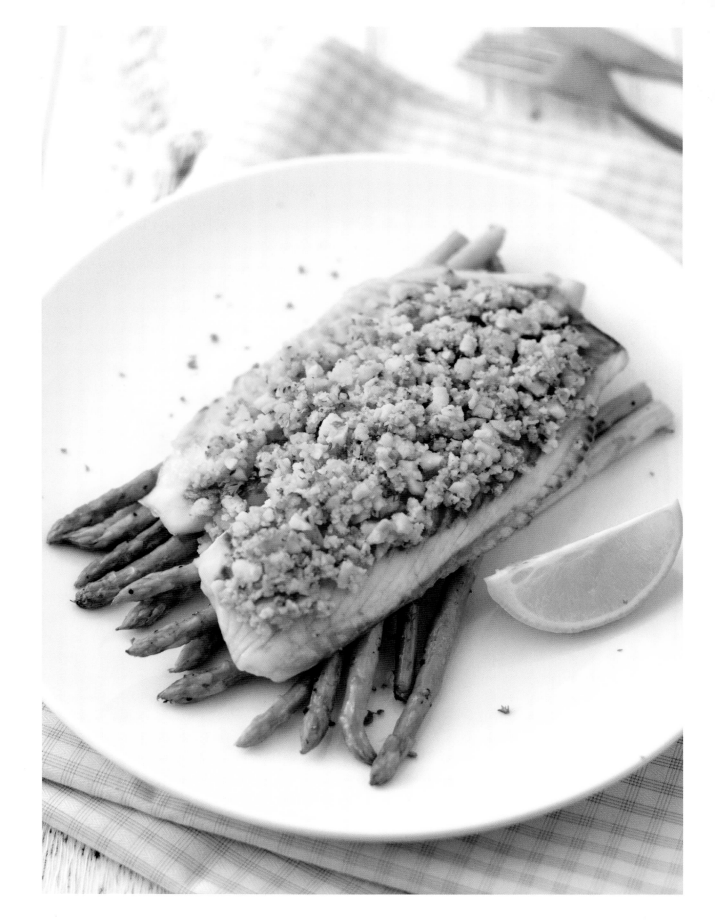

FRIED TUNA PATTIES

PREP TIME: 5 MINUTES • COOK TIME: 20 MINUTES • YIELD: 6 PATTIES (2 PER SERVING)

Tuna salad is a great choice for a quick keto meal, but if you crave a little more variety, these delicious pan fried patties are a great option.

2 large eggs

1 tablespoon fresh lemon juice

¼ cup grated Parmesan cheese

¼ cup golden flaxseed meal

2 tablespoons chopped fresh parsley

2 teaspoons Old Bay seasoning

1 (12-ounce) can white tuna, in water

¼ cup finely chopped onions

¼ teaspoon salt

¼ cup avocado oil, for frying

Lemon wedges, for serving (optional)

tip: Serve with the low-carb dipping sauce of your choice for added fat!

1 In a bowl, beat the eggs with the lemon juice.

2 Stir in the Parmesan cheese, flaxseed meal, parsley, and Old Bay seasoning.

3 Drain the tuna well, removing as much of the water as possible. Add the drained tuna and onions to the Parmesan mixture and mix well. Season with salt and pepper to taste.

4 Shape the tuna mixture into 6 patties.

5 Heat the oil in a large skillet over medium heat. When hot, add half of the patties and fry until golden brown, 3 to 5 minutes per side, then set on a paper towel–lined dish to soak up any excess oil. Repeat with the remaining patties.

6 Serve with lemon wedges, if desired.

per serving:

CALORIES: 305 | FAT: 18 g | PROTEIN: 31 g | TOTAL CARBS: 5 g | NET CARBS: 2 g

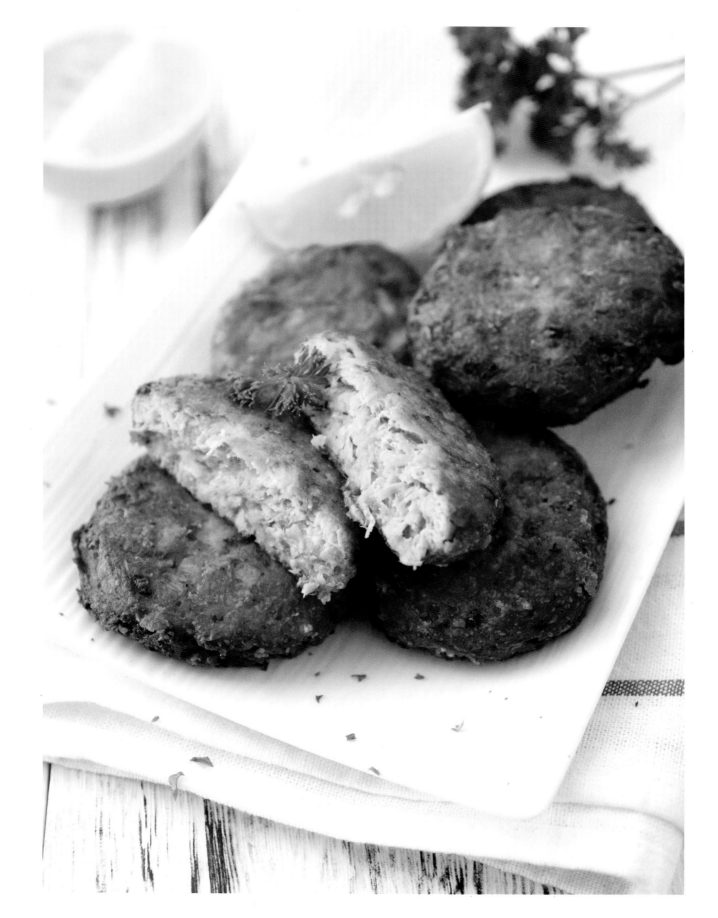

GREEK SALAD
WITH GRILLED SALMON

⏱ ⃠ ◍ PREP TIME: 15 MINUTES • COOK TIME: 8 MINUTES • YIELD: 4 SERVINGS

A fresh and flavorful salad perfect for any day of the week!

Salad

2 medium heads romaine lettuce, chopped

½ medium cucumber, chopped

¾ cup cherry tomatoes, halved

¾ cup crumbled feta cheese

½ cup pitted Kalamata olives

½ cup thinly sliced red onions

1 teaspoon dried ground oregano

Pinch of salt

Pinch of ground black pepper

Dressing

¼ cup extra-virgin olive oil

¼ cup red wine vinegar

1 large clove garlic, minced

2 teaspoons onion powder

2 teaspoons dried ground oregano

Salt and pepper

Salmon

4 (6-ounce) skin-on salmon fillets

1 tablespoon extra-virgin olive oil

Salt and pepper

1 tablespoon avocado oil or other cooking oil of choice, for the grill grates

Fresh dill, for garnish (optional)

1 In a large bowl, combine all the salad ingredients and toss. Divide the salad among 4 bowls and set aside.

2 Make the dressing: Place the olive oil, vinegar, garlic, oregano, and onion powder in a bowl and whisk to combine. Season with salt and pepper to taste and set aside.

3 Rinse the salmon and pat dry. Brush the salmon with the olive oil and season with salt and pepper.

4 Preheat a grill to medium-high heat, then brush the hot grill grates with the avocado oil.

5 Place the salmon skin side up on the grill, close the grill lid, and cook for 2 minutes. Flip the salmon and cook skin side down for 5 to 6 minutes, until the internal temperature reaches 145°F.

6 Allow the salmon to rest for a few minutes, then place a fillet on top of each salad. Whisk the salad dressing again and drizzle it over the salads. Garnish with fresh dill, if desired, and enjoy!

per serving:

CALORIES: 588 | FAT: 41.7 g | PROTEIN: 42 g | TOTAL CARBS: 10.3 g | NET CARBS: 7.8 g

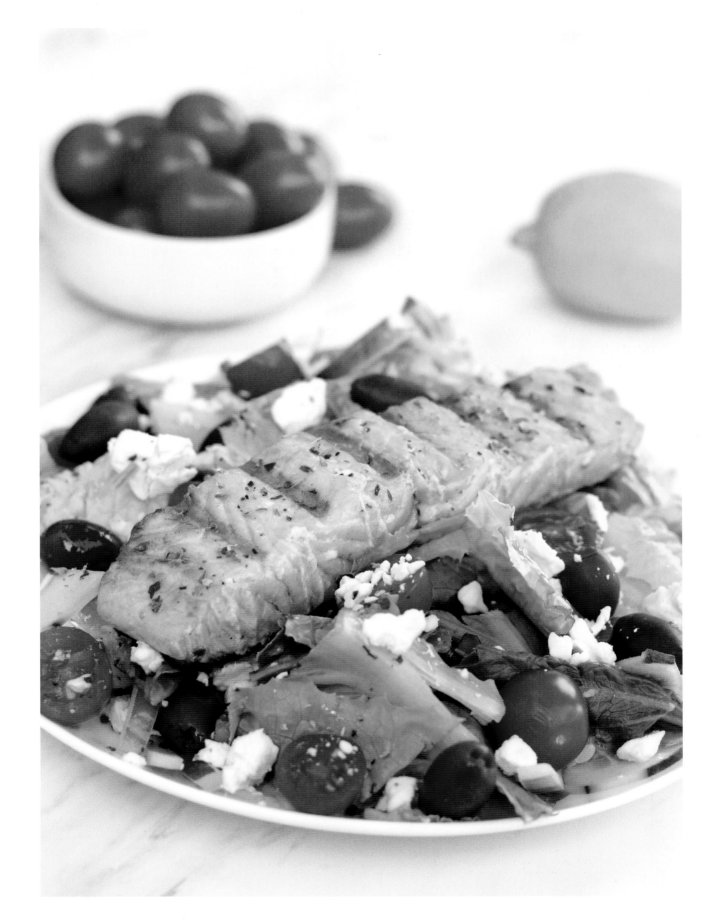

LOW-CARB CRAB CAKES

PREP TIME: 15 MINUTES, PLUS TIME TO REFRIGERATE • COOK TIME: 10 MINUTES
YIELD: 4 CRAB CAKES (1 PER SERVING)

I love crab cakes, but often they are full of breadcrumbs, so I set out to make a delicious keto-friendly version. These simple crab cakes are pan-fried until golden brown and ready in under 30 minutes!

1 large egg

¼ cup mayonnaise

1 green onion, chopped, plus extra for garnish (optional)

1 teaspoon Old Bay seasoning

1 tablespoon Dijon mustard

1 tablespoon chopped fresh parsley

1½ teaspoons fresh lemon juice

1 pound fresh lump crabmeat

¼ cup golden flaxseed meal

2 to 3 tablespoons avocado oil, for frying

Spring mix greens or arugula, for serving (optional)

Lemon wedges, for serving (optional)

note: Pairs well with Aioli (page 72).

1 In a large mixing bowl, combine the egg and mayonnaise and whisk until smooth. Add the green onion, Old Bay seasoning, mustard, parsley, and lemon juice and mix well.

2 Sort through the crabmeat to ensure that no shells remain in the meat. Then add the crabmeat to the bowl with the egg mixture and gently mix with a spoon until well blended. Be sure to mix gently so that you don't break up the crabmeat too much.

3 Gently fold in the flaxseed meal.

4 Refrigerate the mixture for 20 to 30 minutes, then use your hands to form it into four 4-ounce patties.

5 Heat the avocado oil in a large skillet over medium-high heat. When hot, add the crab cakes and pan-fry for 4 to 5 minutes on each side, until golden brown and warm throughout.

6 Serve immediately. If desired, serve each crab cake over a bed of spring mix or arugula with lemon wedges on the side and garnished with extra green onions.

per serving:

CALORIES: 331 | FAT: 22 g | PROTEIN: 28 g | TOTAL CARBS: 3.8 g | NET CARBS: 1.75 g

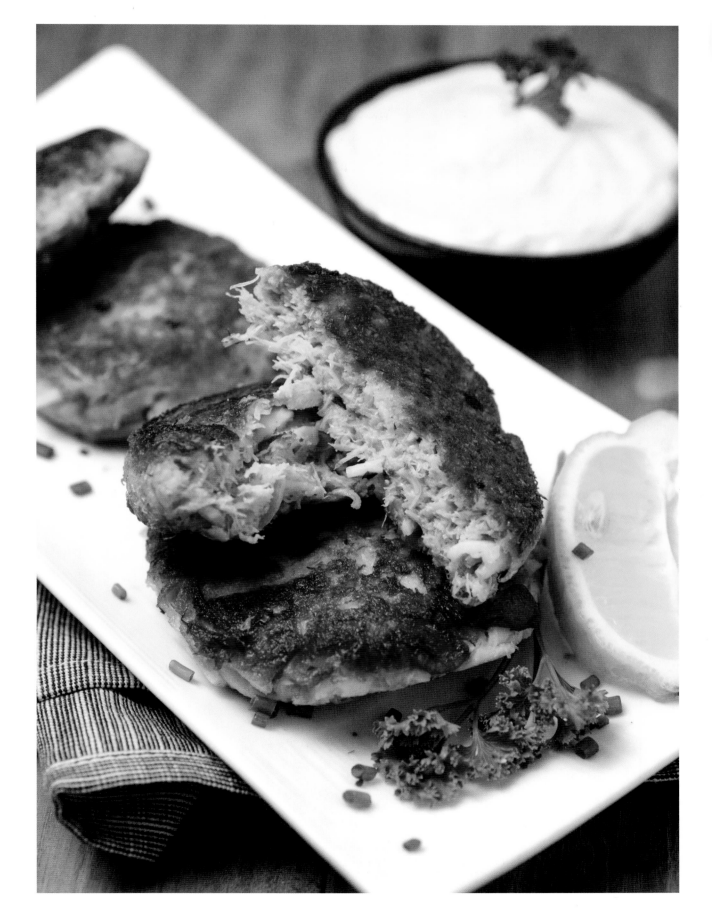

PARMESAN—CRUSTED SALMON BAKE WITH ASPARAGUS

🕐 PREP TIME: 15 MINUTES • COOK TIME: 15 MINUTES • YIELD: 4 SERVINGS

Moist and flaky salmon with a delicious Parmesan crust, paired with asparagus, all in under 30 minutes!

1½ to 2 pounds asparagus (6 to 8 spears per serving)

3 tablespoons coconut oil, melted but not hot

1 teaspoon garlic powder

⅓ cup grated Parmesan cheese

¼ cup plus 2 tablespoons mayonnaise

1 clove garlic, pressed

4 salmon fillets (about 6 ounces each), rinsed and patted dry

Finely chopped fresh dill or dill sprigs, for garnish (optional)

1 lemon, sliced, for serving (optional)

1. Preheat the oven to 350°F.

2. Rinse the asparagus and trim or snap off the tough end of each spear.

3. Place the asparagus, coconut oil, and garlic powder in a zip-top plastic bag, seal, and shake lightly to coat the asparagus.

4. In a bowl, mix the Parmesan cheese, mayonnaise, and pressed garlic.

5. Lay out 4 rectangular pieces of parchment paper, large enough to fit the asparagus and fish with plenty of paper remaining on the sides and ends to fold into packets and seal. Divide the seasoned asparagus evenly among the sheets of parchment.

6. Place the fillets on top of the asparagus, skin side down. Top the salmon with the mayonnaise mixture.

7. Fold the parchment paper over the fish and seal on all sides. The packet should look like a calzone.

8. Place the packets on a rimmed baking sheet and bake for 12 to 15 minutes, until the internal temperature of the salmon reaches 145°F.

9. Garnish with fresh dill and lemon slices, if desired.

per serving:

CALORIES: 477 | FAT: 33.3 g | PROTEIN: 38.5 g | TOTAL CARBS: 7.25 g | NET CARBS: 3.8 g

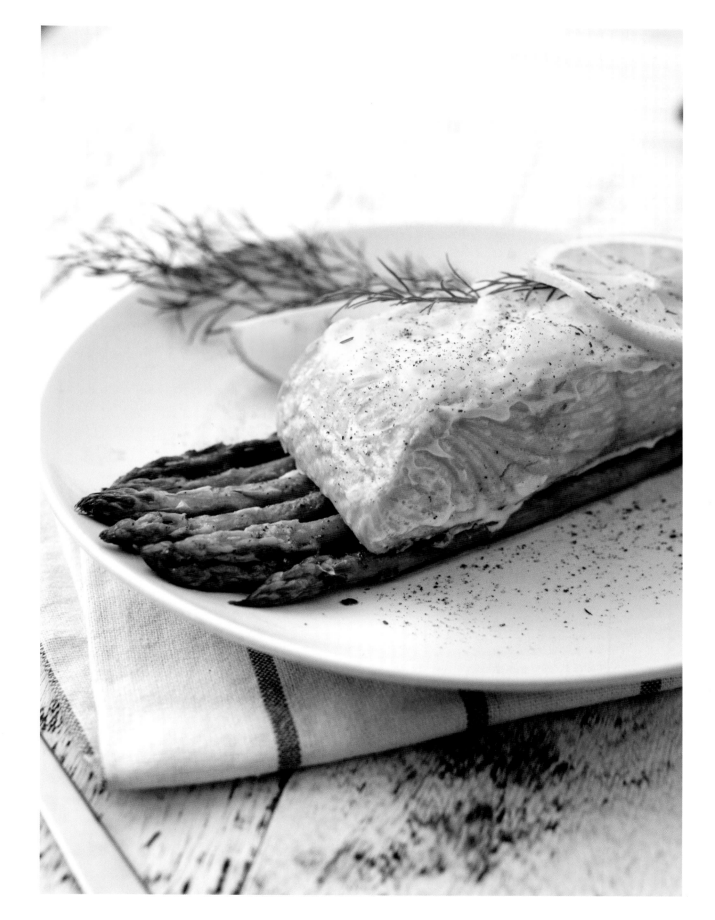

PESTO SHRIMP KABOBS

PREP TIME: 5 MINUTES, PLUS 30 MINUTES TO MARINATE • COOK TIME: 8 MINUTES • YIELD: 4 SERVINGS

Shrimp kabobs are a great alternative to chicken or steak kabobs and cook in only 4 to 8 minutes! These are great on their own or served with Mashed Cauliflower (Fauxtatoes) (page 246).

1 pound large shrimp, peeled and deveined

⅓ cup pesto, homemade (page 70) or store-bought

2 tablespoons unsalted butter

Pinch of garlic powder

Salt and pepper

Lemon slices, for garnish (optional)

Special Equipment

• 6 wood or metal skewers (soak wood skewers in water for 30 minutes before grilling to prevent them from catching fire on the grill)

1 Place the shrimp and pesto in a large zip-top plastic bag or bowl and mix well to coat the shrimp. Place in the refrigerator to marinate for 30 minutes, then thread the shrimp onto wood or metal skewers.

2 Preheat a grill to medium heat. Place the skewers on the grill and grill for 2 to 4 minutes on each side, until the shrimp have turned pink; do not overcook or they will become rubbery.

3 Place the butter and garlic powder in a small microwave-safe bowl and melt in the microwave, 15 to 20 seconds.

4 Drizzle each kabob with ½ tablespoon of the melted garlic butter. Season with salt and pepper to taste and garnish with lemon slices, if desired.

per serving:

CALORIES: 297 | FAT: 18 g | PROTEIN: 30.5 g | TOTAL CARBS: 1.3 g | NET CARBS: 1.3 g

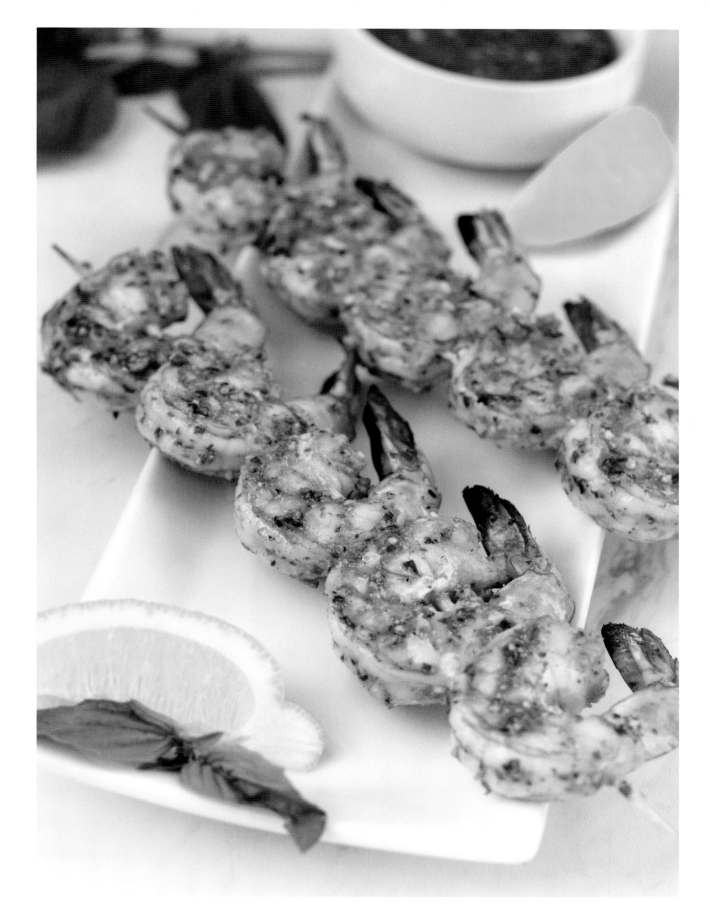

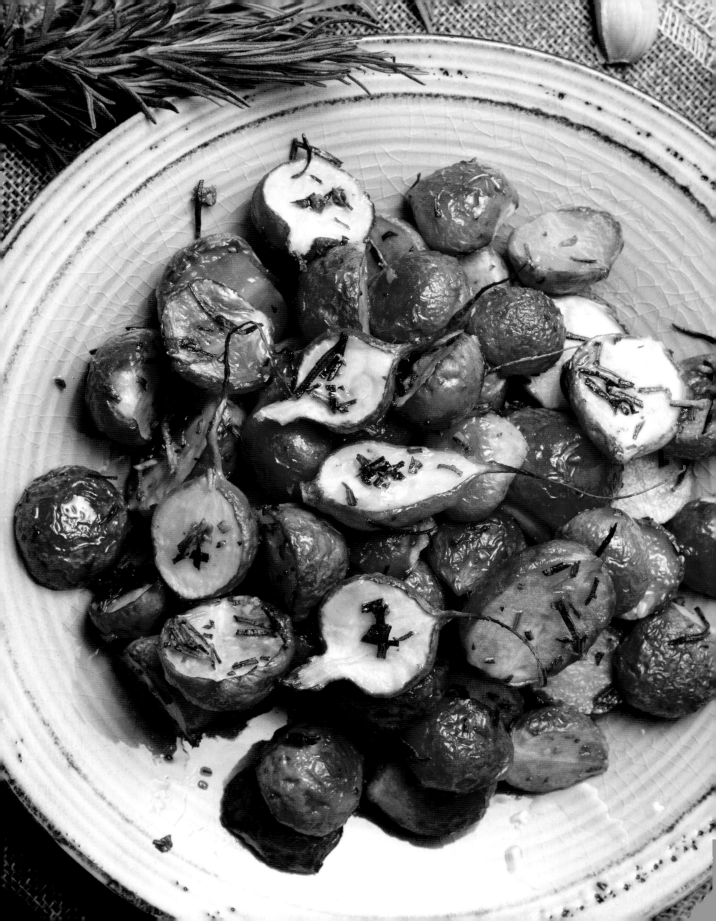

SOUPS AND SIDES

ARUGULA SALAD

 PREP TIME: 10 MINUTES • YIELD: 4 SERVINGS

A simple salad with lots of flavor and crunch!

Salad

6 cups baby arugula

1 avocado, diced

½ cup cherry tomatoes, halved

⅓ cup shaved Parmesan cheese

¼ cup thinly sliced red onions

¼ cup pili nuts or pine nuts

Dressing

3 tablespoons extra-virgin olive oil

1 tablespoon red wine vinegar

1 small clove garlic, pressed or minced

Salt and pepper, to taste

1   Place all the salad ingredients in a large bowl and gently toss.

2   In a small bowl, stir together the dressing ingredients. Toss the salad with the dressing right before serving.

per serving:

CALORIES: 275 | FAT: 23.8 g | PROTEIN: 8.8 g | TOTAL CARBS: 9 g | NET CARBS: 4 g

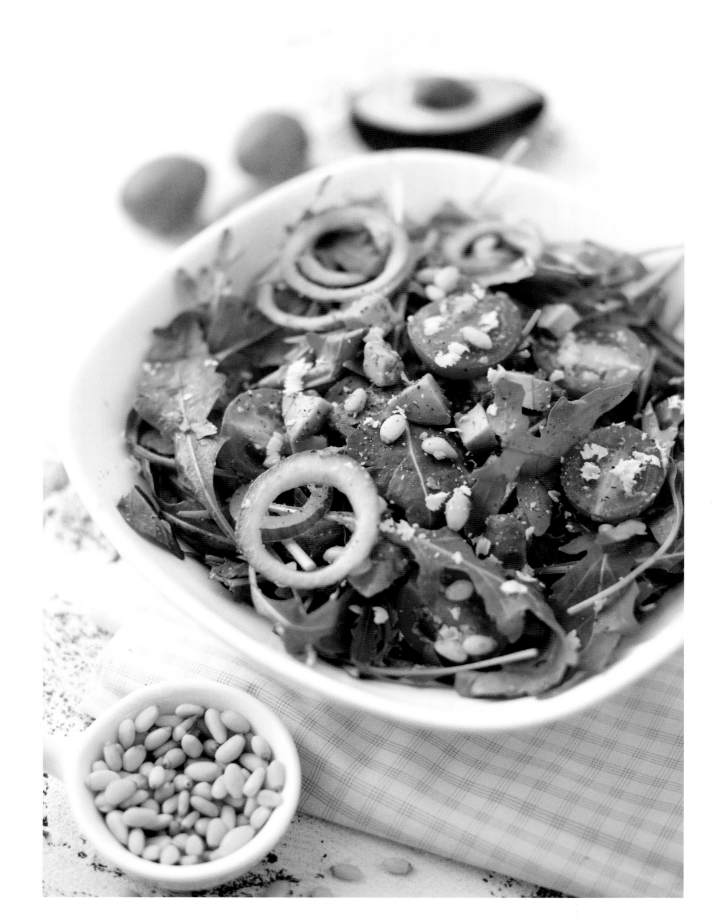

CAPRESE SALAD WITH AVOCADO

 PREP TIME: 10 MINUTES • YIELD: 5 SERVINGS (2 STACKS PER SERVING)

2 medium tomatoes, each cut into 5 slices

Coarse salt (I use pink Himalayan or sea salt)

6 ounces fresh mozzarella, cut into 10 slices

2 avocados, cut into 30 thin slices

3 to 4 large basil leaves, chopped, plus additional leaves for garnish

¼ cup extra-virgin olive oil or avocado oil

1 lime, halved

Ground black pepper

Italian seasoning (optional)

1   Lay the tomato slices on a serving plate and sprinkle with salt. On top of each tomato, stack a mozzarella slice, 3 avocado slices, and some chopped basil.

2   Drizzle with the oil and squeeze some lime juice over the top. Sprinkle with pepper and Italian seasoning, if using. Garnish each stack with a basil leaf, if desired.

per serving:

CALORIES: 283 | FAT: 25.6 g | PROTEIN: 7.6 g | TOTAL CARBS: 8 g | NET CARBS: 3.4 g

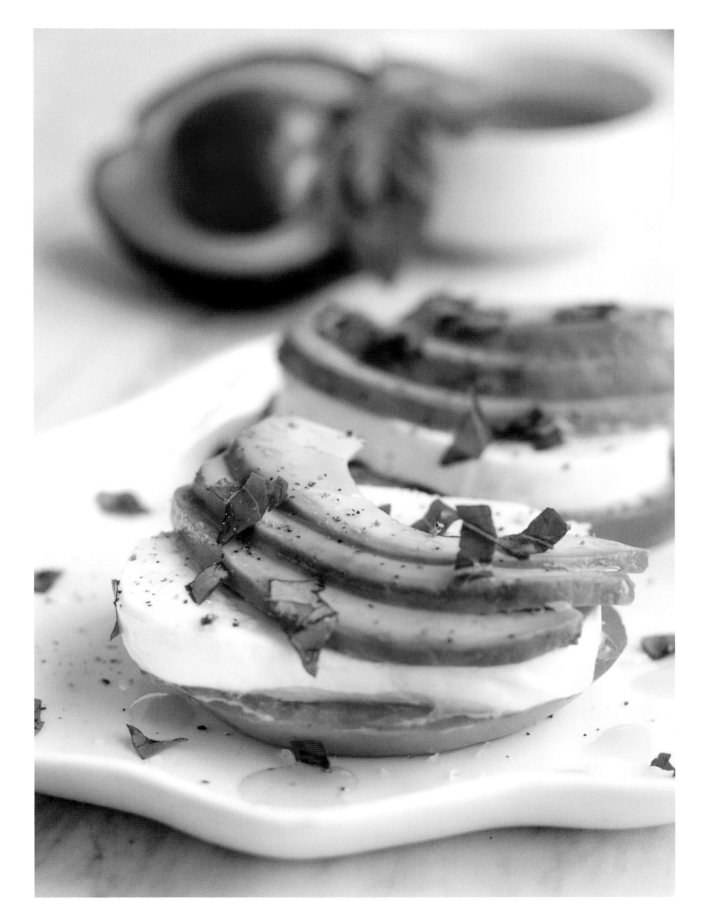

MIKE'S CUCUMBER SALAD WITH FETA

⏱ ⊘ ◐ PREP TIME: 10 MINUTES • YIELD: 5 SERVINGS

Our good friend Mike always prepares this fresh and delicious cucumber salad at his barbecues. I love that it's quick and simple to make, and it pairs perfectly with a variety of proteins, like chicken, burgers, or steak!

2 medium-large cucumbers

½ cup thinly sliced red onions

4 ounces feta cheese, crumbled

Salt and pepper

Dressing

¼ cup extra-virgin olive oil

1 tablespoon red wine vinegar

1 tablespoon Swerve confectioners'-style sweetener

½ teaspoon dried ground oregano

1 Peel the cucumbers as desired and cut in half lengthwise, then slice.

2 In a medium-sized bowl, toss the cucumbers with the onions. Add the feta and gently toss to combine.

3 Make the dressing: Place all the ingredients in a small bowl and whisk to combine.

4 Serve right away or place in the refrigerator to chill before serving. To serve, gently toss the salad with the dressing and season to taste with salt and pepper.

per serving:

CALORIES: 171 | FAT: 15.4 g | PROTEIN: 4.6 g | TOTAL CARBS: 6.4 g | NET CARBS: 3.6 g

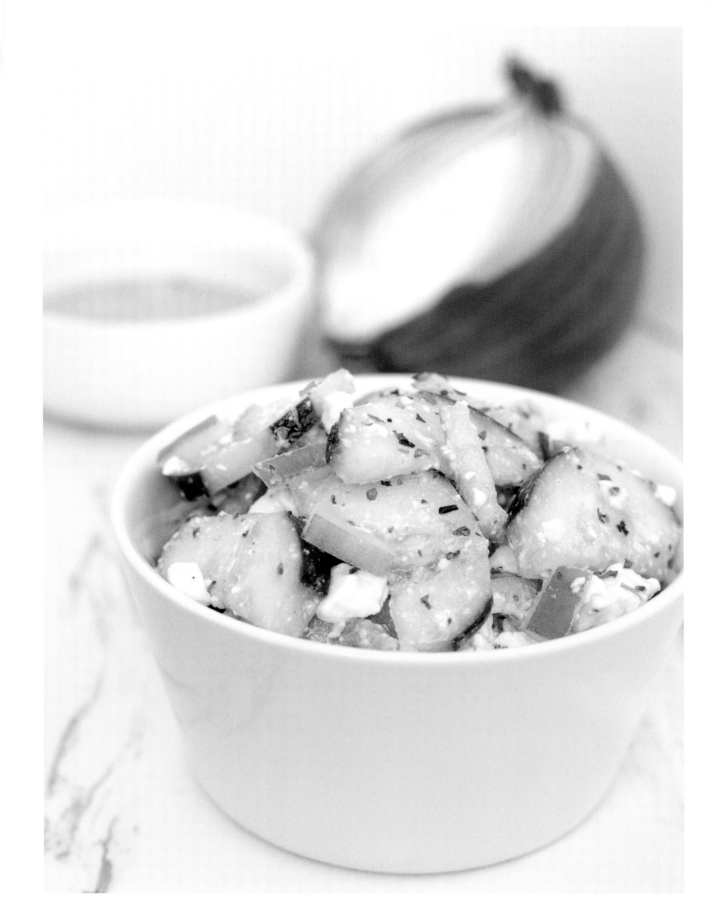

SPINACH COBB SALAD

🕐 PREP TIME: 15 MINUTES • YIELD: 4 SERVINGS

This salad is loaded with everything you could ever want in a salad, from crispy bacon and creamy avocado to pecans for a nice crunch! Toss the salad ingredients together for a quick meal, as described below, or take a little extra time to arrange the ingredients artfully, as shown in the photo opposite.

8 cups baby spinach

4 slices bacon, pan-fried and chopped

3 large eggs, hard-boiled and sliced

10 grape tomatoes, halved

2 avocados, sliced or cubed

½ medium red onion, thinly sliced

½ cup sliced white mushrooms

⅓ cup chopped pecans

Ground black pepper

¾ cup ranch or blue cheese dressing

1 In a large bowl, gently toss the spinach, bacon, hard-boiled eggs, tomatoes, avocados, onion, mushrooms, and pecans. Season with pepper to taste.

2 Top with the dressing just before serving.

per serving:

CALORIES: 403 | FAT: 34.5 g | PROTEIN: 13 g | TOTAL CARBS: 11.2 g | NET CARBS: 7.5 g

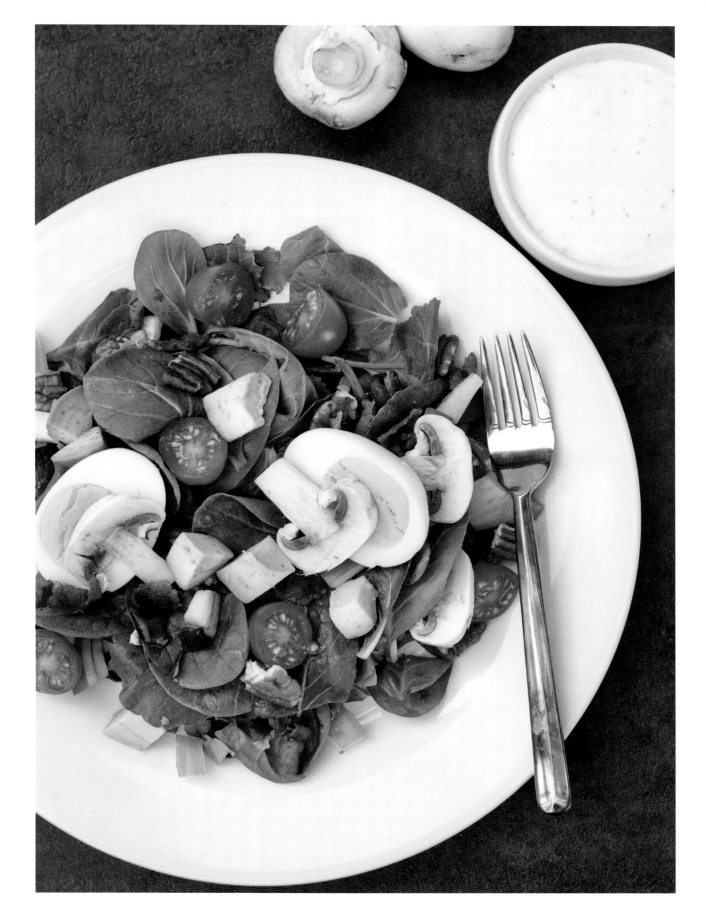

EGG DROP SOUP

PREP TIME: 5 MINUTES • COOK TIME: 5 MINUTES • YIELD: 4 SERVINGS

A delicious and simple soup made with only six ingredients and ready in 10 minutes for a light lunch or starter course.

4 cups chicken broth

2 tablespoons unsalted butter

3 large eggs

Salt and pepper

1 green onion, sliced, for garnish

1. In a medium-sized pot over high heat, bring the chicken broth and butter to a boil.

2. Crack the eggs into a bowl, beat with a fork, and set aside.

3. Once the broth is boiling, slowly stir in the beaten eggs, then remove the pot from the heat. Season with salt and pepper to taste.

4. Serve garnished with the sliced green onion.

per serving:

CALORIES: 155 | FAT: 9.5 g | PROTEIN: 9.5 g | TOTAL CARBS: 1 g | NET CARBS: 1 g

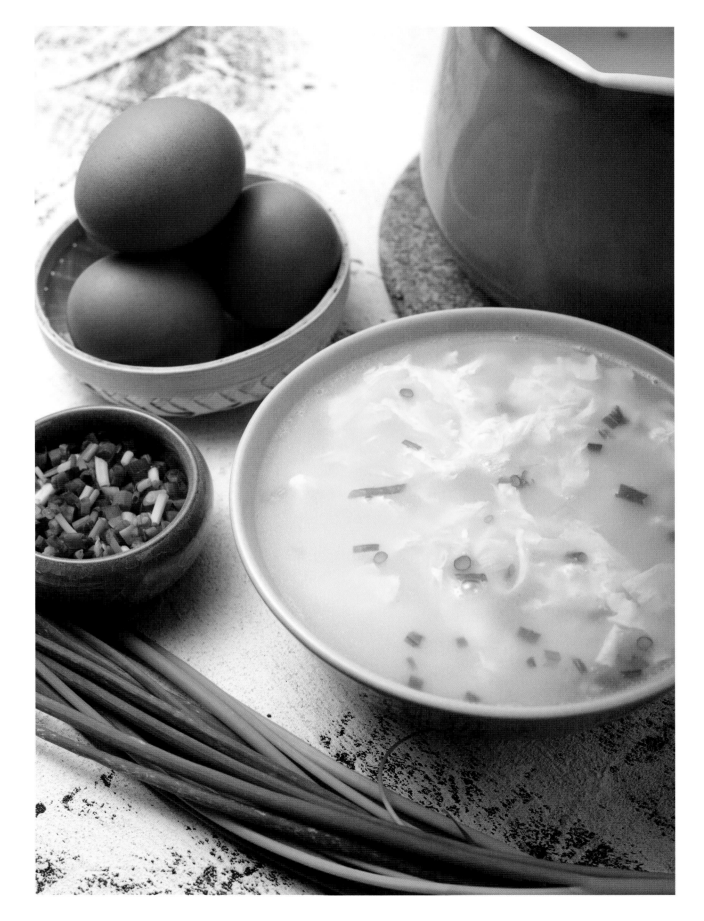

SLOW COOKER LOADED CAULIFLOWER SOUP

PREP TIME: 15 MINUTES • COOK TIME: 4 OR 8 HOURS
YIELD: 10 CUP SERVINGS (1 CUP EACH) OR 5 BOWL SERVINGS (2 CUPS EACH)

By now you know that cauliflower is a fan favorite in the keto community. Cauliflower is the perfect ingredient for this creamy and delicious soup that practically makes itself.

10 slices bacon (see tip)

2 large or 3 small heads cauliflower

4 cups chicken broth

½ large yellow onion, chopped (about 1⅓ cups)

3 cloves garlic, pressed

¼ cup (½ stick) salted butter

2 cups shredded cheddar cheese, plus extra for garnish

1 cup heavy whipping cream

Salt and pepper

Snipped fresh chives or sliced green onions, for garnish (optional)

tip: Use precooked bacon or bacon crumbles as a shortcut.

1 Fry the bacon in a large skillet over medium heat. Transfer to a paper towel–lined plate, allow to cool, and then chop. Set aside in the refrigerator.

2 Core the heads of cauliflower and cut the cauliflower into florets. Place the florets in a food processor and chop into small to medium-sized pieces. (Don't rice it.)

3 In a large slow cooker (I use a 5½-quart slow cooker), combine the chicken broth, onion, garlic, butter, and cauliflower. Stir, cover, and cook on high for 4 hours or on low for 8 hours.

4 Once the cauliflower is tender, switch the slow cooker to the keep warm setting and use a whisk to stir and mash the cauliflower to a smooth consistency.

5 Add about three-quarters of the chopped bacon, the cheese, and the cream. Season with salt and pepper to taste. Stir well until the cheese is melted.

6 Serve garnished with additional cheese, the remaining bacon, and chives or green onions, if desired.

per serving:

CALORIES: 282 | FAT: 22 g | PROTEIN: 12 g | TOTAL CARBS: 8 g | NET CARBS: 6 g

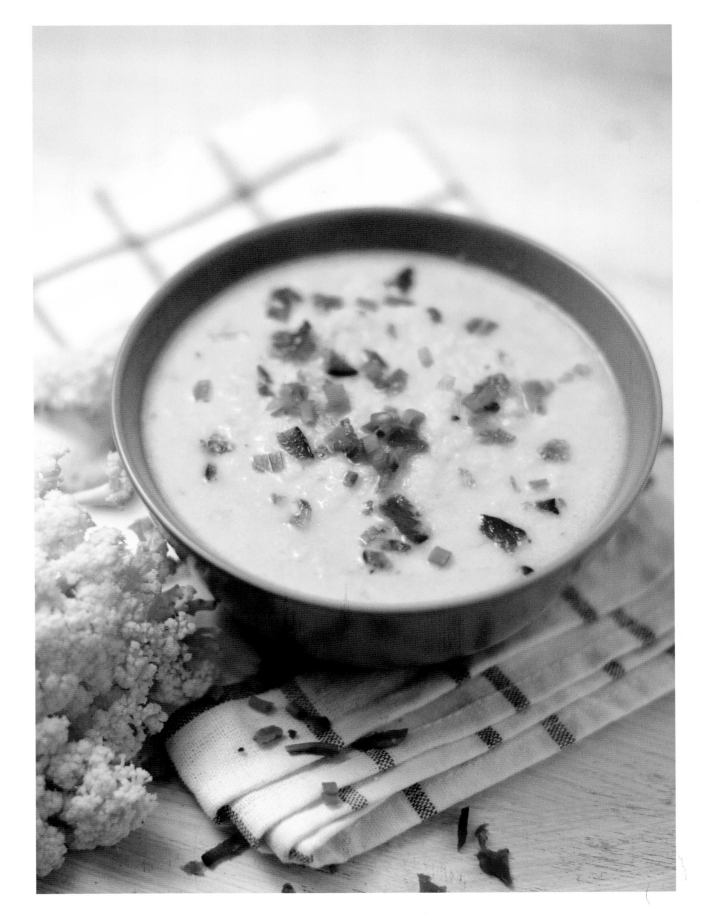

CAULIFLOWER RICE–THREE WAYS

PREP TIME: 5 MINUTES • COOK TIME: 11 MINUTES • YIELD: 4 SERVINGS EACH

Who knew that cauliflower could be transformed into so many different dishes? Cauliflower rice is a handy alternative to regular white or brown rice, and it can be flavored in a variety of ways. These are three of my favorites.

BASIC CAULIFLOWER RICE

1 medium head cauliflower

2 tablespoons unsalted butter

1 clove garlic, minced

Salt and pepper

1 Core the cauliflower and set the florets aside.

2 Use a food processor or grater to rice the cauliflower. (Be careful not to chop it too finely if using a food processor.)

3 In a large skillet over medium-high heat, melt the butter. Add the garlic and sauté for 1 minute. Add the riced cauliflower, reduce the heat to medium, and cook for 10 minutes or until the cauliflower rice is crisp-tender and warm throughout. Season with salt and pepper to taste.

per serving:

CALORIES: 81.3 | FAT: 6 g | PROTEIN: 2.3 g | TOTAL CARBS: 6 g | NET CARBS: 3.5 g

FRIED CAULIFLOWER RICE

1 medium head cauliflower

3 tablespoons unsalted butter, divided

1 clove garlic, minced

Salt and pepper

3 large eggs

4 green onions, thinly sliced, plus extra for garnish

2 to 3 tablespoons soy sauce (see note)

2 tablespoons sesame seeds, plus extra for garnish

1 teaspoon Sriracha sauce (optional)

Mick's Spicy Aioli (page 78), for serving (optional)

note: Gluten-free soy sauce is available if you are avoiding gluten.

1 Core the cauliflower and set the florets aside.

2 Use a food processor or grater to rice the cauliflower. (Be careful not to chop it too finely if using a food processor.)

3 In a large skillet over medium-high heat, melt 2 tablespoons of the butter. Add the garlic and sauté for 1 minute. Add the riced cauliflower, reduce the heat to medium, and cook for 10 minutes or until the cauliflower rice is crisp-tender and warm throughout. Season with salt and pepper to taste.

4 In a separate pan, melt the remaining 1 tablespoon of butter and scramble the eggs. Add the cooked eggs to the cauliflower rice.

5 Add the green onions, soy sauce, sesame seeds, and Sriracha sauce, if using, and toss to combine. Serve as is or top with Spicy Aioli. Garnish with sliced green onions and sesame seeds.

per serving:

CALORIES: 170 | FAT: 11.8 g | PROTEIN: 8.5 g | TOTAL CARBS: 9.2 g | NET CARBS: 6 g

CILANTRO LIME CAULIFLOWER RICE

1 medium head cauliflower

2 tablespoons unsalted butter

1 clove garlic, minced

Salt and pepper

¼ cup chopped fresh cilantro, plus extra for garnish

Juice of 1 lime

Lime wedges, for garnish (optional)

1 Core the cauliflower and set the florets aside.

2 Use a food processor or grater to rice the cauliflower. (Be careful not to chop it too finely if using a food processor.)

3 In a large skillet over medium-high heat, melt the butter. Add the garlic and sauté for 1 minute. Add the riced cauliflower, reduce the heat to medium, and cook for 10 minutes, until the cauliflower rice is crisp-tender and warm throughout. Season with salt and pepper to taste.

4 Remove from the heat and add the cilantro and lime juice. Stir to incorporate, then garnish with cilantro and lime slices, if desired.

per serving:

CALORIES: 84 | FAT: 6 g | PROTEIN: 2.3 g | TOTAL CARBS: 6.7 g | NET CARBS: 4.2 g

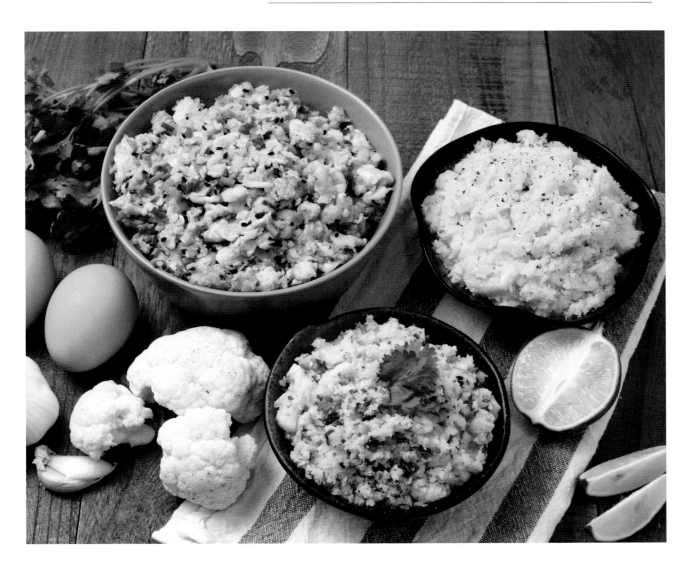

CREAMED SPINACH

PREP TIME: 5 MINUTES • COOK TIME: 5 MINUTES • YIELD: 4 SERVINGS

Sometimes you need a quick and easy side dish. While there are many ways to make creamed spinach, this method is quick and delicious!

1 tablespoon unsalted butter

1 clove garlic, minced

9 ounces fresh spinach, chopped

2 ounces cream cheese

½ cup grated Parmesan cheese

2 tablespoons heavy whipping cream

Salt and pepper

1 In a large pot over medium heat, combine the butter and garlic. Sauté, stirring frequently, for 3 to 4 minutes, until fragrant.

2 Add the spinach and cream cheese and use a spatula to combine.

3 Stir in the Parmesan cheese and cream. Bring to a simmer and cook, stirring, for about 1 minute to reduce a bit.

4 Remove from the heat and season with salt and pepper to taste before serving.

per serving:

CALORIES: 172 | FAT: 14 g | PROTEIN: 7 g | TOTAL CARBS: 4 g | NET CARBS: 2.5 g

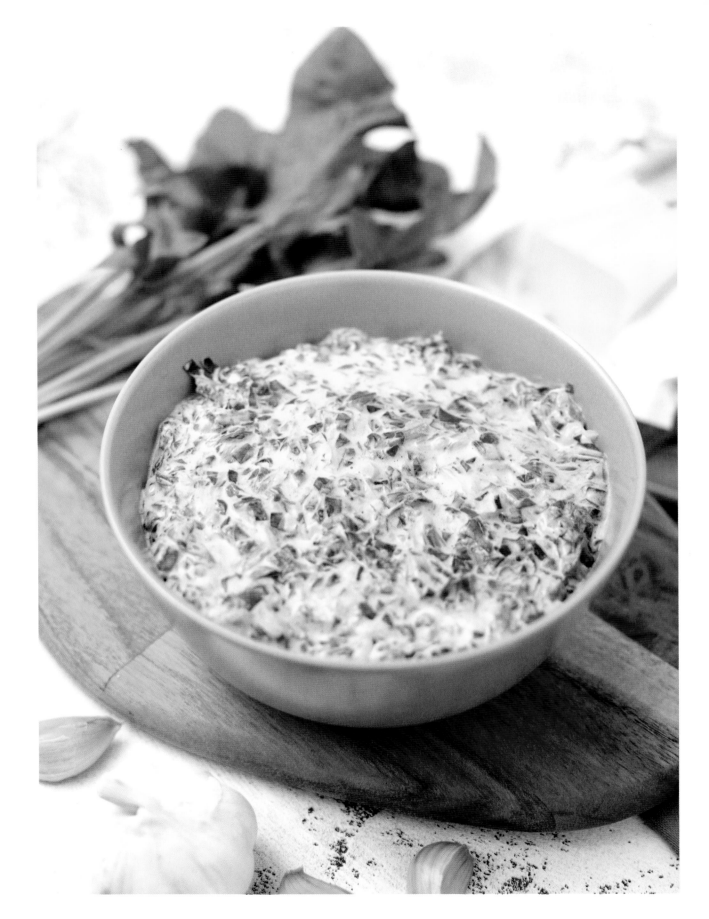

MASHED CAULIFLOWER (FAUXTATOES)

PREP TIME: 5 MINUTES • COOK TIME: 20 MINUTES • YIELD: 4 SERVINGS

With recipes like this, who needs potatoes? The key to success with mashed cauliflower is to boil the cauliflower for an extended period. When you allow the cauliflower to get super-tender, there is no need for a food processor; you can easily stir and mash the cauliflower into the perfect smooth consistency using a potato masher or whisk.

1 medium head cauliflower

Salt

3 ounces cream cheese, softened

3 tablespoons unsalted butter, softened

2 tablespoons heavy whipping cream

½ teaspoon garlic powder

Pepper

1   Core and stem the cauliflower and chop the cauliflower into small pieces.

2   Bring a large pot of salted water to a boil. Add the cauliflower and cook until tender, about 20 minutes. Drain.

3   In a large bowl, combine the cream cheese and butter. Add the drained cauliflower and use a whisk or potato masher to blend well and mash into a puree.

4   Stir in the cream and garlic powder and season to taste with salt and pepper.

per serving:

CALORIES: 205 | FAT: 18.3 g | PROTEIN: 3.8 g | TOTAL CARBS: 7 g | NET CARBS: 4.5 g

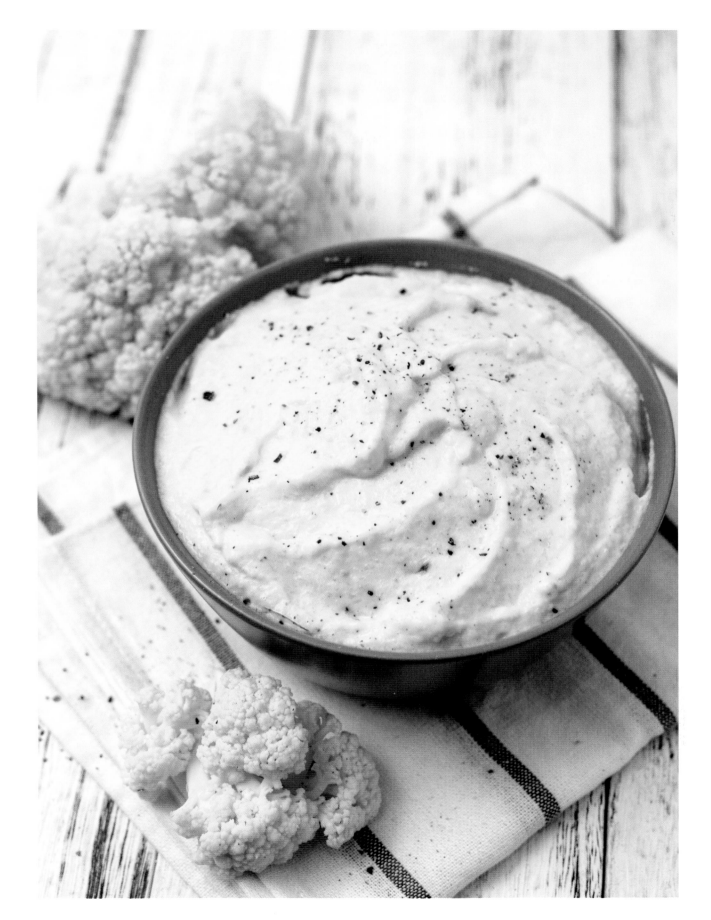

ROASTED BROCCOLI

PREP TIME: 10 MINUTES • COOK TIME: 20 MINUTES • YIELD: 4 SERVINGS

A simple and delicious alternative to basic steamed broccoli.

1½ pounds broccoli, cut into bite-sized florets

¼ cup extra-virgin olive oil

Juice of ½ lemon

2 cloves garlic, minced

Salt and pepper

Red pepper flakes (optional)

1 Preheat the oven to 400°F.

2 In a large mixing bowl, combine the broccoli, oil, lemon juice, and garlic and toss until well coated. Season lightly with salt, black pepper, and red pepper flakes, if using.

3 Pour onto a rimmed baking sheet and spread out in a single layer. Bake for 18 to 20 minutes, until lightly golden brown.

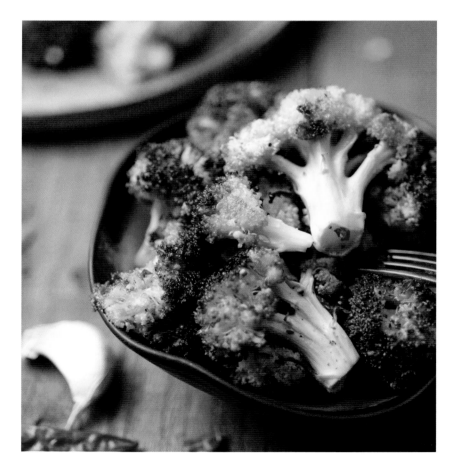

per serving:

CALORIES: 133 | FAT: 14 g | PROTEIN: 1 g | TOTAL CARBS: 3.6 g | NET CARBS: 2.5 g

ROASTED RADISHES

PREP TIME: 15 MINUTES • COOK TIME: 35 MINUTES • YIELD: 4 SERVINGS

If you are missing potatoes, give this recipe a try. These roasted radishes remind me of little red potatoes and are just as easy to prepare, yet they are low in carbs!

2 to 3 bunches radishes (1 to 1½ pounds), trimmed and halved (or quartered if large)

¼ cup avocado oil or other cooking oil of choice

1 clove garlic, pressed, or ½ teaspoon garlic powder

1 tablespoon chopped fresh rosemary

Salt

1. Preheat the oven to 425°F. Line a baking dish with parchment paper.

2. In a medium-sized mixing bowl, combine the radishes and oil and toss well. Add the garlic and rosemary, season lightly with salt, and toss again.

3. Pour the seasoned radishes into the lined baking dish and spread out in an even layer. Roast for 15 minutes, flip the radishes over, and roast for another 15 to 20 minutes, or until lightly golden brown. If desired, turn the oven to broil and broil the radishes for 2 to 3 minutes for extra crunch.

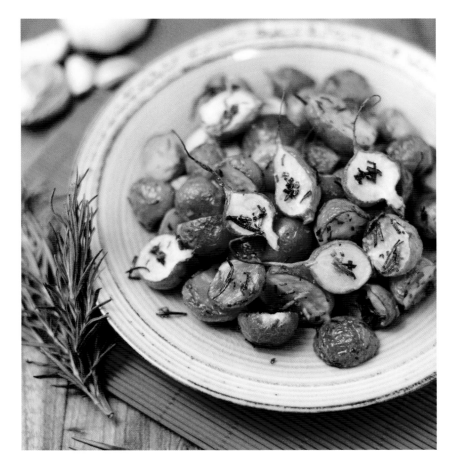

per serving: CALORIES: 133 | FAT: 14 g | PROTEIN: 0.5 g | TOTAL CARBS: 1.8 g | NET CARBS: 1.3 g

SIMPLY ROASTED BRUSSELS SPROUTS

PREP TIME: 5 MINUTES • COOK TIME: 35 MINUTES • YIELD: 4 SERVINGS

My good friends Jessica and Dan introduced me to cooking Brussels sprouts this way, and I haven't looked back since! Perfectly seasoned and roasted golden brown, these Brussels are super-easy to make and absolutely delicious.

1 pound Brussels sprouts, trimmed and halved lengthwise

3 tablespoons coconut oil, melted

Salt and pepper

Mick's Spicy Aioli (page 78), for serving (optional)

1 Preheat the oven to 350°F. Line a rimmed baking sheet with parchment paper.

2 In a large bowl, combine the Brussels sprouts and melted coconut oil. Toss to coat.

3 Pour the oiled Brussels sprouts onto the lined baking sheet in a single layer. Season lightly with salt and pepper.

4 Bake for 35 minutes, or until lightly golden in color. Serve with spicy aioli, if desired.

per serving:

CALORIES: 139 | FAT: 10.8 g | PROTEIN: 3 g | TOTAL CARBS: 10.3 g | NET CARBS: 6 g

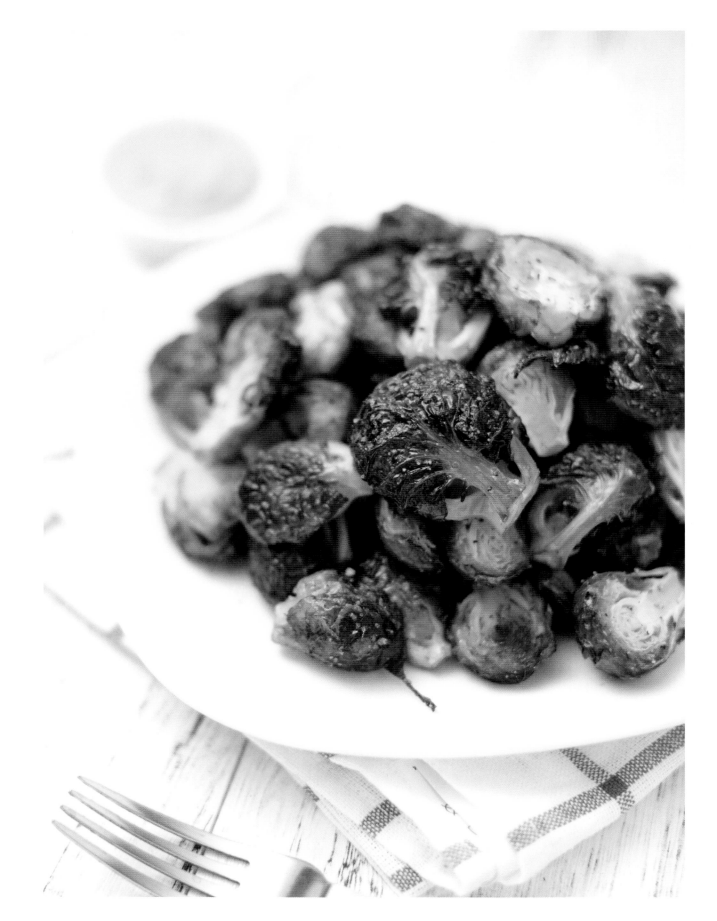

TWICE-BAKED CAULIFLOWER CASSEROLE

PREP TIME: 5 MINUTES • COOK TIME: 45 MINUTES • YIELD: 9 SERVINGS

"Twice-baked cauliflower" is a play on words, as its ingredients mimic those in a twice-baked potato. This recipe is the epitome of home-cooked comfort food, and it's on a weekly rotation in our house. I hope you love it as much as we do!

6 slices bacon (see tip)

1 large head cauliflower

Salt

½ cup sour cream

4 ounces cream cheese, softened

⅓ cup grated Parmesan cheese

¼ cup chopped green onions, plus extra for garnish

1 teaspoon garlic powder, or 1 or 2 cloves garlic, pressed

Pepper

1 cup shredded cheddar cheese

tip: You can use a small bag of precooked bacon bits or pieces (nitrate-free if possible) instead of frying the bacon if you're in a hurry!

1 Fry the bacon in a large skillet over medium heat. Transfer to a paper towel–lined plate, allow to cool, and then chop.

2 Core the cauliflower and chop the florets into small pieces.

3 In a large pot of boiling salted water, boil the cauliflower until soft, 15 to 18 minutes for a chunkier texture or 20 to 22 minutes for a super-smooth texture.

4 Meanwhile, in a large mixing bowl, combine the sour cream, cream cheese, Parmesan cheese, green onions, garlic powder, and two-thirds of the bacon.

5 Preheat the oven to 350°F.

6 Drain the cauliflower well, then pour the cauliflower over the cream cheese mixture in the bowl. Mash with a potato masher or whisk until the consistency is to your liking. Season to taste with salt and pepper.

7 Spread the cauliflower mixture evenly in an 8-inch square casserole dish. Top with the cheddar cheese and remaining bacon.

8 Bake for 15 to 20 minutes, until the cheese is melted. Garnish with chopped green onions before serving.

per serving:

CALORIES: 230 | FAT: 20 g | PROTEIN: 9 g | TOTAL CARBS: 6 g | NET CARBS: 4 g

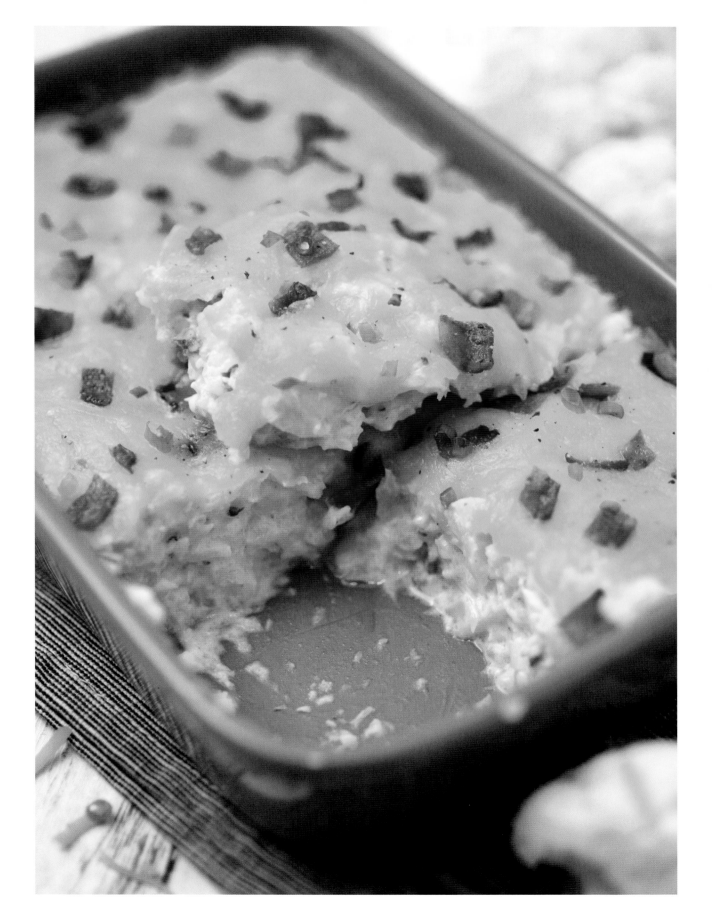

ZOODLES (SPIRALIZED ZUCCHINI NOODLES)

⏱ ⊘ ◐ PREP TIME: 5 MINUTES • COOK TIME: 1 TO 5 MINUTES • YIELD: 2 SERVINGS

Zucchini noodles, also known as zoodles, are the perfect substitute for pasta. They can be eaten plain or topped with sauce. My favorite way to prepare them is to add Alfredo sauce, pesto, or marinara to the pan with the zoodles as they cook.

2 to 3 medium zucchini

2 tablespoons unsalted butter

1 small clove garlic, pressed

Salt and pepper

Special Equipment
• Spiral slicer

1 Rinse the zucchini and cut off both ends. Using a spiral slicer, turn the zucchini to create noodles.

2 Preheat a large skillet over medium heat. Add the butter and garlic and cook for just under a minute. Add the zucchini noodles and toss to coat in the garlic butter.

3 Cook for 1 to 5 minutes, depending on how well cooked you like your zoodles. Season with salt and pepper to taste and serve.

per serving:

CALORIES: 137 | FAT: 12 g | PROTEIN: 2.5 g | TOTAL CARBS: 6.5 g | NET CARBS: 4.5 g

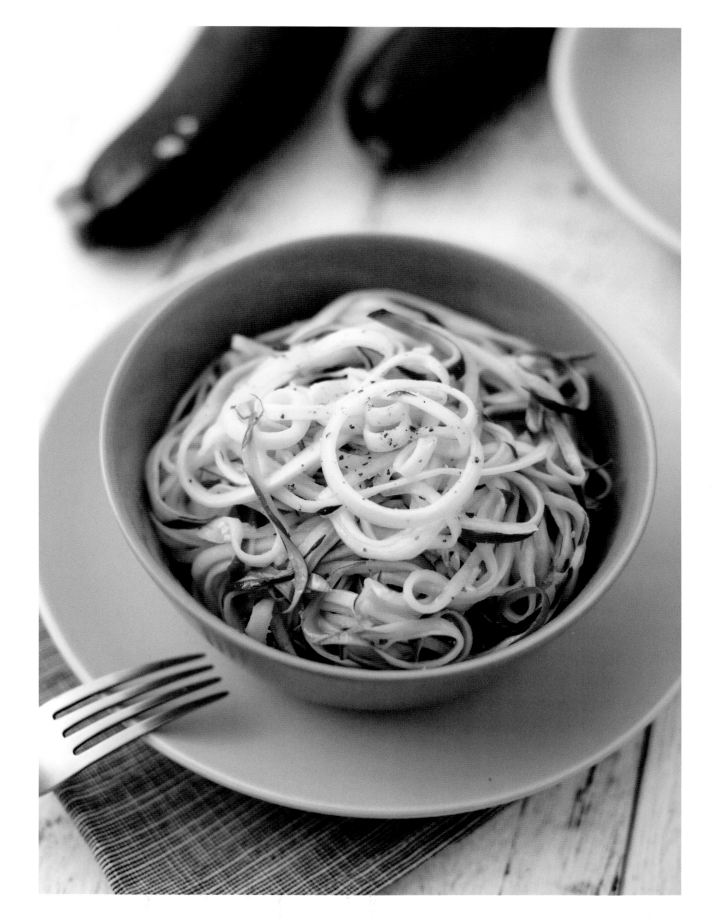

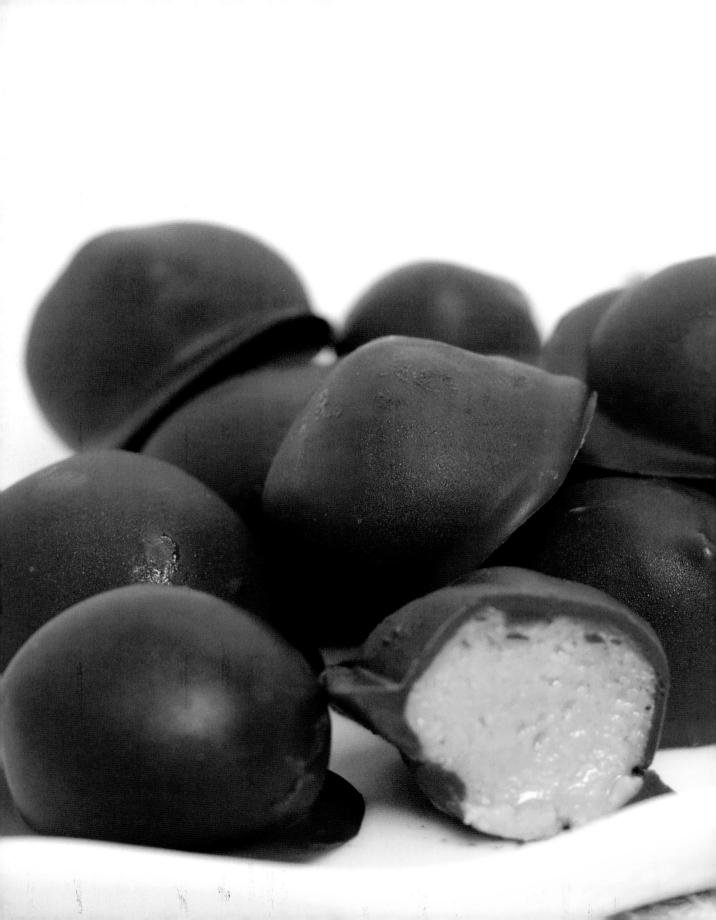

DESSERTS AND DRINKS

BROWNIES

PREP TIME: 10 MINUTES • COOK TIME: 40 MINUTES • YIELD: 16 SERVINGS

Serve these warm and moist brownies as is or top them with Keto Whipped Cream (page 290) or a scoop of sugar-free vanilla ice cream.

¾ cup blanched almond flour

½ cup Swerve confectioners'-style sweetener

¼ cup unsweetened cocoa powder

1 teaspoon baking powder

¼ teaspoon salt

3 ounces cream cheese, softened

¼ cup (½ stick) unsalted butter, melted

2 large eggs, beaten

1 teaspoon vanilla extract

⅓ cup stevia-sweetened chocolate chips (see note)

Confectioners'-style Swerve sweetener, for dusting (optional)

note: I use Lily's baking chips.

1 Preheat the oven to 325°F. Spray an 8-inch square baking pan with nonstick cooking spray.

2 In a medium-sized mixing bowl, combine the dry ingredients and whisk to blend.

3 Add the cream cheese, melted butter, eggs, and vanilla. Mix until well blended. Fold in the chocolate chips.

4 Pour the batter evenly into the prepared pan and smooth the top. Bake for 35 to 40 minutes, until a toothpick inserted in the center comes out clean. Let cool.

5 Dust with sweetener, if desired, then cut into 2-inch squares.

per serving:

CALORIES: 96 | FAT: 8.6 g | PROTEIN: 2.7 g | TOTAL CARBS: 8 g | NET CARBS: 1.7 g

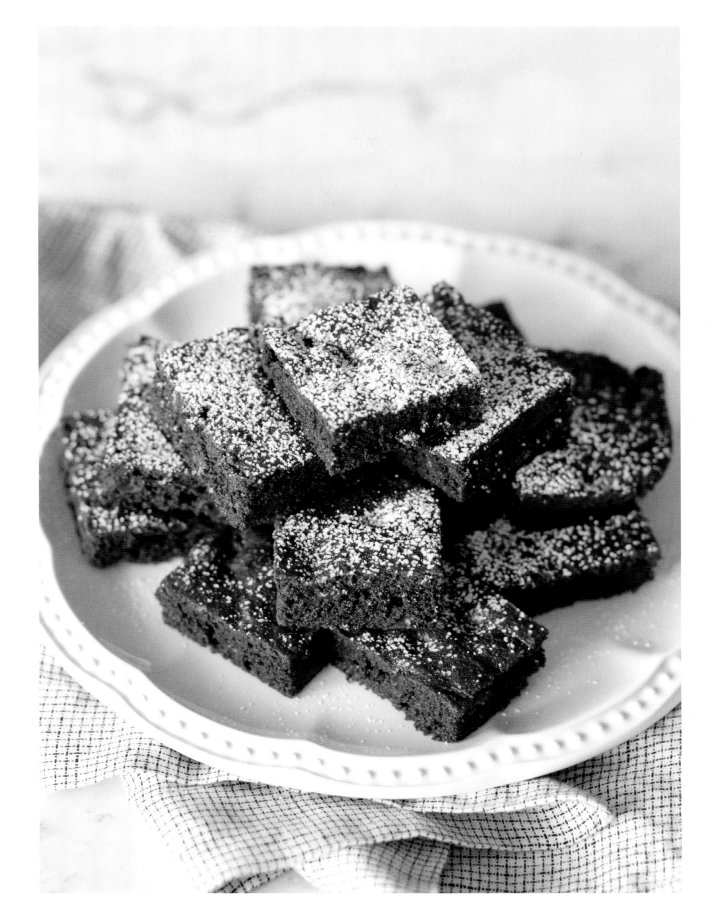

CHIA SEED PUDDING

Chia seed pudding has a unique texture and is packed with fiber, calcium, antioxidants, and omega-3s! I generally prepare this recipe in the evening so that the pudding is ready to enjoy for breakfast or as a snack the next day.

1 cup unsweetened vanilla almond milk

1½ tablespoons Swerve confectioners'-style sweetener

¼ cup chia seeds

A few fresh blueberries, for topping (optional)

note: Sometimes the chia seeds settle toward the bottom of the glass. An hour or two before consuming the pudding, stir well to help distribute the chia seeds evenly.

1 In a blender, combine the almond milk and sweetener and blend for 1 minute.

2 Place the chia seeds in a 12-ounce glass, then pour the almond milk mixture over the top.

3 Stir well, cover with plastic wrap, and refrigerate overnight.

4 Divide between two bowls or glasses and serve topped with a few blueberries, if desired.

per serving:

CALORIES: 135 | FAT: 7.5 g | PROTEIN: 6.5 g | TOTAL CARBS: 15.3 g | NET CARBS: 0 g

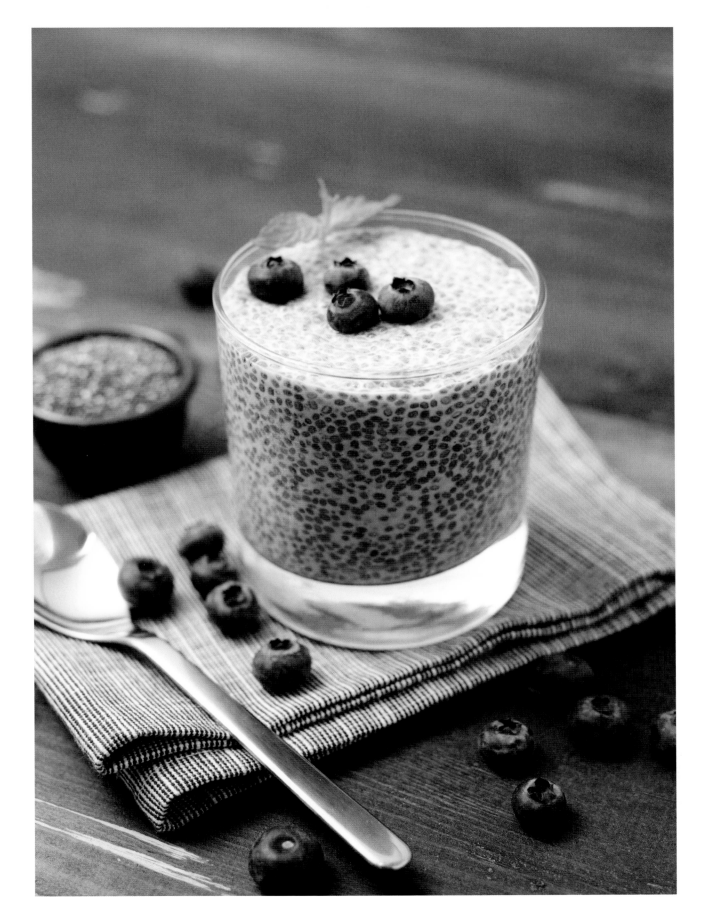

CHOCOLATE AVOCADO PUDDING

PREP TIME: 5 MINUTES, PLUS 30 MINUTES TO CHILL • YIELD: 2 SERVINGS

The key to making this pudding extra-delicious is selecting a perfectly ripe avocado. If your avocado is too ripe or under-ripe, the avocado flavor will stand out too much. With that in mind, may the avocado odds be ever in your favor! Also, it's worth mentioning that I've served this dessert to a number of my friends, some who aren't big fans of avocado, and most couldn't even taste the avocado.

1 avocado, soft but not super ripe, halved and pitted

2 tablespoons heavy whipping cream

2 tablespoons Swerve confectioners'-style sweetener

1 heaping tablespoon unsweetened cocoa powder

½ teaspoon vanilla extract

Keto Whipped Cream (page 290), for topping (optional)

1   Scoop the flesh of the avocado into a bowl. Add the rest of the ingredients and blend with a hand mixer until smooth. Place in the refrigerator to chill for 30 minutes.

2   Serve topped with fresh whipped cream, if desired.

per serving:

CALORIES: 175 | FAT: 16 g | PROTEIN: 2 g | TOTAL CARBS: 16 g | NET CARBS: 2.5 g

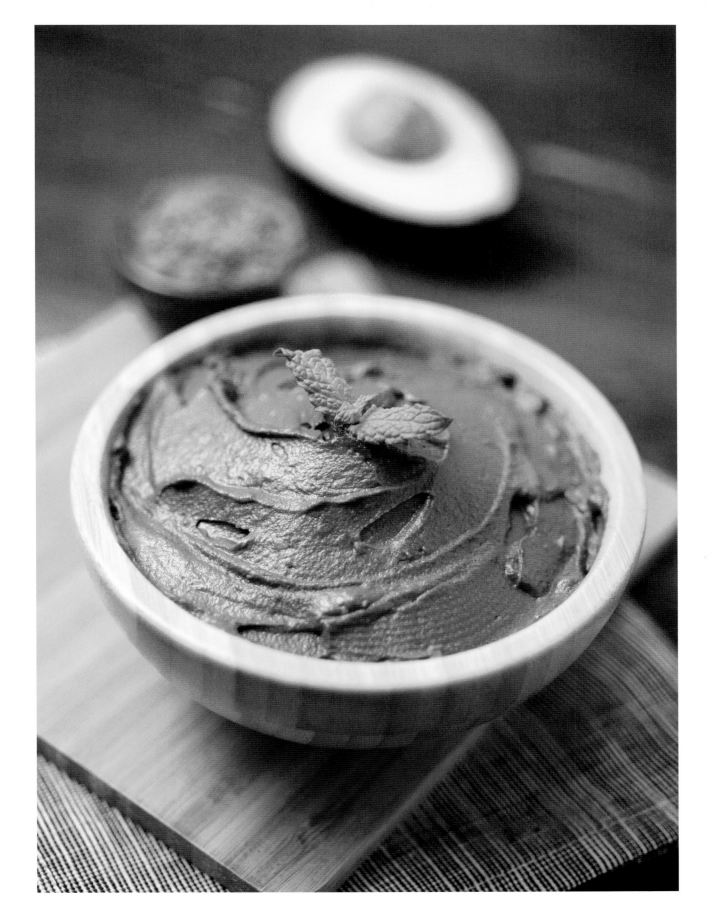

CHOCOLATE CHIP COOKIES FOR TWO

🕥 PREP TIME: 5 MINUTES • COOK TIME: 14 MINUTES • YIELD: 2 COOKIES (1 PER SERVING)

Moderation is a term that can be oversimplified; for example, before starting keto, I would buy a box of cookies, and my idea of moderation was to eat only one-third of the box instead of the entire box. As a person who has struggled with overeating, I enjoy making some recipes smaller so that they yield only one or two servings. With this in mind, I created this easy recipe for when you want just one or two cookies, without the temptation of an entire batch.

1 large egg yolk

1 tablespoon salted butter, melted

¼ teaspoon vanilla extract

⅓ cup blanched almond flour

1½ to 2 tablespoons Swerve confectioners'-style sweetener (see notes)

⅛ teaspoon baking powder

Pinch of salt

2 tablespoons stevia-sweetened chocolate chips (see notes)

notes: Use 1½ tablespoons of Swerve for semisweet cookies, or 2 tablespoons for sweet cookies. Try them both ways and see which version you like better!

I use Lily's baking chips.

It is important to press these cookies into shape before baking, as the dough doesn't expand like typical cookie dough.

1 Preheat the oven to 350°F. Line a small baking sheet with parchment paper.

2 In a medium-sized mixing bowl, combine the egg yolk, melted butter, and vanilla and stir with a fork until blended. Add the almond flour, sweetener, baking powder, and salt and mix well with a spoon. Fold in the chocolate chips.

3 Make 2 balls out of the dough and place the balls on the lined baking sheet. Press each ball into a 3-inch circle. Bake for 12 to 14 minutes, until golden brown.

4 Transfer the cookies to a wire rack to cool for 15 minutes; they will firm up as they cool.

per serving:

CALORIES: 209 | FAT: 19.3 g | PROTEIN: 6 g | TOTAL CARBS: 11.3 g | NET CARBS: 2.5 g

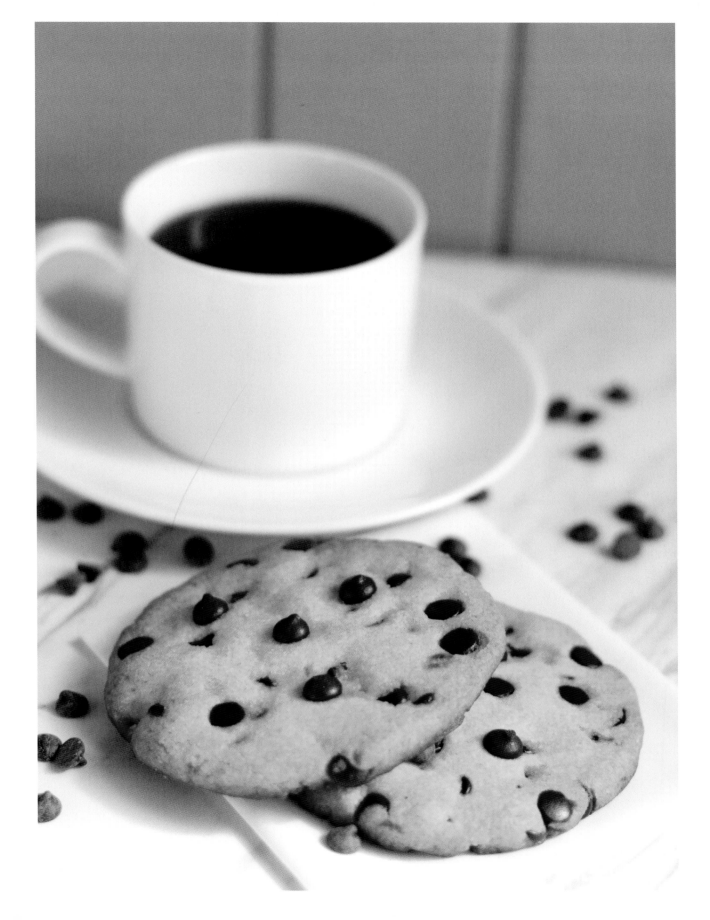

CHOCOLATE CHIP MUG CAKE

🕐 PREP TIME: 5 MINUTES • COOK TIME: 1 MINUTE • YIELD: 1 SMALL CAKE (2 SERVINGS)

You know those nights when you get a sweet tooth but don't feel like making a big mess or cooking for an army? Yeah, I feel you. This delicious little mug cake is quick, easy, and sure to hit the spot!

3 tablespoons blanched almond flour

1½ tablespoons Swerve confectioners'-style sweetener

1 tablespoon coconut flour

1 tablespoon unsweetened cocoa powder

¼ teaspoon baking powder

Dash of salt

1 large egg

1 tablespoon unsalted butter, softened

1 teaspoon avocado oil

1 tablespoon stevia-sweetened chocolate chips (see note)

Keto Whipped Cream (page 290), for topping (optional)

note I use Lily's baking chips.

1 Place the dry ingredients in a mug and mix with a fork until blended.

2 Add the egg, butter, and avocado oil, then stir with a fork until well mixed. Mix in the chocolate chips. Use a spoon to smooth the top.

3 Microwave for 1 minute, or until a toothpick inserted in the center comes out clean. (You might need to adjust the cooking time based on the power of your microwave.)

4 Invert the mug over a plate, pop out the cake, and slice in half. Enjoy as is for breakfast, or top with whipped cream for a dessert.

per serving, without whipped cream:

CALORIES: 202 | FAT: 17 g | PROTEIN: 6.5 g | TOTAL CARBS: 15.5 g | NET CARBS: 4 g

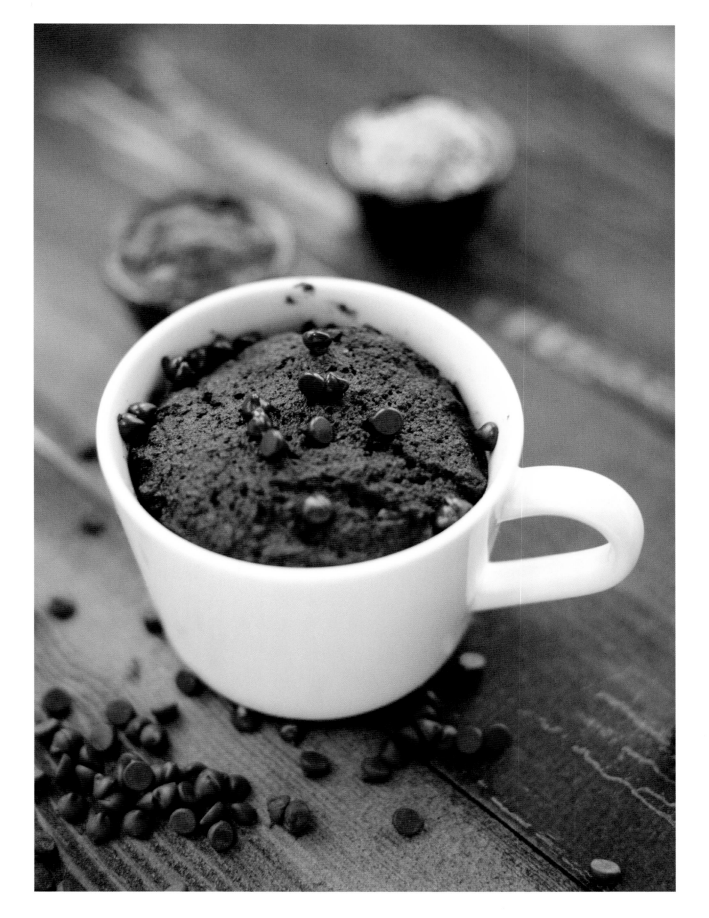

CHOCOLATE-COVERED MACADAMIA NUT FAT BOMBS

PREP TIME: 5 MINUTES, PLUS 30 MINUTES TO FREEZE • COOK TIME: ABOUT 1 MINUTE
YIELD: 8 FAT BOMBS (2 PER SERVING)

Macadamia nuts are arguably one of the most ketogenic nuts, since they are high in fat and low in carbs. The only thing that could possibly make them better is—you guessed it—chocolate! These fat bombs are salty, sweet, and absolutely delicious.

¼ cup stevia-sweetened chocolate chips (see note)

1 tablespoon MCT oil

Coarse salt (I use pink Himalayan or sea salt)

24 raw macadamia nut halves

Special Equipment

• Truffle mold, mini muffin pan, or 8 mini baking cups

note: I use Lily's baking chips. These chocolate chips are dairy-free but are manufactured using equipment that may come into contact with dairy, so those with dairy allergies should be cautious.

1 In a small microwave-safe dish, microwave the chocolate chips for 50 seconds or until melted. Stir until smooth, then add the MCT oil and a pinch of coarse salt; mix until blended.

2 Place 3 macadamia nut halves in each of 8 wells of a truffle mold or mini muffin pan or in each of 8 mini baking cups. Spoon some of the chocolate mixture into each well or baking cup, completely covering the nuts. Sprinkle additional salt over the chocolate.

3 Transfer the mold or baking cups to the freezer for a minimum of 30 minutes, until the chocolate is solid.

4 Store extras in a zip-top plastic bag in the freezer for up to 6 months.

per serving:

CALORIES: 182 | FAT: 19.3 g | PROTEIN: 2 g | TOTAL CARBS: 9.3 g | NET CARBS: 2.75 g

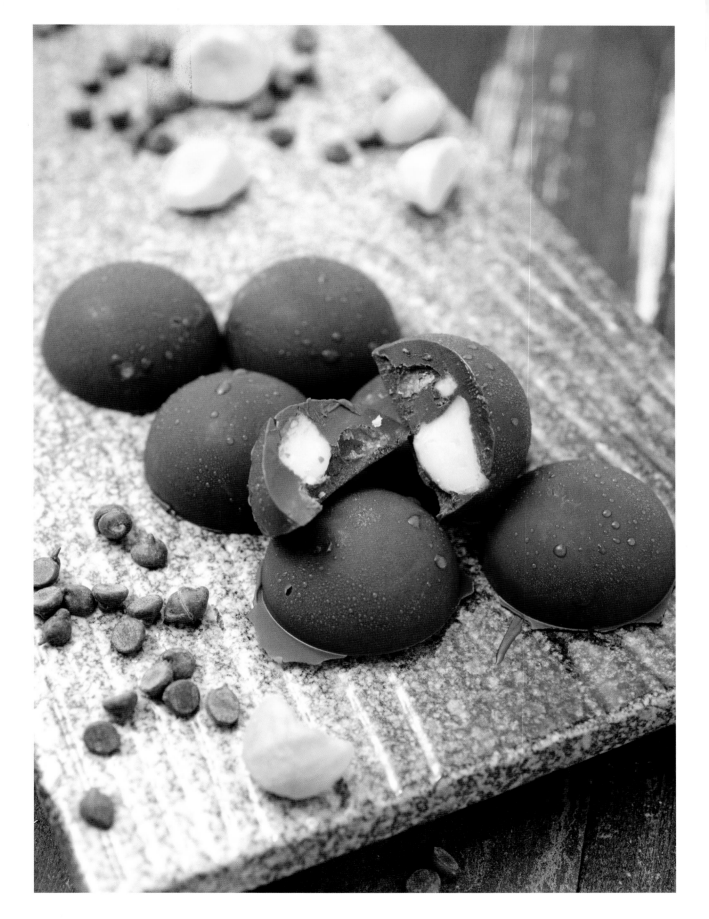

CHOCOLATE-COVERED STRAWBERRIES

PREP TIME: 5 MINUTES, PLUS 10 MINUTES TO CHILL • COOK TIME: 1 MINUTE
YIELD: 10 STRAWBERRIES (5 PER SERVING)

Who doesn't love a fresh chocolate-covered strawberry? These sweet bites are ready to enjoy in under 20 minutes and require only three simple ingredients!

10 medium-sized fresh strawberries

¼ cup stevia-sweetened chocolate chips (see note)

1½ teaspoons MCT oil

note: I use Lily's baking chips. These chocolate chips are dairy-free but may have been manufactured using equipment that also comes into contact with dairy, so those with dairy allergies should be cautious.

1 Rinse the strawberries and pat dry.

2 Place the chocolate chips in a small microwave-safe bowl and microwave until fully melted, about 1 minute. Add the MCT oil to the melted chocolate and stir until smooth.

3 Line a small rimmed baking sheet or plate with parchment paper. Dip the bottom three-quarters of each strawberry into the melted chocolate mixture and place on the parchment paper. Repeat until all the strawberries are coated.

4 Place in the refrigerator for 10 to 15 minutes to harden the chocolate shell before eating. Store covered in the refrigerator for up to 3 days.

per serving:

CALORIES: 92.5 | FAT: 8.5 g | PROTEIN: 1.5 g | TOTAL CARBS: 14.5 g | NET CARBS: 5.5 g

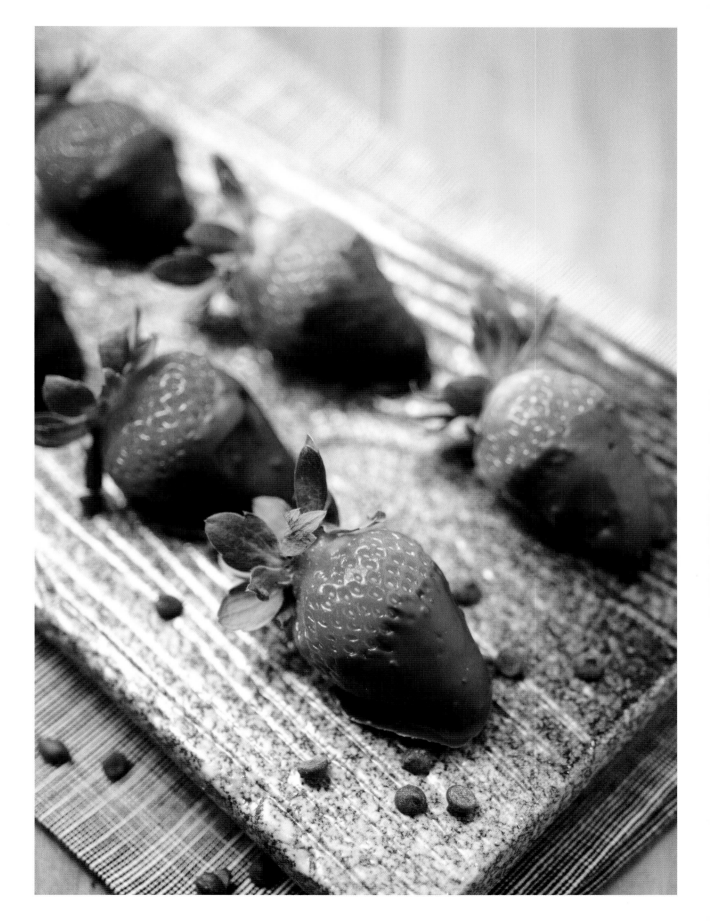

POP-POP'S CHOCOLATE PEANUT BUTTER BITES

PREP TIME: 5 MINUTES, PLUS 40 MINUTES TO CHILL • COOK TIME: 1 MINUTE
YIELD: 10 BITES (2 PER SERVING)

I have fond memories of making peanut butter pie and chocolate peanut butter balls with my grandfather when I was a child. I developed this quick and easy recipe in his honor, and they taste just like peanut butter cups!

¼ cup natural peanut butter (no sugar added; only peanuts and salt)

2½ tablespoons Swerve confectioners'-style sweetener

2 tablespoons blanched almond flour

¼ teaspoon vanilla extract

¼ cup stevia-sweetened chocolate chips (see note)

1½ teaspoons MCT oil

note: I use Lily's baking chips. These chocolate chips are dairy-free but may have been manufactured using equipment that also comes into contact with dairy, so those with dairy allergies should be cautious.

1. Line a plate or small rimmed baking sheet with parchment paper.

2. In a small bowl, mix the peanut butter, sweetener, almond flour, and vanilla until smooth.

3. Form the peanut butter mixture into 10 small balls and place them on the parchment-lined plate. Place the plate in the freezer for 30 minutes.

4. After 30 minutes, place the chocolate chips in a small microwave-safe bowl and microwave until fully melted, about 45 seconds. Add the MCT oil to the melted chocolate and mix well.

5. Remove the peanut butter balls from the freezer. Dip the balls one at a time into the melted chocolate. Use a spoon to gently roll the balls in the chocolate until they're fully covered. Place the chocolate-coated balls on the parchment paper–lined plate.

6. Place the chocolate-coated balls in the freezer for 10 to 15 minutes, until the chocolate is solid. Store extras in a zip-top plastic bag in the freezer for up to 6 months.

per serving:

CALORIES: 122 | FAT: 10.8 g | PROTEIN: 4.2 g | TOTAL CARBS: 7 g | NET CARBS: 2.6 g

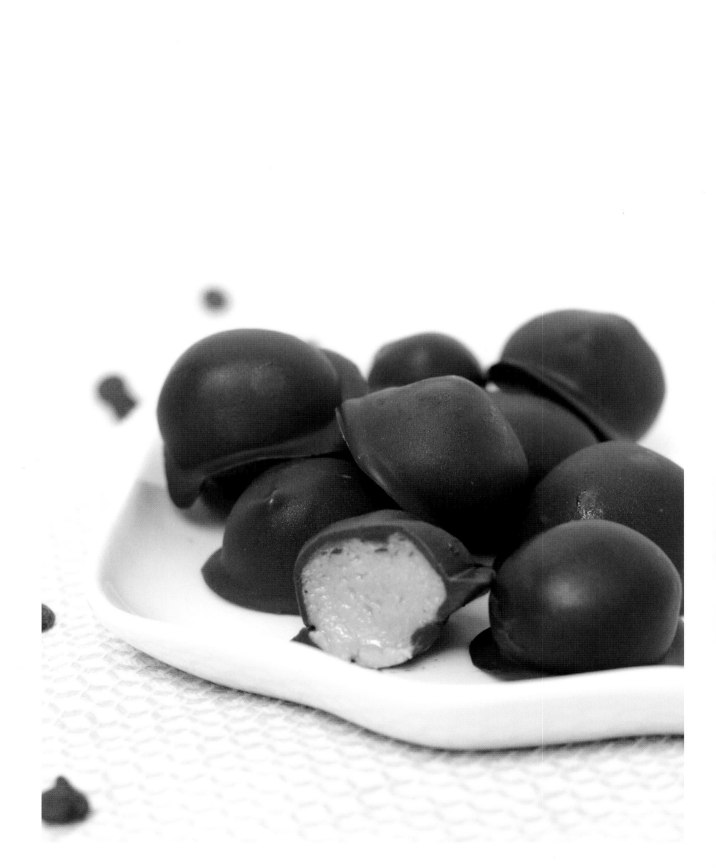

MINI CHEESECAKES

PREP TIME: 15 MINUTES, PLUS 1 HOUR TO CHILL • COOK TIME: 18 MINUTES
YIELD: 8 MINI CHEESECAKES (1 PER SERVING)

Cheesecake is one of the simplest and most delicious desserts to prepare on a low-carb, high-fat diet. These mini cheesecakes are the perfect size for a sensible treat. Enjoy as is or top them with fresh berries or Keto Whipped Cream (page 290).

Crust

½ cup plus 2 tablespoons almond meal

1 tablespoon Swerve confectioners'-style sweetener

1 tablespoon unsalted butter, melted

Cheesecake Filling

1 (8-ounce) package cream cheese, softened

⅓ cup Swerve confectioners'-style sweetener

1 large egg

1½ teaspoons fresh lemon juice

1½ teaspoons vanilla extract

Sliced strawberries, for garnish (optional)

1 Preheat the oven to 350°F. Place 8 paper liners in a standard-size muffin pan.

2 In a small bowl, combine the crust ingredients and mix by hand until well blended. Sprinkle a thin layer of the crust mixture into each paper liner or tartlet pans and press until smooth and even.

3 In a medium-sized bowl, combine the cheesecake filling ingredients and blend with a hand mixer until smooth. Pour the filling evenly into the paper liners, on top of the crust, filling the liners almost to the top.

4 Bake for 15 to 18 minutes, until the cheesecakes are set. Remove from the oven and let cool to room temperature in the pan before removing. Refrigerate for 1 to 2 hours before serving.

5 Serve garnished with sliced strawberries, if desired.

per serving:

CALORIES: 175 | FAT: 16 g | PROTEIN: 3.8 g | TOTAL CARBS: 12.8 g | NET CARBS: 1.8 g

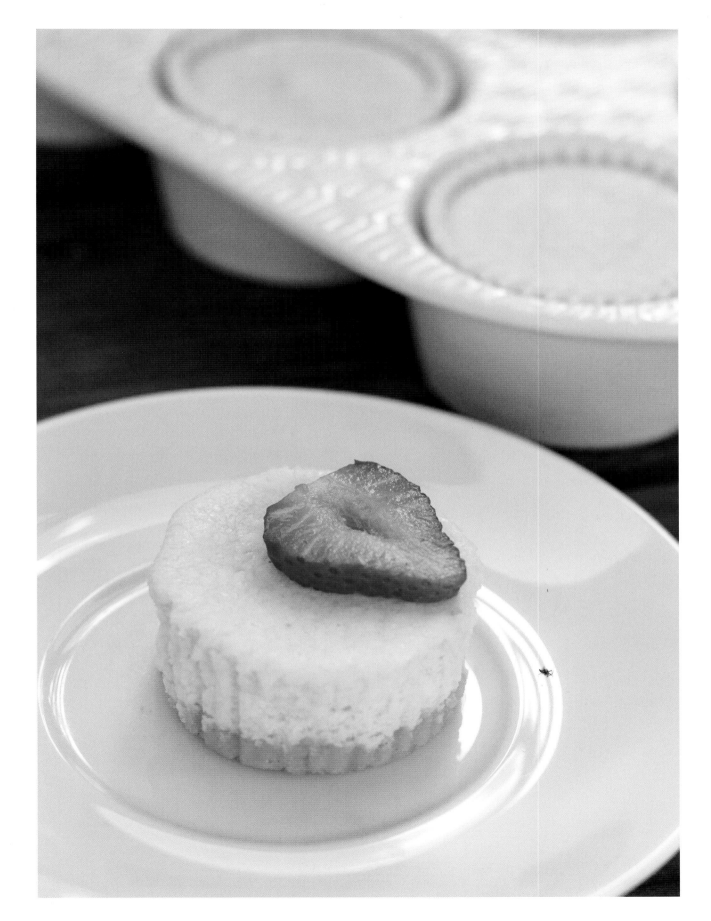

RASPBERRY CHEESECAKE FAT BOMBS

PREP TIME: 10 MINUTES, PLUS 45 MINUTES TO FREEZE • YIELD: 30 FAT BOMBS (3 PER SERVING)

A fat bomb is a bite-sized snack that is high in healthy fat and low in carbs. Fat bombs can be sweet, savory, and everything in between! They are great for a quick and filling snack or treat.

12 fresh raspberries

6 ounces cream cheese, softened

¼ cup MCT oil

2 tablespoons unsalted butter

½ teaspoon vanilla extract

3 tablespoons Swerve confectioners'-style sweetener

Special Equipment

· Silicone truffle mold(s) with at least 30 cavities (optional)

1 In a large mixing bowl, combine all the ingredients and mix with a fork until smooth.

2 Distribute the cheesecake mixture evenly among 30 cavities of a truffle mold(s). (Alternatively, use a spoon to dollop bite-sized portions of the mixture onto a sheet of parchment paper.) Freeze for 45 minutes or until set.

3 Store extras in the freezer for up to 3 weeks.

per serving:

CALORIES: 122 | FAT: 13.3 g | PROTEIN: 1.2 g | TOTAL CARBS: 0.9 g | NET CARBS: 0.8 g

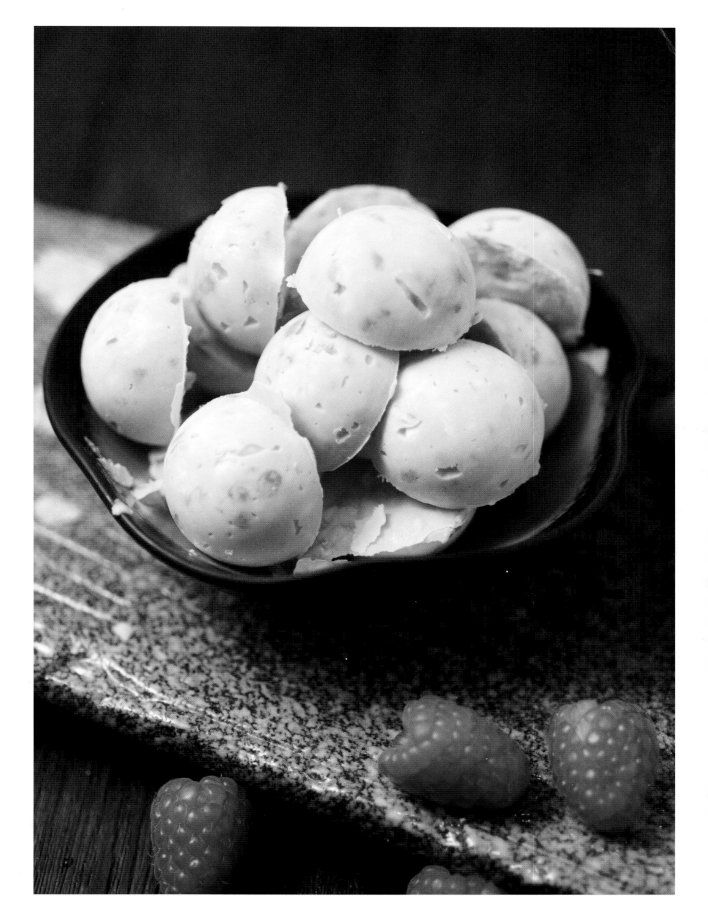

SNICKERDOODLE CUPCAKES

🕧 PREP TIME: 10 MINUTES • COOK TIME: 12 MINUTES • YIELD: 6 CUPCAKES

No sugar, but spice and everything nice! These snickerdoodle cupcakes are moist and decadent and topped with a delicious cinnamon cream cheese frosting.

Cupcake Batter

½ cup blanched almond flour

1 tablespoon coconut flour

½ teaspoon baking powder

¼ cup Swerve confectioners'-style sweetener

3 ounces cream cheese, softened

1 large egg

1 teaspoon vanilla extract

Frosting

2 ounces cream cheese, softened

2 tablespoons unsalted butter, softened

1½ tablespoons Swerve confectioners'-style sweetener

¼ teaspoon ground cinnamon, plus extra for garnish (optional)

¼ teaspoon vanilla extract

1. Preheat the oven to 350°F. Line 6 wells of a standard-size muffin pan with cupcake liners.

2. In a large bowl, whisk together the almond flour, coconut flour, baking powder, and sweetener.

3. Add the cream cheese, egg, and vanilla and mix with a hand mixer until well blended. Pour the batter evenly into the cupcake liners, filling each about three-quarters full. Bake for 12 minutes or until a toothpick inserted in the center comes out clean. Let cool completely before frosting.

4. Make the frosting: In a separate bowl, combine all the frosting ingredients and blend with the hand mixer until smooth.

5. Top each cooled cupcake with the frosting. Dust lightly with cinnamon, if desired.

per cupcake:

CALORIES: 188 | FAT: 17 g | PROTEIN: 4.8 g | TOTAL CARBS: 12 g | NET CARBS: 2.2 g

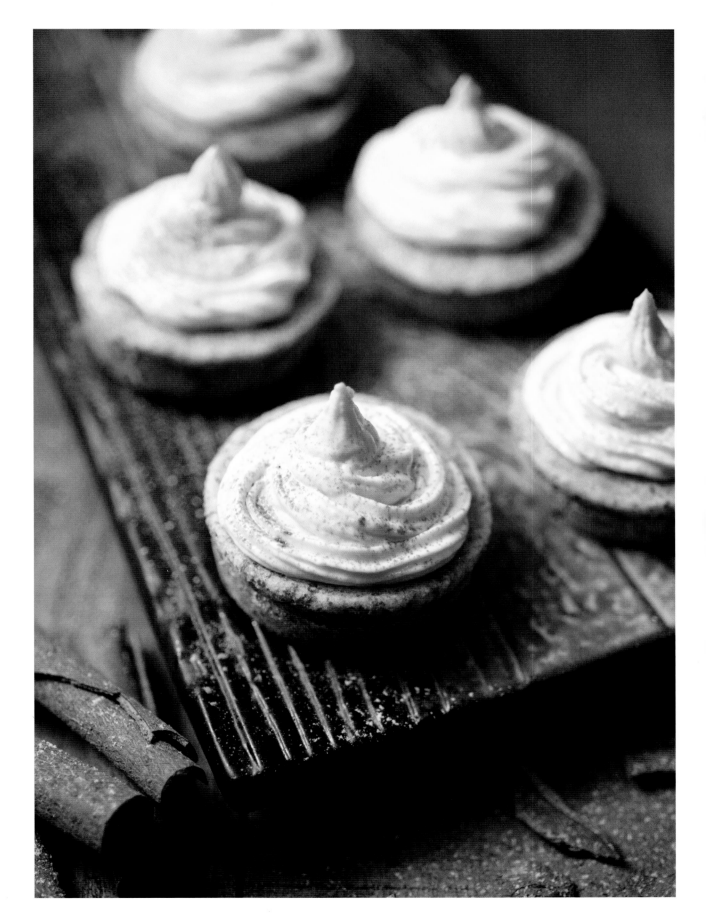

STRAWBERRY CREAM ICE POPS

Ø PREP TIME: 5 MINUTES, PLUS 3 HOURS TO FREEZE • YIELD: 6 POPS

Ice pops are loved by kids and adults alike. This strawberry cream version is easy to make and great for a quick dessert!

8 fresh strawberries, hulled and quartered

1 cup heavy whipping cream

½ cup unsweetened almond milk

2 ounces cream cheese, softened

2½ tablespoons Swerve confectioners'-style sweetener

½ teaspoon vanilla extract

Special Equipment
• 6 standard-size ice pop molds

1 Place the strawberries and cream in a blender and blend until the cream starts to form peaks.

2 Add the almond milk, cream cheese, sweetener, and vanilla and blend until smooth. Pour into ice pop molds and freeze for at least 3 hours.

3 To remove the ice pops from the molds, run the molds under hot water. Store extras in the freezer for up to 3 weeks.

per ice pop:

CALORIES: 175 | FAT: 16.5 g | PROTEIN: 1 g | TOTAL CARBS: 8 g | NET CARBS: 3.8 g

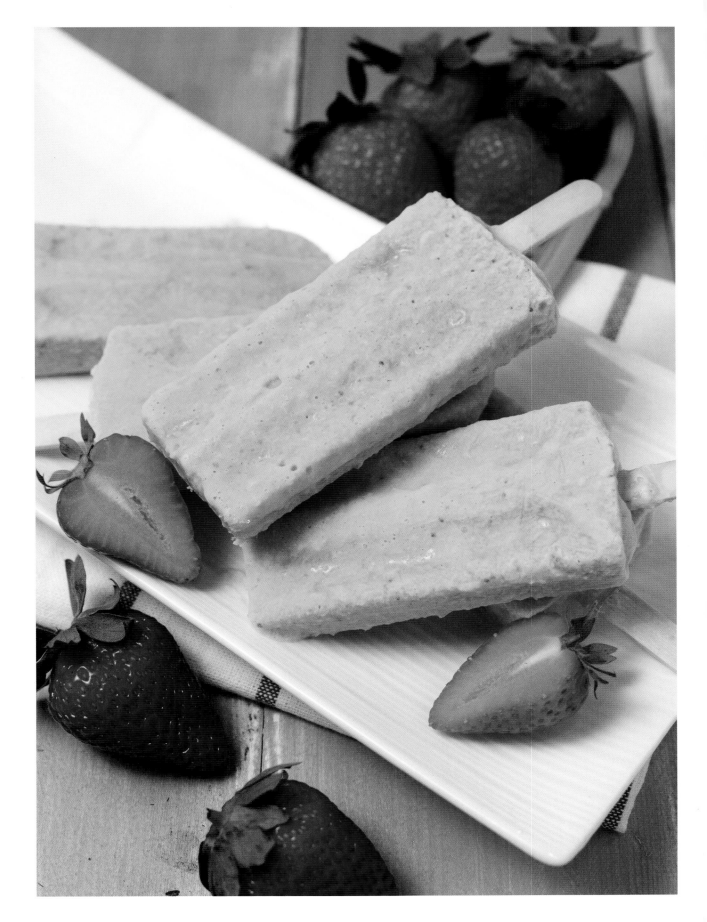

MORNING COFFEE

🕐 ⊘ ◖ PREP TIME: 5 MINUTES (NOT INCLUDING TIME TO BREW COFFEE) • YIELD: 1 SERVING

Growing up, I remember my dad looking forward to his coffee each morning. I never fully understood it until I grew up and had my own child. (Hello, sleep deprivation!) Boy, do I love my coffee now! I often get asked what I put in my coffee each morning, so here's my recipe.

1½ cups brewed coffee, hot

2 tablespoons heavy whipping cream

1 tablespoon MCT oil

1 or 2 drops vanilla extract (optional)

Stevia or other keto-friendly sweetener of choice, to taste (optional)

Pour the hot coffee into a mug. Add the cream, MCT oil, vanilla (if using), and sweetener (if using). Stir well with a spoon or, for a frothier drink, use a milk frother. Serve.

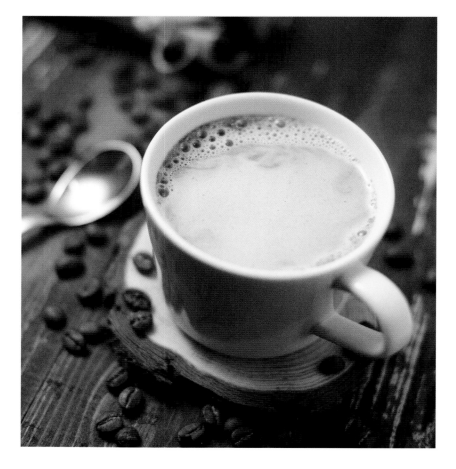

per serving:

CALORIES: 202 | FAT: 24 g | PROTEIN: 0 g | TOTAL CARBS: 2 g | NET CARBS: 2 g

MINT, CUCUMBER, AND LIME-INFUSED WATER

PREP TIME: 5 MINUTES, PLUS AT LEAST 1 HOUR TO INFUSE • YIELD: 2 QUARTS

We all know that staying hydrated is important, but let's face it, drinking plain water can be boring sometimes. Infused water is a great way to add a little flavor while staying away from sugar, artificial sweeteners, and artificial flavors.

2 quarts water

1 cup sliced cucumbers

10 to 12 fresh mint leaves, muddled

1 lime, thinly sliced

Fresh mint sprigs, for garnish (optional)

tip: Flavored sparkling water, such as LaCroix, is another great option for flavored water without any sugar.

1 Place all the ingredients in a pitcher and allow to infuse for at least 1 hour before drinking. Serve with fresh mint sprigs, if desired.

2 Store in an airtight container (such as a mason jar, water bottle, or jug) in the refrigerator for up to a week.

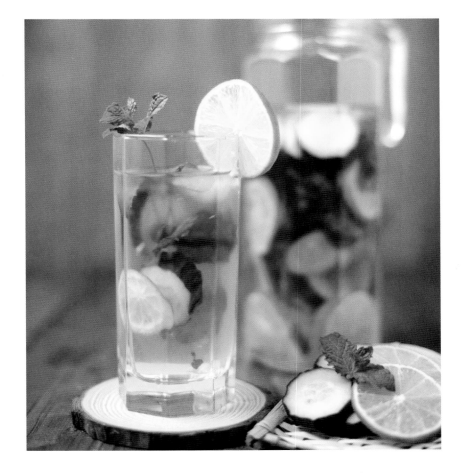

per serving: CALORIES: 0 | FAT: 0 g | PROTEIN: 0 g | TOTAL CARBS: 0 g | NET CARBS: 0 g

COLD-BREW MINT COFFEE

PREP TIME: 5 MINUTES • YIELD: 1 SERVING

I've always loved coffee, and this iced mint coffee is by far one of my favorite drinks, especially on a hot day. The mint adds a refreshing and flavorful spin on traditional iced coffee, and as a bonus, mint has been shown to aid in digestion.

10 to 15 fresh mint leaves, plus extra for garnish

Stevia or other keto-friendly sweetener of choice

Ice (see tip)

1½ cups cold-brewed coffee, homemade or store-bought

3 tablespoons heavy whipping cream

tip: To prevent the coffee from getting watered down, freeze brewed coffee in ice cube trays and use coffee ice cubes instead of regular ice cubes.

1 Rinse the mint leaves and place them in a glass. Add sweetener to taste.

2 Using a spoon or muddler, press down lightly on the leaves and give it a few gentle twists.

3 Add ice to the glass, then pour in the coffee and cream and stir. (For a frothier consistency, you can blend the coffee and cream with a milk frother before adding them to the cup.)

4 Garnish with a few mint leaves.

per serving:

CALORIES: 152 | FAT: 15 g | PROTEIN: 0 g | TOTAL CARBS: 3 g | NET CARBS: 3 g

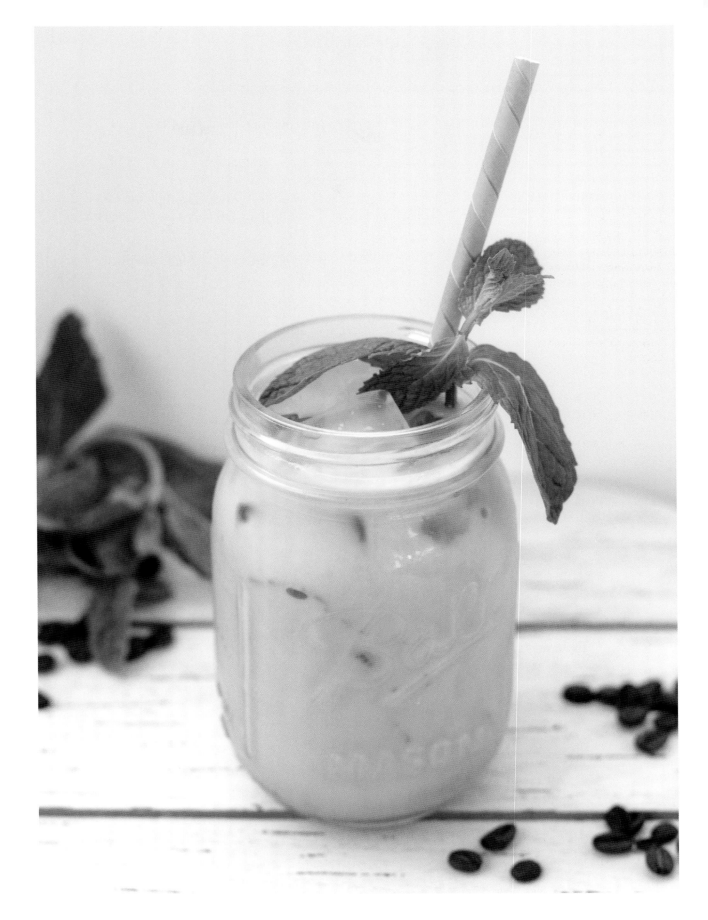

KETO HOT CHOCOLATE

Hot chocolate always makes me feel warm and cozy. Now you can enjoy the same great taste without all the unnecessary sugar!

1 cup unsweetened almond milk

2 tablespoons heavy whipping cream

2 tablespoons Swerve confectioners'-style sweetener

1 tablespoon unsweetened cocoa powder, plus extra for dusting (optional)

Keto Whipped Cream (page 290), for serving (optional)

1 In a small saucepan over medium heat, combine all the ingredients. Whisk well for 2 to 3 minutes or until the desired temperature is reached.

2 Serve topped with whipped cream and a dusting of cocoa powder, if desired.

per serving:

CALORIES: 142 | FAT: 14 g | PROTEIN: 2 g | TOTAL CARBS: 24 g | NET CARBS: 3 g

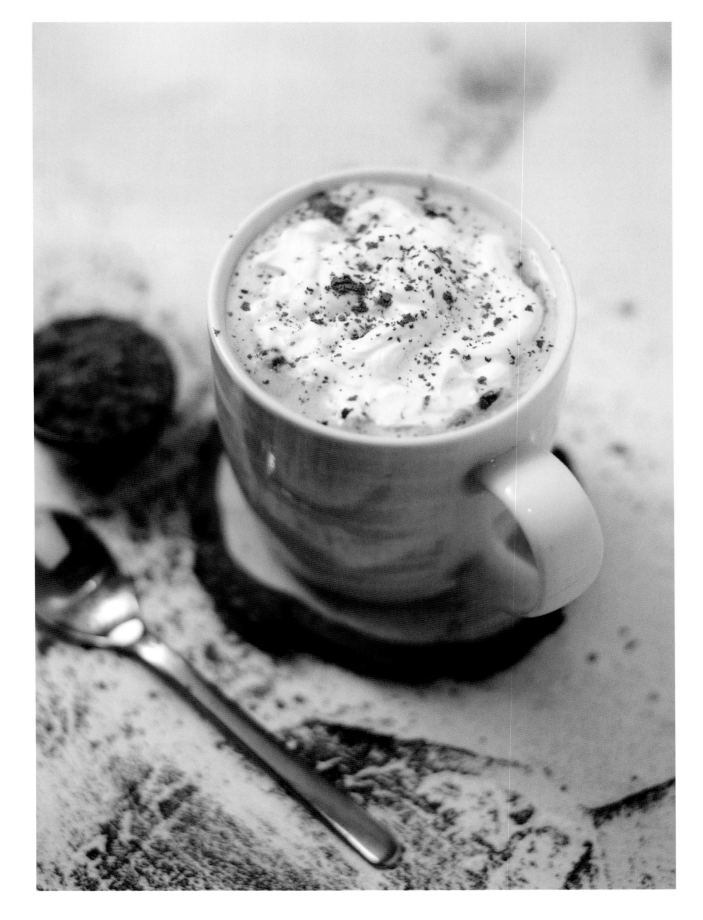

STRAWBERRY VANILLA SMOOTHIE

⏱ ⊘ PREP TIME: 10 MINUTES • YIELD: 1 SERVING

My daughter, Olivia, and I love to make smoothies together! This strawberry smoothie is perfect for breakfast on the go, or whenever you want a fruity and refreshing drink.

1 cup unsweetened vanilla-flavored or plain unsweetened almond milk

1 scoop sugar-free/low-carb protein powder (I use Quest Vanilla Milkshake flavor)

3 frozen strawberries

1 tablespoon heavy whipping cream

1 tablespoon MCT oil

4 to 6 ice cubes

1 fresh strawberry, for garnish (optional)

Place all the ingredients in a blender and blend until smooth. If desired, slice a whole strawberry in half lengthwise, but not all the way through, and hang it from the rim of the glass.

per serving:

CALORIES: 292 | FAT: 22 g | PROTEIN: 23 g | TOTAL CARBS: 8 g | NET CARBS: 5 g

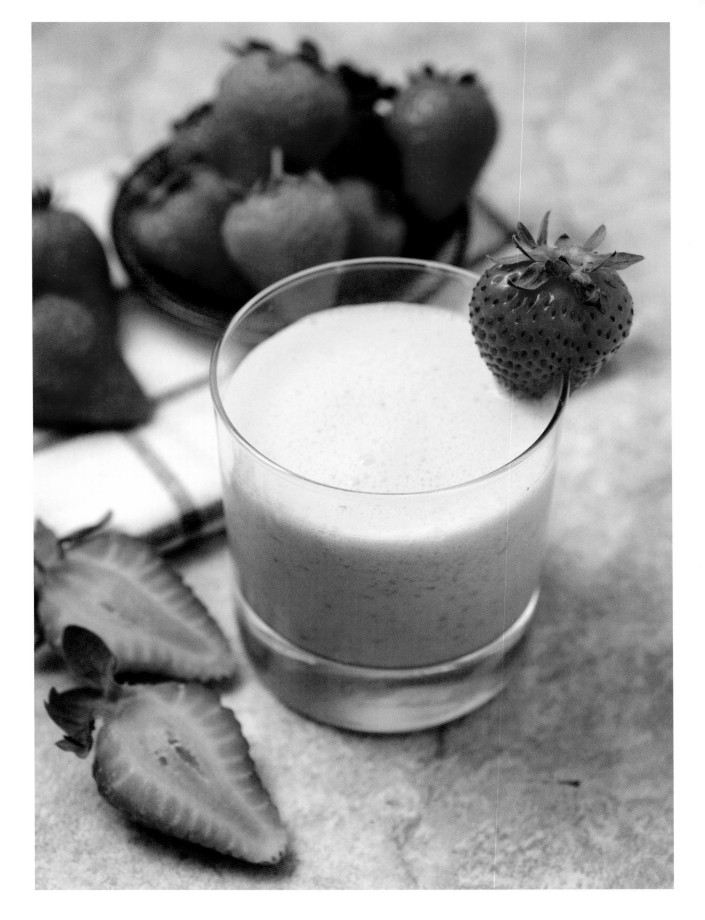

KETO WHIPPED CREAM

 PREP TIME: 5 MINUTES • YIELD: 6 SERVINGS

Whipped cream is so easy to make, and it's the perfect topping for cheesecake, hot chocolate, or even fresh strawberries!

⅔ cup heavy whipping cream

1 tablespoon plus 1 teaspoon Swerve confectioners'-style sweetener

1 teaspoon vanilla extract

note: Pairs well with Brownies (page 258), Chocolate Avocado Pudding (page 262), Keto Hot Chocolate (page 286), Chocolate-Covered Strawberries (page 270), and just about any other keto dessert!

Place all the ingredients in a medium-sized mixing bowl and blend with a hand mixer until stiff peaks form, 3 to 4 minutes.

per serving:

CALORIES: 89.6 | FAT: 8.8 g | PROTEIN: 0 g | TOTAL CARBS: 3.8 g | NET CARBS: 1.8 g

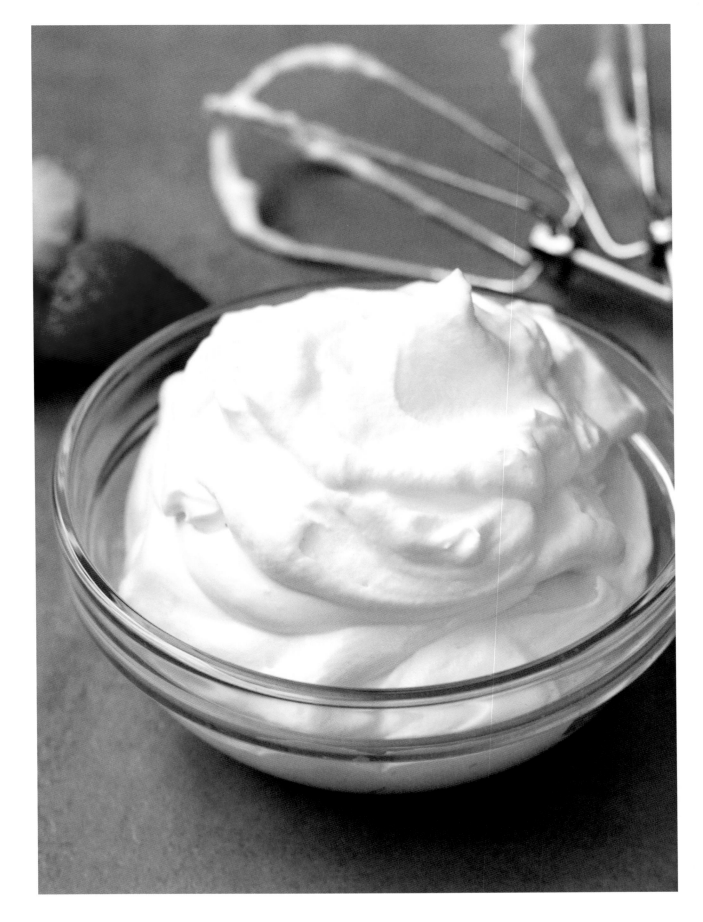

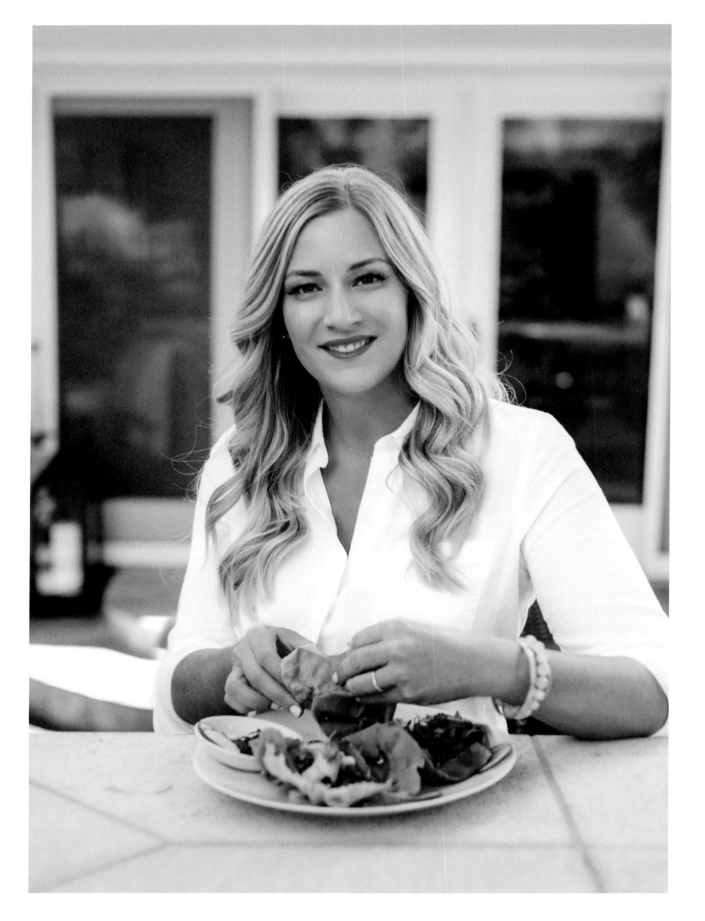

CHAPTER 4

30-Day Meal Plan

Meal plans can be great tools for mapping out and planning for the week(s) ahead, especially when you are just starting out on keto and are still getting used to this way of eating. The plan outlined in this chapter contains a full thirty days of ketogenic breakfasts, lunches, and dinners. However, please don't feel like this is a locked-in plan that you have to follow to a tee. Feel free to swap out recipes to better suit your lifestyle, budget, and food preferences. Keto isn't one-size-fits-all, so set things up in a way that works for you!

Also, while you are following this plan, feel free to enjoy meals out. Keto is a lifestyle change, and although home-cooked meals are great, it's not realistic or necessary to eat at home 24/7. See page 301 for tips and recommendations for eating keto on the go.

I recommend adding nonstarchy veggies or salad greens to as many of your meals as possible. Cook your veggies and dress your salads with healthy fats like avocado oil, butter, ghee, and coconut oil. (See page 42 for more on healthy versus unhealthy fats.)

Whether or not you are following my 30-day plan, often it's best to plan your meals and go shopping for the next one to two weeks. Buying in bulk and freezing food for later use can save you a lot of money and time! When meal planning, try to plan for enough food so that you will have leftovers for lunch or dinner the next day; doing so will save you a lot of effort. You'll notice that my plan makes generous use of leftovers for breakfast and lunch. Let's be real: most of us don't have the time to prepare and cook three meals a day. Utilizing leftovers is a great shortcut!

Depending on how many people you are feeding, the recipes as written may or may not make enough food for the leftovers needed for the meal plan. Make sure to check the serving size of each recipe and make a double or triple batch if necessary so that you have enough food for everyone.

As far as how many times to eat in a day, that is totally up to you. I've set up the meal plan to include three meals a day because that is what most of us are used to, but I encourage you to listen to your body and see what works best for you. Some people find that two ketogenic meals a day is plenty.

Last but not least, don't get too caught up in the idea of "perfection" and think that you have to eat all grass-fed, pastured, organic, and home-cooked food, with no processed foods allowed whatsoever. While there is no argument that choosing high-quality ingredients is important, a lot of people can't afford or stick to such strict guidelines. There are some days when I wake up, grab my Morning Coffee (see page 282) and a Quest bar, and run out the door. While a focus on whole, organic food is best, it's okay to find a balance. Remember, the most perfect plan isn't perfect at all if it's not livable or affordable. It should also be said that not all processed foods are bad. In fact, because of the ketogenic diet and other approaches that focus on clean eating, many thoughtful and ethical food companies are making products from quality ingredients. Let's face it: sometimes life gets busy, and it's helpful to have some grab-and-go foods handy. Be sure to research ingredients and make smart choices (say no to maltitol, for example). You can find some of my favorite keto-friendly products and brands on page 314.

Remember: progress, not perfection. Make this lifestyle livable, and the stress (and weight) will melt away! That being said, don't be afraid to try new things, challenge your comfort zones, and work on developing new and improved healthy habits.

If following the meal plan feels like too much pressure, feel free to skip it. However, at the very least, I do recommend having keto-friendly snacks and other food options at home as well as at work. I've found that people (myself included!) often make less-ideal choices when they find themselves both hungry and unprepared.

Here are some easy snack options to pair with the meal plan:

- Avocado slices
- Bone broth (great for electrolytes!)
- Celery or broccoli with ranch dip
- Cheese (sliced or Cheese Crisps, page 128)
- Coffee or tea with MCT oil or coconut oil
- Fat bombs (pages 268 and 276)
- Jerky (check for added sugars)
- Nuts (see page 56 for recommendations)
- Olives
- Pickles
- Pork rinds
- Sliced meats (pepperoni, prosciutto, and so on)

	Breakfast	Lunch	Dinner
DAY 01	102 Easy Egg Scramble with avocado slices	154 BLTA Lettuce Wraps	252 Grilled chicken thighs and Twice-Baked Cauliflower Casserole
DAY 02	110 Sausage, Egg, and Cheese Breakfast Bake	LEFTOVER LEFTOVER Grilled chicken thighs and Twice-Baked Cauliflower Casserole	190 Chicken and Broccoli Alfredo Bowls
DAY 03	LEFTOVER Sausage, Egg, and Cheese Breakfast Bake	LEFTOVER Chicken and Broccoli Alfredo Bowls	178 250 Sunny-Side-Up Burgers and Simply Roasted Brussels Sprouts
DAY 04	108 Quick and Easy Capicola Egg Cups with sliced avocado	Egg salad in butter lettuce wraps with tomato	206 243 Tina's Slow Cooker Salsa Chicken Lettuce Wraps and Cilantro Lime Cauliflower Rice
DAY 05	LEFTOVER Quick and Easy Capicola Egg Cups with sliced avocado	LEFTOVER LEFTOVER Tina's Slow Cooker Salsa Chicken Lettuce Wraps and Cilantro Lime Cauliflower Rice	188 Chicken Caesar Salad (or substitute steak or shrimp for the chicken)
DAY 06	100 Olivia's Cream Cheese Pancakes and bacon	120 78 Sweet and Spicy Fried Shrimp over arugula with Mick's Spicy Aioli	162 134 Fajita Kabobs with Guacamole

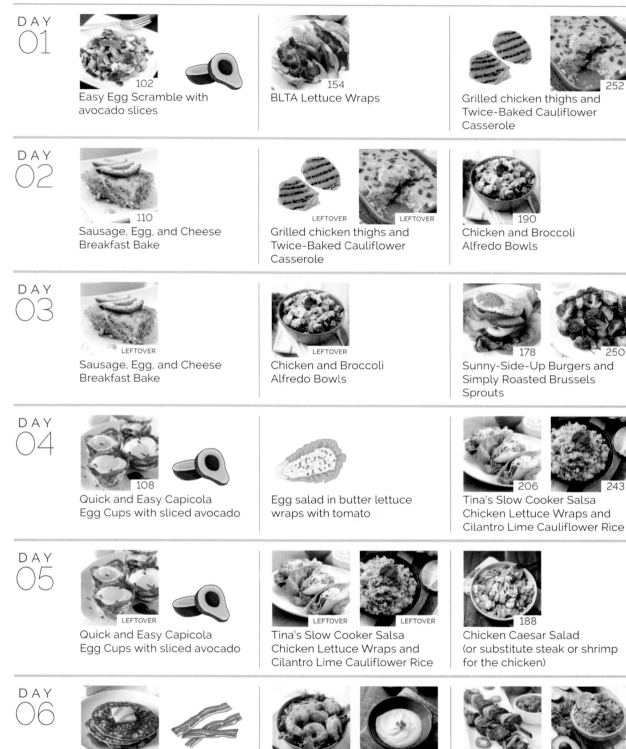

Breakfast	Lunch	Dinner

DAY 07

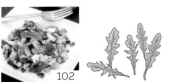
102
Easy Egg Scramble with baby arugula

 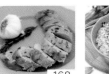
LEFTOVER   LEFTOVER
Fajita Kabobs with Guacamole

168   244
Lemon Garlic Pork Tenderloin and Creamed Spinach

DAY 08

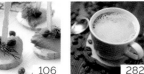
106   282
Lox and Cream Cheese Sliders with Morning Coffee

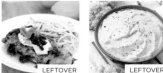
LEFTOVER   LEFTOVER
Lemon Garlic Pork Tenderloin and Creamed Spinach

208   246
Tuscan Chicken and Mashed Cauliflower or Zoodles

DAY 09

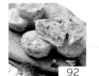
92
Broccoli, Bacon, and Cheese Egg Muffins

LEFTOVER   LEFTOVER
Tuscan Chicken and Mashed Cauliflower or Zoodles

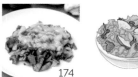
156
Keto Chili with side salad

DAY 10

LEFTOVER
Broccoli, Bacon, and Cheese Egg Muffins

174
Bunless Philly Cheesesteaks with side salad

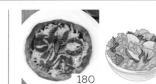
192   249
Chicken Cordon Bleu and Roasted Radishes

DAY 11

94
Chili Egg Scramble (use leftover Keto Chili)

LEFTOVER   LEFTOVER
Chicken Cordon Bleu and Roasted Radishes

180
Quick and Easy Personal Pizza with side salad and ranch

DAY 12

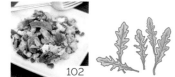
102
Easy Egg Scramble with baby arugula

160
Chili Cheese Dogs (use leftover Keto Chili)

224
Parmesan-Crusted Salmon Bake with Asparagus

	Breakfast	Lunch	Dinner

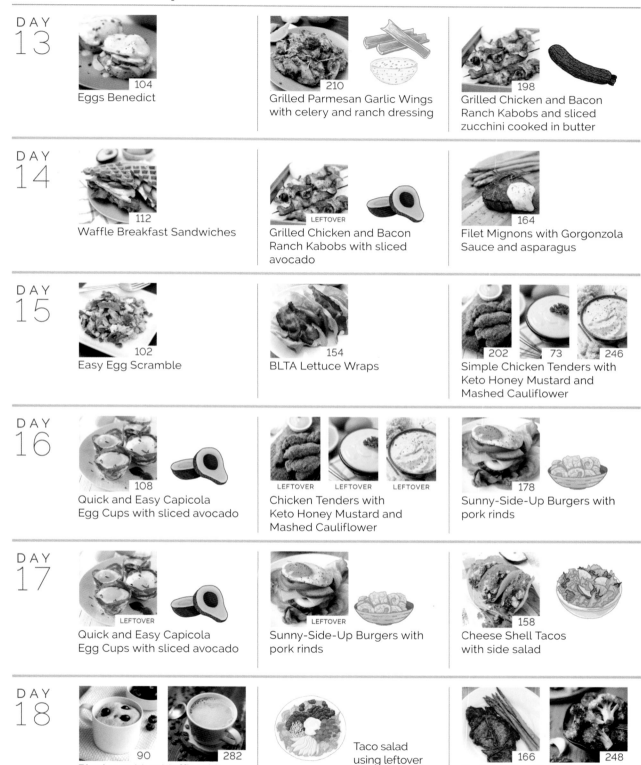

DAY 13

104
Eggs Benedict

210
Grilled Parmesan Garlic Wings with celery and ranch dressing

198
Grilled Chicken and Bacon Ranch Kabobs and sliced zucchini cooked in butter

DAY 14

112
Waffle Breakfast Sandwiches

LEFTOVER
Grilled Chicken and Bacon Ranch Kabobs with sliced avocado

164
Filet Mignons with Gorgonzola Sauce and asparagus

DAY 15

102
Easy Egg Scramble

154
BLTA Lettuce Wraps

202 73 246
Simple Chicken Tenders with Keto Honey Mustard and Mashed Cauliflower

DAY 16

108
Quick and Easy Capicola Egg Cups with sliced avocado

LEFTOVER LEFTOVER LEFTOVER
Chicken Tenders with Keto Honey Mustard and Mashed Cauliflower

178
Sunny-Side-Up Burgers with pork rinds

DAY 17

LEFTOVER
Quick and Easy Capicola Egg Cups with sliced avocado

LEFTOVER
Sunny-Side-Up Burgers with pork rinds

158
Cheese Shell Tacos with side salad

DAY 18

90 282
Blueberry Mug Muffin with Morning Coffee

Taco salad using leftover meat from Cheese Shell Tacos, cheese, lettuce, tomato, onion, and sour cream

166 248
Garlic Butter–Basted Rib-eye and Roasted Broccoli

	Breakfast	**Lunch**	**Dinner**

DAY 19

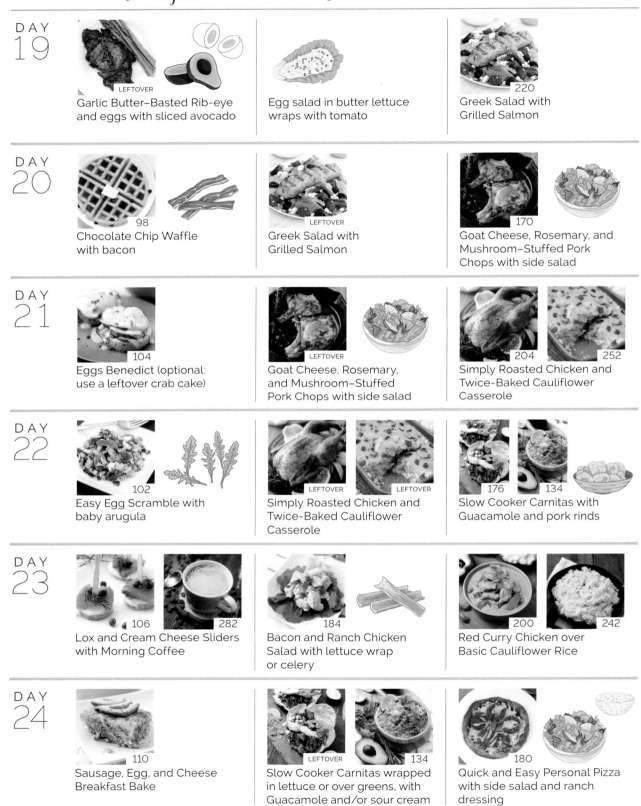

LEFTOVER
Garlic Butter–Basted Rib-eye and eggs with sliced avocado

Egg salad in butter lettuce wraps with tomato

220
Greek Salad with Grilled Salmon

DAY 20

98
Chocolate Chip Waffle with bacon

LEFTOVER
Greek Salad with Grilled Salmon

170
Goat Cheese, Rosemary, and Mushroom–Stuffed Pork Chops with side salad

DAY 21

104
Eggs Benedict (optional: use a leftover crab cake)

LEFTOVER
Goat Cheese, Rosemary, and Mushroom–Stuffed Pork Chops with side salad

204   252
Simply Roasted Chicken and Twice-Baked Cauliflower Casserole

DAY 22

102
Easy Egg Scramble with baby arugula

LEFTOVER   LEFTOVER
Simply Roasted Chicken and Twice-Baked Cauliflower Casserole

176   134
Slow Cooker Carnitas with Guacamole and pork rinds

DAY 23

106   282
Lox and Cream Cheese Sliders with Morning Coffee

184
Bacon and Ranch Chicken Salad with lettuce wrap or celery

200   242
Red Curry Chicken over Basic Cauliflower Rice

DAY 24

110
Sausage, Egg, and Cheese Breakfast Bake

LEFTOVER   134
Slow Cooker Carnitas wrapped in lettuce or over greens, with Guacamole and/or sour cream

180
Quick and Easy Personal Pizza with side salad and ranch dressing

	Breakfast	Lunch	Dinner

DAY 25

LEFTOVER
Sausage, Egg, and Cheese Breakfast Bake

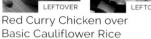
LEFTOVER   LEFTOVER
Red Curry Chicken over Basic Cauliflower Rice

156
Keto Chili with side salad

DAY 26

94
Chili Egg Scramble (use leftover Keto Chili)

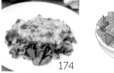
174
Bunless Philly Cheeseteaks with side salad

162   134
Fajita Kabobs with Guacamole

DAY 27

104
Eggs Benedict

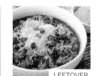
LEFTOVER
Keto Chili with side salad

226   246
Pesto Shrimp Kabobs and Mashed Cauliflower

DAY 28

96
Biscuits and Gravy

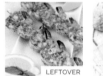
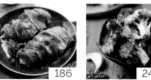
LEFTOVER   LEFTOVER
Pesto Shrimp Kabobs and Mashed Cauliflower

186   248
Bacon-Wrapped Cheesy Chicken and Roasted Broccoli

DAY 29
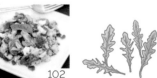
102
Easy Egg Scramble with baby arugula

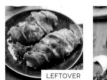
LEFTOVER   LEFTOVER
Bacon-Wrapped Cheesy Chicken and Roasted Broccoli

236
Spinach Cobb Salad with ranch dressing

DAY 30
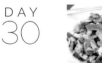
102
Easy Egg Scramble

154
BLTA Lettuce Wraps

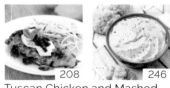
208   246
Tuscan Chicken and Mashed Cauliflower or Zoodles

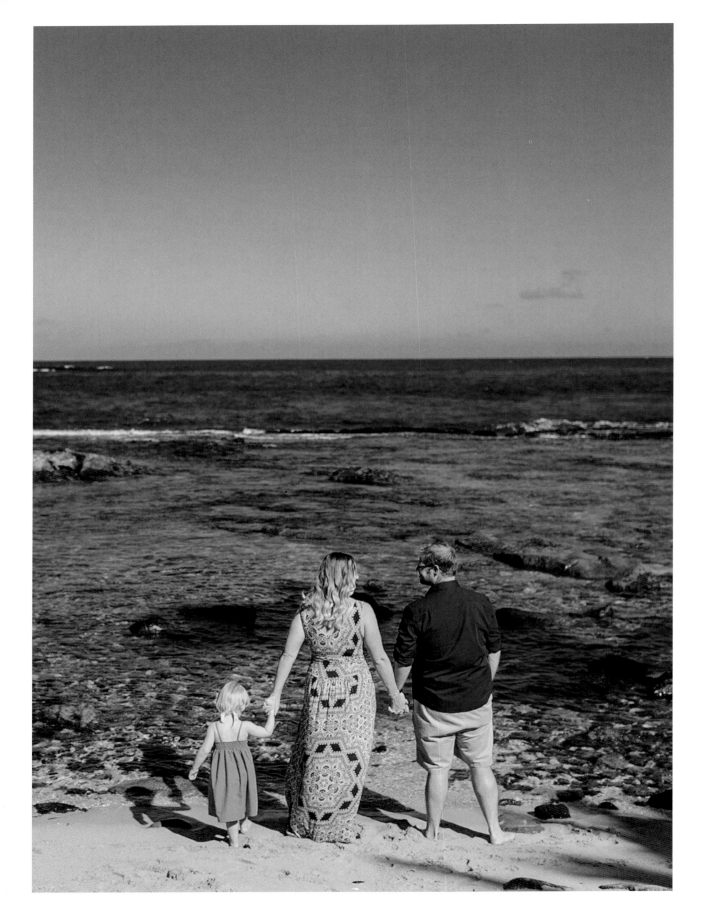

CHAPTER 5:

Taking Keto on the Road

It's true that cooking at home is usually the cheapest and healthiest option—which is why Chapter 3 of this book includes more than 100 delicious keto recipes. However, as I've said, this is a lifestyle change, and not many of us have the time or the desire to cook every single meal ourselves. In this chapter, I've collected my best tips for eating out and snacking on the go without sabotaging your ketogenic lifestyle.

DINING OUT ON KETO

One of the great things about the ketogenic diet is that you can find something keto-friendly to eat at almost any restaurant. I've been on a number of diets in the past that made it nearly impossible to dine out, which I now realize wasn't livable or realistic. But on keto, no matter where you go, you can almost always find something on the menu, either as presented or with a few simple modifications. Here are some of my favorite finds:

- **American:** Bunless burgers, sandwiches without the bread, bunless cheesesteaks, salads, side of avocado, side of pickles, sautéed veggies. If the restaurant serves breakfast, you can order eggs, bacon or sausage, and cheese; just ask for no bread/biscuit/muffin.

- **BBQ:** Pulled pork, brisket, sausage, ribs, smoked chicken, collard greens or other nonstarchy veggies, salads. The trick is to ask for no barbecue sauce on your meat. If you want to be extra-careful, you can even ask if the seasonings/rubs are sugar-free.

- **Breakfast/brunch:** Omelets, eggs Benedict (substitute avocado slices for the English muffin), eggs with bacon and avocado, steak and eggs.

- **Burger joints:** The majority will allow you to pass on the bun and give you a lettuce wrap if you ask. Be sure to have them leave off the ketchup, and add mayo if you like. Some burger places offer grilled chicken as an alternative, which you can eat with ranch dressing or on a salad (no croutons, and choose either ranch or Caesar dressing).

- **Chinese:** Egg drop soup, chicken with mushrooms, beef or chicken and broccoli, garlic prawns. Watch for sugar in sauces; feel free to ask about ingredients before ordering.

- **German:** Sausage, bunless burgers, sauerkraut, salads.

- **Greek:** Kabobs and Greek salads are great choices. Also, tzatziki sauce is usually pretty low in carbs.

- **Indian:** Tandoori chicken, kabobs, roasted eggplant (without breading).

- **Italian:** Chicken Alfredo (substitute broccoli or asparagus for the pasta), steak and veggies, antipasto salad. Remember that a lot of Italian dishes, such as meatballs, contain breadcrumbs, so watch out for hidden carbs.

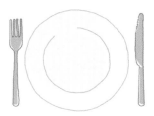

- **Japanese steakhouse:** One of my favorites! Chicken, steak, shrimp, scallops, or lobster; skip the rice and ask for extra veggies (often mushrooms, zucchini, and onion; I ask for light onion). Skip the orange ("yum yum") sauce, as it's not low-carb. Brown ginger sauce is usually low in carbs—feel free to ask, or simply use a little soy sauce. Also, meals generally come with a clear broth soup and a salad with ginger dressing. (The ginger dressing at my local place has 2 grams of carbs per tablespoon, so use it sparingly or skip it altogether.)

- **Mexican (sit-down):** Fajitas (skip the tortillas); taco salad with no beans and no tortilla bowl or tortilla pieces; carnitas with a side of guacamole; avocado stuffed with chicken, beef, or shrimp.

- **Mexican (fast-casual):** Burrito bowl without dressing. Pick a protein and then add toppings—I like fajita veggies, pico de gallo, cheese, sour cream, and guacamole. Another option is to order several tacos or one large burrito with no beans or rice and ask for no shells/tortillas; they will serve it in a bowl or on a plate.

- **Seafood:** Shrimp (not breaded), scallops, fish (not breaded), oysters, crab (but not imitation crabmeat; 3 ounces has 14 grams of carbs!), lobster, salads, nonstarchy veggies.

- **Sub/sandwich shops:** Many offer lettuce-wrapped subs; Jimmy John's calls this an Unwich.

- **Sushi:** Sashimi, rolls with cucumber wraps (no rice, and sugar-free sauces only), miso soup, salad. Skip the imitation crabmeat.

- **Thai:** Non-breaded garlic prawns with veggies instead of rice, Tom Kha Gai (coconut milk soup with chicken), red curry (ask if it contains added sugar).

- **Vietnamese:** Pho; select a protein (I get rare beef) and ask for no noodles. The server will bring you sprouts, jalapeño, and fresh basil to add. Some restaurants will even give you veggies (broccoli, cabbage, and so on) instead of noodles.

- **Wing restaurants:** Chicken wings (not breaded; sometimes called "naked" wings) are a good choice. Stay away from sweet sauces; stick to Buffalo sauce or dry rubs without sugar. Dip the wings in ranch or blue cheese dressing and enjoy them with a side of celery.

tip: *I find it really helpful to let the server know upfront that I would prefer not to be served a bread basket, chips and salsa, or pitas and hummus. It's better not to have the temptation in front of you, especially when you're hungry! If you're out with friends who aren't low-carb, then obviously this won't work. In that case, if you're feeling tempted, I recommend ordering a side salad (skip the croutons) with ranch or blue cheese dressing, or ordering a keto-friendly appetizer that you can enjoy before your meal.*

NAVIGATING COFFEE SHOPS

Here are some safe options to order from your favorite barista:

- Coffee (black)
- Coffee (hot or iced) with half-and-half
- Coffee (hot or iced) with heavy whipping cream
- Americano with half-and-half
- Americano with heavy whipping cream
- Espresso
- Hot tea
- Iced tea (unsweetened)
- Sparkling water

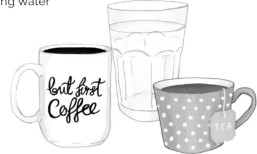

All of the above can be paired with your preferred low-carb sweetener. Some coffee shops, including Starbucks, offer sugar-free syrups; these are sweetened with sucralose (Splenda). I personally don't add syrups to my coffee, but if you enjoy them, just be sure to use them in moderation.

And here are some low-carb snacks often sold at coffee shops:

- Breakfast sandwiches (just remove the bread)
- Hard-boiled eggs
- Meat and cheese plates
- Moon Cheese
- Salads (remove any croutons and stick to low-carb dressings)
- Salted almonds

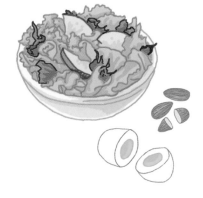

ROAD TRIP SNACKS FROM CONVENIENCE STORES

 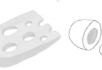

Beverages: water, sparkling water (sugar-free), unsweetened hot or iced tea, coffee

Cheese

Hard-boiled eggs

Jerky *(check the carb count)*

Nuts

Pickles

Pork rinds

Quest bars

Snack recipes from this book that travel well in a small cooler:

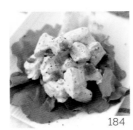
130

Callie's Creamy Herb Dip with veggies

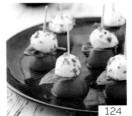
124

Caprese Skewers

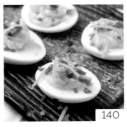
260

Chia Seed Pudding

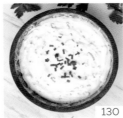
184

Bacon and Ranch Chicken Salad

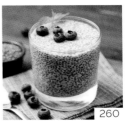
140

Loaded Deviled Eggs

Snack recipes from this book that travel well without a cooler:

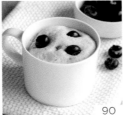
90

Blueberry Mug Muffin

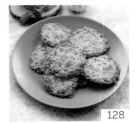
128

Cheese Crisps

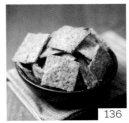
136

Keto Crackers

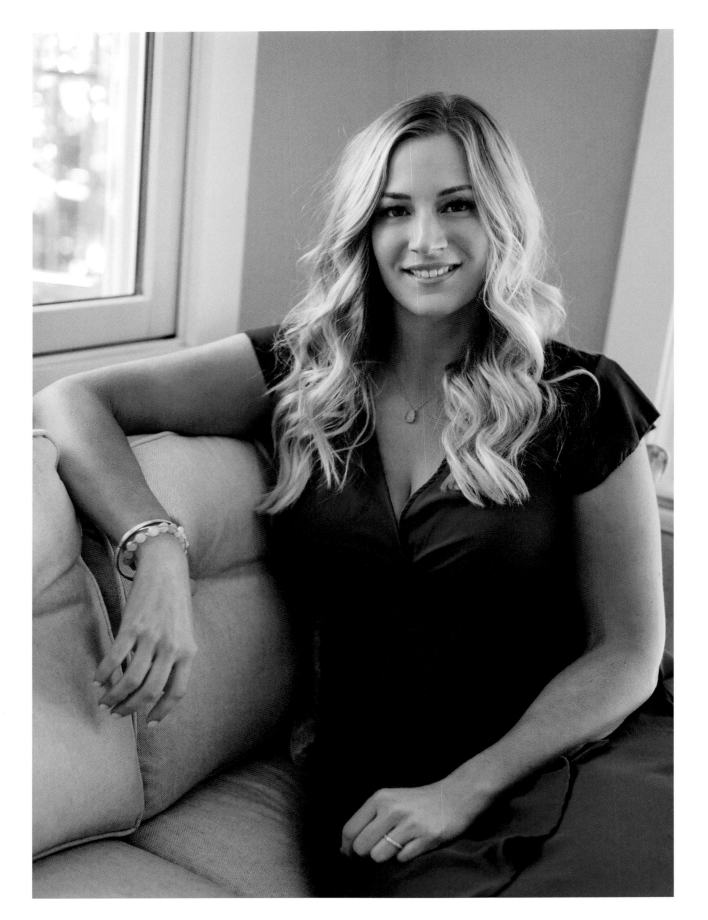

Closing Inspiration

When I was approached to write this book, my initial thought was, "Who, me? I'm just a regular, normal, everyday person!" And in that moment, something clicked. For far too long, we've been led to believe that in order to change our lives, we need to be something more than who we are. Whether it's in the form of obtaining an academic degree, buying a product, taking a pill, drinking a shake, or following a program, these things can reinforce the idea that we simply can't do it on our own. My goal is to inspire you to see that you already have all the tools you need. The key to lasting weight loss is rarely found by looking outward, because the solution and everything you need to implement it is already within you.

At any moment, you can decide to change the direction of your life. The ability to succeed doesn't depend on perfection, but on the choices you make when faced with the ups and downs of real life. A lot of us tend to compare ourselves to a level of perfection that truly doesn't exist. We get caught up in the idea that everything in our lives has to be flawless in order for us to be successful. But the truth is that no one is perfect; we are all just figuring things out day by day. Try to recognize and stop the vicious cycle of comparison. Strive to be better each day, keep an open mind, and be kind to yourself.

I encourage you to spend time retraining your inner voice to focus on self-love; when negative thoughts trickle into your mind, replace them with more supportive, uplifting, and kind ones. We are often our own worst critics, and those negative thoughts can derail your success and diminish your self-worth. The key to weight loss is often mind over matter; it's small, livable steps done consistently over time. So enjoy each step, push the boundaries of your comfort zone, and get invested in the process. After all, the ketogenic lifestyle isn't a punishment. It's a new opportunity—an investment in your health, your happiness, and, most importantly, your life.

Although this is the end of the book, my hope is that this is just the beginning of a new path for you. I hope you know that regardless of what has happened in your past, you are capable of anything you set your heart and mind to. I encourage you not to compare yourself to others; you are unique, and the struggles and successes you've faced throughout your life will further prepare you for the journey ahead. There will be days when it feels like you have a mountain to move, but I have no doubt that you will move it. In your journey you will face setbacks, and when you do, I hope you dig deep and overcome those, too. Remember, progress, not perfection.

You are enough, and change is possible.

Lots of love,

Suzanne Ryan

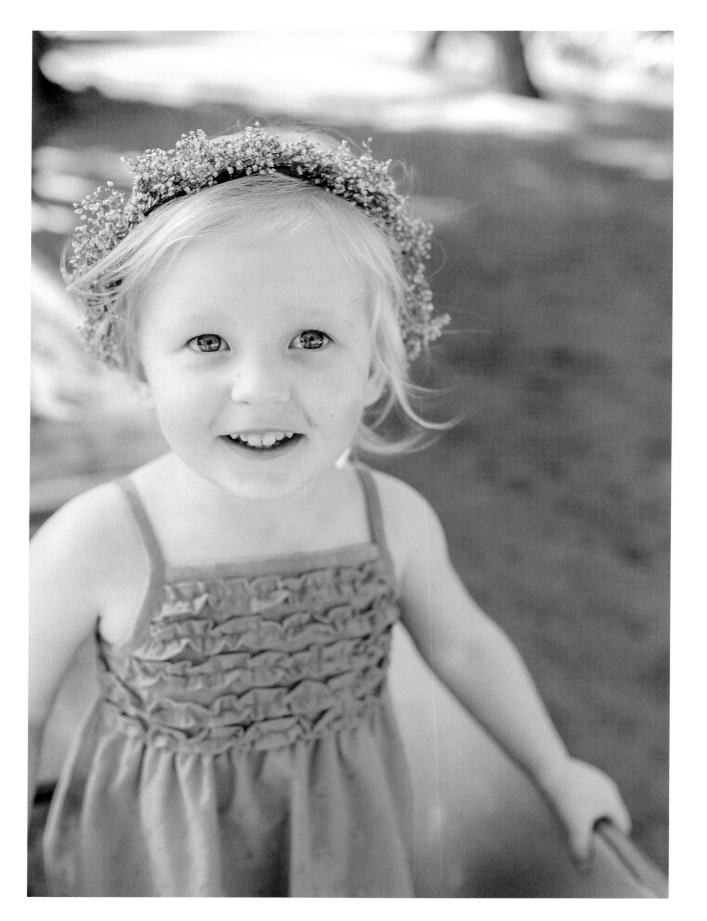

Gratitude

To the keto community: Where do I begin? You all have been by my side through thick and thin. I wouldn't be where I am today without your endless love and support. I'm so thankful for each and every one of you. Thank you for being the most amazing support system! I promise to pay it forward and help as many people as possible!

Mick, I couldn't ask for a more loving and supportive husband. Thank you for loving me at every size, through ups and downs, and for always making me feel loved. Thank you for countless hours editing YouTube videos, working on the blog, and being the best recipe tester! You are my rock, my always and forever. I love you!

Olivia, my sweet little girl, you have absolutely changed my life for the better. You are the most kind, caring, and beautiful child, and I'm honored to be your mom. Thank you for teaching me so much about love, life, and happiness. You truly complete our family, and I'm thankful for every day with you by my side.

Dad, not a single day goes by that I don't feel thankful to have you as my father. Thank you for showing me how important it is to be compassionate and caring. I love that even more than being my dad, you are one of my very best friends. I love you more than I could ever put into words.

Mom, thank you for encouraging me to chase my dreams. You helped me see that I could turn my pain into something positive and helpful. Thank you for always being a phone call away. I love you very much!

John and Cher, I love you both very much. I'm so thankful to have you both in my life. John, thank you for always looking out for me. Throughout my life I've always known that you cared deeply for me, and that truly means the world to me. Thank you for all your help with my blog!

Jack, Joni, and Jennifer, thank you for being such positive and constant influences in my life. I'm so thankful for your love, encouragement, and support. Lots of love to Luke, Riley, and Trey! Joni, thank you for never giving up on me. You believed in my ability to change before I did, and I'll never forget that. I love you!

Emily, my second mom, thank you for loving me, believing in me, and testing all my recipes. I'm so thankful to have you in my life. I love you!

Callie and Tina, my two lifelong best friends, thank you for being the most amazing, uplifting, and loyal friends and for being there for me every step of the way. I love you both to the moon and back!

Mike and Karin, I miss you every single day. Thank you for your friendship, support, and endless laughs.

Jessica, thank you so much for being such an amazing friend and for the countless hours talking about life, raising kids, keto, design ideas, and more. I'm beyond thankful for your friendship.

Melissa, Kristen, and Rachel, I loved keto before I met you, but I love it even more for bringing the three of you into my life. It's priceless to have friends who totally understand the same struggles. I'm so proud of all of you, and I'm thankful for your friendship.

Colleen Pugh, I can't thank you enough for your beautiful drawings throughout this book. I'm so thankful that keto brought us together. Congratulations on your weight loss and health improvements—I'm so proud of you!

Jennifer Skog and Chelsea Foster, thank you both for the cover of this book! Jennifer, I'm someone who has always struggled with feeling beautiful, but you made me feel truly beautiful from the inside out. Thank you for your photography and positive impact on my life. Chelsea, I love our "quick" design calls that end up lasting for hours. Thank you for all your hard work to make everything look gorgeous!

Bill Staley and Hayley Mason, thank you for the gorgeous back cover photograph. I had such a great time working with both of you.

The Victory Belt Team: Erich, Lance, Susan, Pam, Holly, Donna, Yordan, and Boryana, thank you from the bottom of my heart for all your hard work to make this book come to life. I couldn't ask for a more caring and thoughtful group of people to work with. Thank you for the countless hours you all spent to make this dream a reality. It means the world to me!

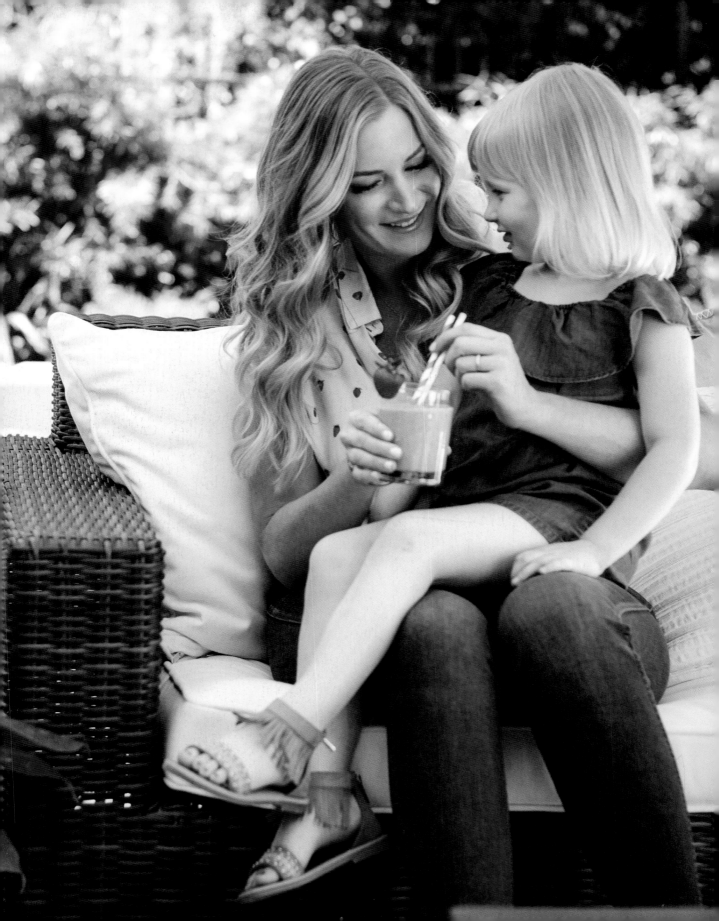

HELPFUL
RESOURCES

ONLINE SUPPORT

Having a support system has been an invaluable part of my success, so I encourage you to connect with others who are on the same path! The ketogenic community is full of helpful and caring people. The following are some great (and free!) places online to find support, encouragement, and friends.

- **Reddit Keto (www.reddit.com/r/keto/):** This is where I got my start. r/keto is an amazing community full of helpful and supportive people! Be sure to read the FAQ and Keto In A Nutshell overview. There is even a chat room where you can connect with others and ask questions.

- **Instagram and Facebook:** Search popular hashtags, such as #keto, #ketogenicdiet, #lchf, #ketofam, and #lowcarb, to find people to connect with. Some choose to use their personal accounts, and others set up whole new accounts specifically for keto. You can choose to be anonymous, an open book, or anything in between—whatever fits your needs and lifestyle best. You can find me on both Instagram (@ketokarma) and Facebook (Keto Karma).

- **YouTube:** A lot of amazing and inspiring people share their personal journeys, recipes, advice, and more on YouTube. Check out my YouTube channel, Keto Karma, at www.youtube.com/ketokarma2015.

RECOMMENDED KETO RECIPE BLOGS AND OTHER ONLINE RESOURCES

In addition to my own blog, *Keto Karma*, there are many great ketogenic recipe/food blogs and resources. Here are a few of my favorites:

- The Applied Science & Performance Institute (theaspi.com)

- Art and Science of Low Carb (www.artandscienceoflowcarb.com)

- Diet Doctor (www.dietdoctor.com)

- Ditch the Carbs (www.ditchthecarbs.com)

- I Breathe I'm Hungry (www.ibreatheimhungry.com)

- Keto Connect (www.ketoconnect.net)

- Peace, Love and Low Carb (peaceloveandlowcarb.com)

- Reddit Keto (www.reddit.com/r/keto/)

RECOMMENDED BOOKS

Here are some of my favorite books for gaining a deeper understanding of the science and research behind the ketogenic diet and its many health benefits.

- *The Art and Science of Low Carbohydrate Living* by Stephen D. Phinney and Jeff S. Volek

- *The Art and Science of Low Carbohydrate Performance* by Stephen D. Phinney and Jeff S. Volek

- *Cholesterol Clarity* by Jimmy Moore with Eric C. Westman

- *Keto Clarity* by Jimmy Moore with Eric C. Westman

- *The Ketogenic Bible* by Jacob Wilson and Ryan Lowery

- *Why We Get Fat and What to Do About It* by Gary Taubes

RECOMMENDED DOCUMENTARIES

I learned so much from these two documentary films that focus on sugar and how it negatively impacts health:

- *Fed Up* (2014): A film about the dangers of sugar and how it has contributed to the obesity epidemic in the United States.

- *That Sugar Film* (2014): An Australian documentary showing one man's journey as he changes his diet to one that is high in sugar, all while eating perceived "healthy" foods, which are often lower in fat but have added sugar.

MY FAVORITE FOOD COMPANIES AND PRODUCTS

These are some of my all-time favorite low-carb companies and products! Let's face it, life gets busy, and it's wonderful to have convenience foods that are thoughtfully made from healthy ingredients.

- **Cali'flour Foods:** Delicious and low-carb premade cauliflower pizza crusts (www.califlourfoods.com)

- **Choc Zero:** Sugar-free chocolate, hot chocolate, keto bark, and dipping chocolate (www.choczero.com)

- **Eating Evolved:** Keto Cups, which are low-carb, high-fat chocolate snack cups (www.eatingevolved.com/collections/keto-cups)

- **Epic:** Bacon Bars, bacon bits, pork rinds, pork cracklings, and more (www.epicbar.com)

- **Front Porch Pecans:** Hands down the best roasted pecans I've ever tried! (www.frontporchpecans.com)

- **Good Dee's:** Delicious and easy keto-friendly mixes, from brownies to muffins to cakes and cookies. My favorite are the blondies—so good! (www.gooddees.com)

- **Keto Krate:** Monthly subscription box for keto snacks (www.ketokrate.com)

- **Know Foods:** A variety of gluten-free and sugar-free foods—breads, wraps, waffles, maple syrup, donuts, cookies, and more (www.knowfoods.com)

- **LaCroix:** Sugar-free sparkling water (lime is my favorite); this was my first step toward cutting out soda (www.lacroix.com)

- **Lily's Chocolate:** Stevia-sweetened chocolate bars and chocolate chips (www.lilyssweets.com)

- **Moon Cheese:** Crunchy cheese balls—I like Cheddar, Gouda, and Pepper Jack (www.mooncheese.com)

- **Natural Calm:** A magnesium and calcium supplement drink that helps balance electrolytes and relieve stress (www.naturalvitality.com/natural-calm/)

- **Oloves:** Pitted olives in on-the-go pouches (www.oloves.com)

- **Pique Tea:** Tea crystals that you can mix with hot or cold water—by far my favorite tea (www.piquetea.com)

- **Primal Palate:** Organic spices, the majority of which are keto-friendly with no added sugar (www.primalpalate.com)

- **Quest Nutrition:** Quest bars (cookie dough and blueberry muffin are my favorite flavors), MCT and coconut powder, and Beyond Cereal Bars (www.questnutrition.com)

- **Real Good Pizza:** Low-carb pizza made with a chicken and cheese-based crust (www.realgoodfoods.com)

- **Sarayo:** A creamy and spicy Sriracha mayo (www.sarayosauce.com)

- **Swerve:** Erythritol-blend sweetener; I prefer the confectioners' style because it blends really nicely (www.swervesweet.com)

- **Zevia:** Stevia-sweetened zero-calorie soda (www.zevia.com)

COMMON KETO TERMS AND ABBREVIATIONS

Here are some of the most common terms and abbreviations you'll see online and elsewhere in regard to the ketogenic diet:

BG: Blood glucose

BMI: Body mass index

BPC: Bulletproof Coffee (a high-fat mixture of coffee and MCT oil or coconut oil and butter or ghee)

CW: Current weight

GI: Glycemic Index (see page 57)

GW: Goal weight

HF: High fat

HWC: Heavy whipping cream

IF: Intermittent fasting

KCKO: Keep Calm Keto On

Keto: Short for ketosis or ketogenic

Lazy Keto: A term coined by the keto community for a very simplistic approach to a ketogenic diet without tracking macros or food intake. (*Note:* There are many approaches to this option.)

LCHF: Low Carb High Fat

Macros: Macronutrients (generally the breakdown of fat, protein, and carbohydrates in foods and drinks)

MCTs: Medium-chain triglycerides (see page 53)

MFP: MyFitnessPal

NK: Nutritional ketosis

NSV: Non-scale victory (something to celebrate that is unrelated to the number on the scale)

SD: Start date (when you started keto)

SV: Scale victory (a celebration of pounds lost)

WOE: Way of eating

CONVERSION CHART

Measurements & Temperatures

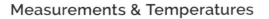

CUP TO TABLESPOONS TO TEASPOONS TO MILLILITERS (ML)

1 cup = 16 tablespoons = 48 teaspoons = 240 ml

¾ cup = 12 tablespoons = 36 teaspoons = 180 ml

⅔ cup = 11 tablespoons = 32 teaspoons = 160 ml

½ cup = 8 tablespoons = 24 teaspoons = 120 ml

⅓ cup = 5 tablespoons = 16 teaspoons = 80 ml

¼ cup = 4 tablespoons = 12 teaspoons = 60 ml

1 tablespoon = 15 ml

1 teaspoon = 5 ml

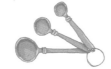
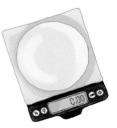

CUP TO FLUID OUNCES (FL. OZ.)

1 cup = 8 fl. oz.

¾ cup = 6 fl. oz.

⅔ cup = 5 fl. oz.

½ cup = 4 fl. oz.

⅓ cup = 3 fl. oz.

¼ cup = 2 fl. oz.

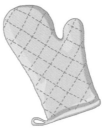

FAHRENHEIT (°F) TO CELSIUS (°C)

500°F = 260°C

475°F = 245°C

450°F = 235°C

425°F = 220°C

400°F = 205°C

375°F = 190°C

350°F = 180°C

325°F = 160°C

300°F = 150°C

275°F = 135°C

250°F = 120°C

225°F = 107°C

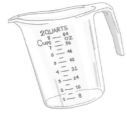

SAFE MINIMUM COOKING TEMPERATURES FOR MEAT AND SEAFOOD

	FOOD	Temperature (°F)	Rest Time*
GROUND MEATS	Beef, lamb, pork, veal	160°F	None
	Turkey, chicken	165°F	None
BEEF, LAMB, VEAL	Steaks, roasts, chops	145°F	3 minutes
PORK	Fresh pork	145°F	3 minutes
	Fresh ham (raw)	145°F	3 minutes
	Precooked ham (to reheat)	140°F	None
POULTRY	Chicken and turkey, whole	165°F	None
	Breasts, roasts	165°F	None
	Thighs, legs, wings	165°F	None
	Duck, goose	165°F	None
SEAFOOD	Finfish	145°F, or cook until flesh is opaque and separates easily with a fork.	None
	Shrimp, lobster, crabs	Cook until flesh is pearly and opaque.	None
	Clams, oysters, mussels	Cook until shells open.	None
	Scallops	Cook until flesh is milky white or opaque and firm.	None

This rest time is for safety purposes. Individual recipes may recommend additional rest time to allow the juices to redistribute throughout the meat, resulting in juicier and tastier meat.

RECIPE INDEX

BASICS

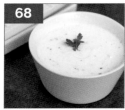

68

Alfredo Sauce

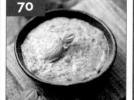

70

Easy Pesto

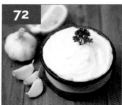

72

Aioli

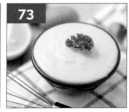

73

Keto
Honey Mustard

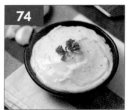

74

Quick and Easy
Caesar Dressing

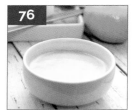

76

Simple Hollandaise

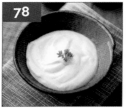

78

Mick's Spicy Aioli

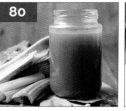

80

Slow Cooker
Beef Bone Broth

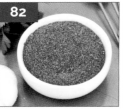

82

Sugar-Free
Taco Seasoning

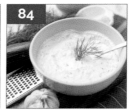

84

Tzatziki Sauce

BREAKFAST

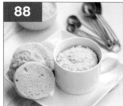

88

60-Second
Mug Biscuits

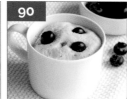

90

Blueberry
Mug Muffin

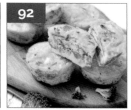

92

Broccoli, Bacon,
and Cheese
Egg Muffins

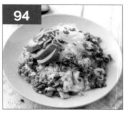

94

Chili Egg Scramble

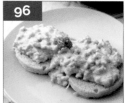

96

Biscuits and Gravy

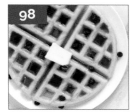

98

Chocolate Chip
Waffle

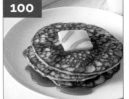

100

Olivia's Cream
Cheese Pancakes

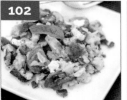

102

Easy Egg Scramble

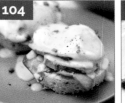

104

Eggs Benedict

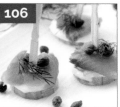

106

Lox and Cream
Cheese Sliders

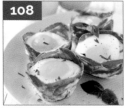

108

Quick and Easy
Capicola Egg Cups

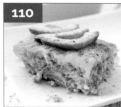

110

Sausage, Egg,
and Cheese
Breakfast Bake

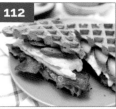

112

Waffle Breakfast
Sandwiches

APPETIZERS AND SNACKS

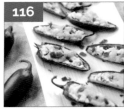
116
Bacon Cheddar
Jalapeño Poppers

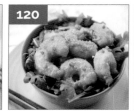
118
Baked Crab Dip

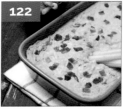
120
Sweet and Spicy
Fried Shrimp

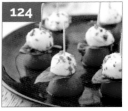
122
Buffalo Chicken Dip

124
Caprese Skewers

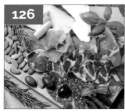
126
Cheese and
Charcuterie Board

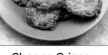
128
Cheese Crisps

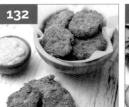
130
Callie's Creamy
Herb Dip

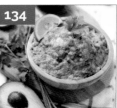
132
Crispy Fried Pickles

134
Guacamole

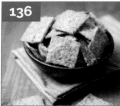
136
Keto Crackers—
Two Ways

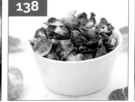
138
Lime Brussels Chips

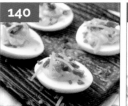
140
Loaded
Deviled Eggs

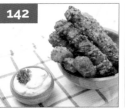
142
Fried Mozzarella
Sticks

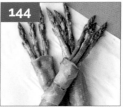
144
Prosciutto-Wrapped
Asparagus

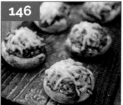
146
Spinach and
Artichoke–Stuffed
Mushrooms

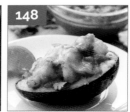
148
Salsa Shrimp-Stuffed
Avocados

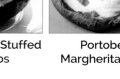
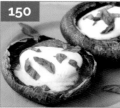
150
Portobello
Margherita Pizzas

BEEF AND PORK

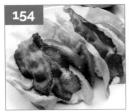

154

BLTA
Lettuce Wraps

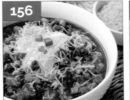

156

Keto Chili

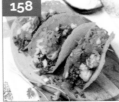

158

Cheese Shell Tacos

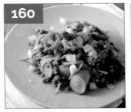

160

Chili Cheese Dogs

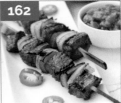

162

Fajita Kabobs

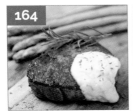

164

Filet Mignons with
Gorgonzola Sauce

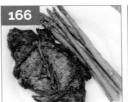

166

Garlic Butter–Basted
Rib-eye

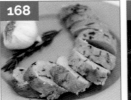

168

Lemon Garlic
Pork Tenderloin

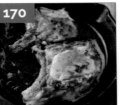

170

Goat Cheese, Rosemary,
and Mushroom Stuffed
Pork Chops

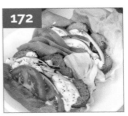

172

Gyro
Lettuce Wraps

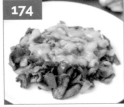

174

Bunless Philly
Cheesesteaks

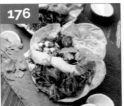

176

Slow Cooker
Carnitas

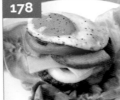

178

Sunny-Side-Up
Burgers

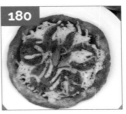

180

Quick and Easy
Personal Pizza

CHICKEN

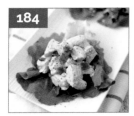

184
Bacon and Ranch
Chicken Salad

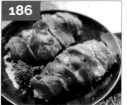

186
Bacon-Wrapped
Cheesy Chicken

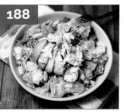

188
Chicken
Caesar Salad

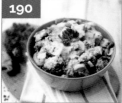

190
Chicken and Broccoli
Alfredo Bowls

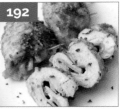

192
Chicken
Cordon Bleu

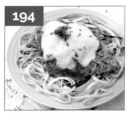

194
Chicken Parmesan

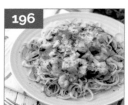

196
Creamy Pesto
Chicken

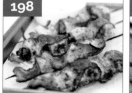

198
Grilled Chicken and
Bacon Ranch Kabobs

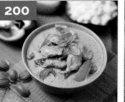

200
Red Curry
Chicken

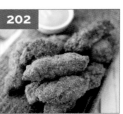

202
Breaded
Chicken Tenders

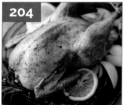

204
Simply Roasted
Chicken

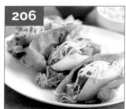

206
Tina's Slow Cooker
Salsa Chicken
Lettuce Wraps

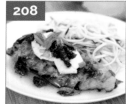

208
Tuscan Chicken

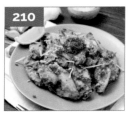

210
Grilled Parmesan
Garlic Wings

SEAFOOD

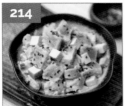

214

Ahi Tuna Poke Bowls
with
Spicy Mayonnaise

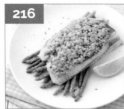

216

Macadamia Nut–
Crusted Tilapia

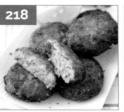

218

Fried Tuna Patties

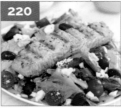

220

Greek Salad with
Grilled Salmon

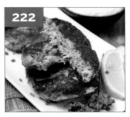

222

Low-Carb
Crab Cakes

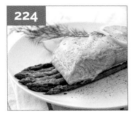

224

Parmesan-Crusted
Salmon Bake
with Asparagus

226

Pesto Shrimp
Kabobs

SOUPS AND SIDES

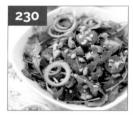
230 Arugula Salad

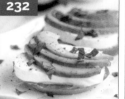
232 Caprese Salad with Avocado

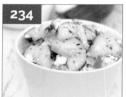
234 Mike's Cucumber Salad with Feta

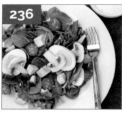
236 Spinach Cobb Salad

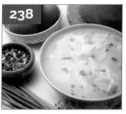
238 Egg Drop Soup

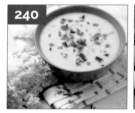
240 Slow Cooker Loaded Cauliflower Soup

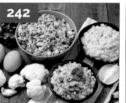
242 Cauliflower Rice— Three Ways

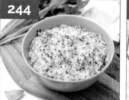
244 Creamed Spinach

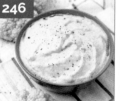
246 Mashed Cauliflower (Fauxtatoes)

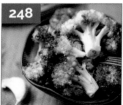
248 Roasted Broccoli

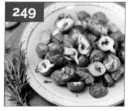
249 Roasted Radishes

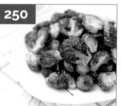
250 Simply Roasted Brussels Sprouts

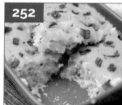
252 Twice-Baked Cauliflower Casserole

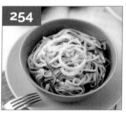
254 Zoodles (Spiralized Zucchini Noodles)

DESSERTS AND DRINKS

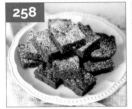
258
Brownies

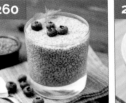
260
Chia Seed
Pudding

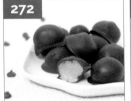
262
Chocolate Avocado
Pudding

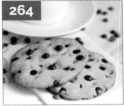
264
Chocolate Chip
Cookies for Two

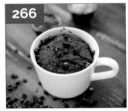
266
Chocolate Chip
Mug Cake

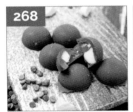
268
Chocolate-Covered
Macadamia Nut
Fat Bombs

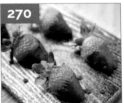
270
Chocolate-Covered
Strawberries

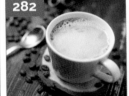
272
Pop-Pop's Chocolate
Peanut Butter Bites

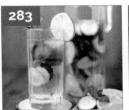
274
Mini Cheesecakes

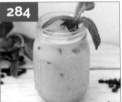
276
Raspberry
Cheesecake
Fat Bombs

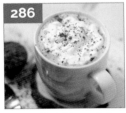
278
Snickerdoodle
Cupcakes

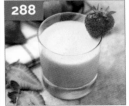
280
Strawberry Cream
Ice Pops

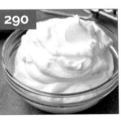
282
Morning Coffee

283
Mint, Cucumber, and
Lime-Infused Water

284
Cold-Brew
Mint Coffee

286
Keto Hot Chocolate

288
Strawberry Vanilla
Smoothie

290
Keto
Whipped Cream

ALLERGEN INDEX

O = option

RECIPES	PAGE	<30 MIN	EGG FREE	NUT FREE	DAIRY FREE
Alfredo Sauce	68	✓	✓	✓	
Easy Pesto	70	✓	✓		
Aioli	72			✓	✓
Keto Honey Mustard	73	✓		✓	✓
Quick and Easy Caesar Dressing	74	✓		✓	
Simple Hollandaise	76	✓		✓	
Mick's Spicy Aioli	78	✓		✓	✓
Slow Cooker Beef Bone Broth	80		✓	✓	✓
Sugar-Free Taco Seasoning	82	✓	✓	✓	✓
Tzatziki Sauce	84		✓	✓	
60-Second Mug Biscuits	88	✓			
Blueberry Mug Muffin	90	✓			
Broccoli, Bacon, and Cheese Egg Muffins	92			✓	
Chili Egg Scramble	94	✓		✓	
Biscuits and Gravy	96	✓			
Chocolate Chip Waffle	98	✓			O
Olivia's Cream Cheese Pancakes	100	✓			
Easy Egg Scramble	102	✓		✓	
Eggs Benedict	104				
Lox and Cream Cheese Sliders	106	✓	✓	✓	
Quick and Easy Capicola Egg Cups	108	✓		✓	O
Sausage, Egg, and Cheese Breakfast Bake	110			✓	
Waffle Breakfast Sandwiches	112	✓		✓	O
Bacon Cheddar Jalapeño Poppers	116		✓	✓	
Baked Crab Dip	118			✓	
Sweet and Spicy Fried Shrimp	120	✓		✓	✓
Buffalo Chicken Dip	122		O	✓	
Caprese Skewers	124		✓	✓	
Cheese and Charcuterie Board	126	✓	✓		
Cheese Crisps	128	✓	✓	✓	
Callie's Creamy Herb Dip	130	✓	✓	✓	
Crispy Fried Pickles	132	✓		✓	
Guacamole	134	✓	✓	✓	O
Keto Crackers-Two Ways	136	✓			
Lime Brussels Chips	138	✓	✓	✓	✓
Loaded Deviled Eggs	140	✓		✓	
Fried Mozzarella Sticks	142			✓	
Prosciutto-Wrapped Asparagus	144	✓	✓	✓	✓
Spinach and Artichoke-Stuffed Mushrooms	146	✓	✓	✓	
Salsa Shrimp-Stuffed Avocados	148	✓	✓	✓	
Portobello Margherita Pizzas	150	✓	✓	✓	
BLTA Lettuce Wraps	154	✓		✓	✓
Keto Chili	156		✓	✓	O
Cheese Shell Tacos	158	✓	✓	✓	
Chili Cheese Dogs	160	✓	✓	✓	
Fajita Kabobs	162		✓	✓	✓
Filet Mignons with Gorgonzola Sauce	164		✓	✓	
Garlic Butter-Basted Rib-eye	166	✓	✓	✓	
Lemon Garlic Pork Tenderloin	168		✓	✓	✓
Goat Cheese, Rosemary, and Mushroom Stuffed Pork Chops	170		✓	✓	
Gyro Lettuce Wraps	172		✓	✓	
Bunless Philly Cheesesteaks	174	✓	✓	✓	O
Slow Cooker Carnitas	176		✓	✓	✓
Sunny-Side-Up Burgers	178	✓		✓	
Quick and Easy Personal Pizza	180	✓			

GENERAL INDEX